# The DISABKIDS questionnaires

## Quality of life questionnaires for children with chronic conditions

## - HANDBOOK -

### The EUROPEAN DISABKIDS GROUP

Silke Schmidt, Corinna Petersen, Holger Mühlan, Marie Claude Simeoni,
David Debensason, Ute Thyen, Esther Müller-Godeffroy, Athanasios Vidalis,
John Tsanakas, Elpis Hatziagorou, Paraskevi Karagianni, Hendrik Koopmann,
Rolanda Baars, John Chaplin, Mick Power, Clare Atherton, Peter Hoare,
Michael Quittan, Othmar Schuhfried and Monika Bullinger

PABST SCIENCE PUBLISHERS
Lengerich, Berlin, Bremen, Miami,
Riga, Viernheim, Wien, Zagreb

*Acknowledgement:*

*The DISABKIDS project was supported by the European Commission (QLG5-CT-2000-00716) within the Fifth Framework Program "Quality of Life and Management of Living Resources".*

Bibliographic information published by Die Deutsche Bibliothek
Die Deutsche Bibliothek lists this publication in the Deutsche Nationalbibliografie; detailed bibliographic data is available in the Internet at <http://dnb.ddb.de>.

*Prof. Dr. Monika Bullinger (Project Coordinator)*
*Dr. Silke Schmidt, Dr. Corinna Petersen*
*Institut und Poliklinik für Medizinische Psychologie*
*Zentrum für Psychosoziale Medizin*
*Universitätsklinikum Hamburg-Eppendorf*
*Martinistr. 52, Haus S 35*
*20246 Hamburg, Germany*
*Tel. ++49 (0) 40 / 42803-6430*
*Fax ++49 (0) 40 / 42803-4940*
*E-mail: bullinge@uke.uni-hamburg.de, sischmid@uke.uni-hamburg.de*

© 2006 Pabst Science Publishers, 49525 Lengerich, Germany

Printing: KM-Druck, 64823 Groß Umstadt, Germany

ISBN 3-89967-166-X

# Table of contents

**APPENDIX**

A-I   THE DISABKIDS QUESTIONNAIRES (english language on page 107pp; all languages
      versions are available on disc)

A-II  REFERENCES DATA (field study sample, see page 168pp)

A-III SPSS SYNTAX FILES *(available on disc)*

# Preface

## Cross-Cultural Instrument Development: The DISABKIDS Project Experience

Cross-cultural issues have been a topic in quality of life research both in terms of the need to address cultural diversity in the quality of life concept, as well as the need to develop assessment instruments, which are sensitive to cultural aspects. Quality of life measures are used increasingly internationally so that assessment instruments have to be available in different languages and for different cultural backgrounds (Anderson et al., 1996; Bullinger, 1996; Schmidt & Bullinger, 2003). Thus, conceptually, methodologically and practically, quality of life research has been confronted with the necessity to incorporate the concept of culture and language in the course of the involvement of the field.

With regard to concepts, two radically different approaches seem to compete, the so-called emic (=referring to intrinsic cultural distinctions) and etic views on quality of life (= referring to external concepts). One approach views quality of life as anthropologically universal; i.e. it can be expected to be represented independently of his or her cultural background. The contrasting view includes the notion that quality of life is highly culturally variable and that the expectation to measure quality of life across cultures with the same instrument is impossible. While the reconciliation of these opposite views could be seen as an empirical question, e.g. by using a specific measure in order to identify cultural diversity or homogeneity, the problem is much more deeply routed. The reason for this is that already in the construction of measures, the respective approach regarding anthropological universality versus differentiation is embedded. For example in Hui and Triandis early work (1985), four components of cross-cultural comparability are noted ranging from conceptual equivalence to metric equivalence. Along these components, a measure can be constructed to either enhance or reduce cross-cultural variability, depending on the theoretical and conceptual starting point of such development work. When reflecting about the concept of culture in quality of life research, several aspects and levels need to be elaborated which have been referred to in earlier work (Schmidt & Bullinger, 2003). These include whether quality of life concept is represented in a specific culture, whether it can be addressed with the methods chosen and whether it leads to an assessment approach which is feasible as well as to results which are interpretable. A review of the literature on cross-cultural quality of life assessment shows wide variation on how this basically radical conceptual question is addressed. While some authors maintain that quality of life can only be assessed within a specific culture and therefore are highly sceptical about any attempt for unification in terms of concepts, measurements and applications, another group of authors is ready to embark on a higher abstraction level, thus viewing a cultural diversity as a variation of the theme.

Concerning measurement approaches, considerable efforts have been made to be sensitive to cross-cultural differences and variations. Anthropology as well as multinational psychiatric epidemiology has been leading the way in cross-cultural assessment methodologies. For example, research on the international prevalence of psychiatric conditions has been dependent on the availability of a measurement instrument that can be used clinically to diagnose and differentiate different forms of the chronic psychiatric conditions worldwide. Concepts of quality of life however, as they concern subjective representations of well-being and function, go beyond the scope of these measures and require specific experiences regarding the cross-cultural assessment methodology. Basically, on the instrument level the question arises whether instruments can be translated from one language to the other *(sequential approach)*, whether they can be compiled from available instruments from different countries *(parallel approach)* or whether they can be constructed jointly by experts from different countries including cultural aspects from the beginning of instrument development *(simultaneous approach)*. The SF-36 Health Survey could be considered as an example for the sequential approach, the early EORTC work as an example of the parallel approach, the development of the WHOQoL questionnaire as an example for a simultaneous approach.

The basic idea of the WHOQoL group started with a definition of facets and dimensions in a group of experts from various countries, thus ensuring already at the conceptual and construction level the variability of cultural representations of quality of life. The work of the WHOQoL group has evolved from the cross-cultural definition of relevant dimensions and facets to the identification of items. Work steps included using focus groups in all languages and countries involved, translating them, sorting them, reducing them and producing longer (WHOQoL 100) and shorter (WHOQoL BREF) versions of a quality of life instrument. The WHOQoL work has been guiding cross-cultural quality of life research in many ways in terms of the methodology of instrument construction but also in the methodology of statistical and psychometric analysis of the questionnaire constructed.

The last decades have brought increasing experiences in developing and testing goal measures cross-culturally. In addition to the WHOQoL work, groups such as the IQoLA group working with the SF-36 or the working groups associated with the Nottingham Health Profile or the EORTC questionnaire have been active in the field. Most of the work concerns generic measures, however, also disease-specific measures have undergone a similar process, however frequently sequential in terms of translating available disease-specific measures in different languages. Independent of the source of the items in the respective approaches, all cross-cultural instrument work has to deal with the item development phase, the translation phase, the psychometric testing phase as well as (if possible) the norming phase.

Guidelines have been published that govern these four steps, mostly related to translation issues but also to the psychometric testing of such measures (e.g. Guillemin and others 1993). With regard to the translation procedure, the recommendation includes having one forward and one backward translation or one or two forward and one backward translation as well as cross-cultural harmonisation of those translations. As concerns item development, the recommendation includes using focus groups to produce the items, and in pilot testing of a questionnaire using cognitive debriefing with the target population to better understand how these items are perceived. As concerns psychometric testing, in addition to the classical indicators of reliability and validity the use of more modern psychometric techniques is recommended. One specific problem in cross-cultural psychometric testing is whether such testing should be done consecutively for each culture involved or whether the data set should be merged and pooled to detect cultural variance in the total item pool. As regards norming, the challenge lies in the question how representative samples from different languages and cultures can be recruited for such a process.

In spite of the intensive work and publication in the cross-cultural Qol area, researchers are mostly involved measuring Qol in adults. To our knowledge there is no study available in which Qol measures for children were constructed cross-culturally in a simultaneous way. This is one of the challenges in developing measures in the paediatric area, which was addressed in a large research project funded by the European Union, the DISABKIDS-project. Owing to the fact that cross culturally developed quality of life instruments for children with chronic conditions are still lacking, the group set out a program which led the process in eleven work steps starting from the literature search and ending in the final report and analysis (see Table P-1).

**Table P-1 Overview on DISABKIDS project work packages**

| Work package | Purpose | Time line |
|---|---|---|
| Work package 1 (WP 1) | Literature Review | Month 0 – 3 |
| Work package 2 (WP 2) | Focus Groups | Month 4 – 6 |
| Work package 3 (WP 3) | Item Development | Month 7 – 9 |
| Work package 4 (WP 4) | Translation | Month 10 – 12 |
| Work package 5 (WP 5) | Pilot Testing | Month 13 – 15 |
| Work package 6 (WP 6) | Pilot Analyses | Month 13 – 15 |
| Work package 7 (WP 7) | Field Testing | Month 19 – 24 |
| Work package 8 (WP 8) | Field Analyses | Month 25 – 27 |
| Work package 9 (WP 9) | Implementation Plan | Month 28 – 30 |
| Work package 10 (WP 10) | Implementation Study | Month 31 – 33 |
| Work package 11 (WP 11) | Final Report, Manual | Month 34 – 36 |

In each of the steps, a specific work program was defined including aims, methods and results as well as deliverables which would subsequently lead to the finally desired product result, i.e. the DISABKIDS questionnaire set. The work steps are described in detail in chapter 3 of the present manual. The stepwise progression in realising all these work packages of the DIS-ABKIDS project resulted in the final phase of the project, in which all information on the questionnaires were provided both in a written report as well as in the present information for using the DISABKIDS tool set. Information will be available on the internet including updates. In addition, language versions of countries not having participated in the project are in preparation by giving interested researchers the possibility to translate and psychometrically test the DISABKIDS tool set in their countries, according to specific rules and regulations and as additional members of the DISABKIDS group. Publications emanating from the project concern both presentation of results at relevant conferences as well publication in relevant journals and books.

Altogether the work of the DISABKIDS group is now available in publications, the internet and presentations and is hopefully used to better understand as well as to have an impact on the quality of life of children with chronic conditions. The present book describes the development and testing of the DISABKIDS tool set and also represents a manual for the use of the questionnaires.

# 1 Introduction

## 1.1 Purpose of the Manual

The health-related quality of life of children and adolescents is increasingly considered a relevant topic for research. Instruments to assess health-related quality of life in children and adolescents of a generic as well as disease- or condition-specific nature are developed and applied in epidemiological surveys, clinical studies, quality assurance, and health economics. Cross-cultural aspects, however, have rarely been addressed. This manual will present a set of instruments to assess Health related Quality of Life (HRQoL) in children with chronic health conditions and their families. These instruments have been developed cross-nationally within the EU-funded project DISABKIDS (QLG5-CT-2000-00716). The DISABKIDS instruments were developed according to international questionnaire development guidelines (cf.Guillemin and others 1993). This manual describes the development, psychometric testing, and final appearance of the DISABKIDS questionnaire modules. Furthermore, it provides reference data and interpretation guidelines.

## 1.2 Outline of Chapters

The manual is divided into different chapters. After an introduction of the DISABKIDS instruments (Chapter 1), the second chapter gives a short overview of health-related quality of life assessment in children and adolescents. Chapter 3 describes the methodology of the DISABKIDS project, while Chapter 4 outlines contents, scoring procedures and core reference data for each of the modules. Chapter 4 also gives instructions for using the DISABKIDS tool set for individual patients in clinical practice and for using the DISABKIDS computer version. In an appendix, reference data is presented using different linear transformations scores, (e.g. T-scores, percentiles) for each of the modules. On a disc included, all questionnaire versions and syntaxes for analysing DISABKIDS modules are provided.

## 1.3 Overview of the DISABKIDS Instruments

The DISABKIDS instruments have been translated and adapted for use in several languages and can be applied by clinicians, researchers, pharmaceutical companies, health care providers, and government agencies to:

- document the HRQoL of children and adolescents,
- describe the impact of a disease or treatment on the child's well-being,

- assess pediatric health outcome measures for use in health economic research,
- give parents and children a voice in health care.

The instruments are available as self- or proxy report forms in paper/ pencil or computer versions. The DISABKIDS instrument tool set includes the following modules:

- DISABKIDS Chronic Generic Measure – long form (DCGM-37)
- DISABKIDS Chronic Generic Measure – short form (DCGM-12)
- DISABKIDS Smiley Measure
- Condition-specific modules for asthma, arthritis, cerebral palsy, cystic fibrosis, dermatitis, diabetes, and epilepsy.

In all, the DISABKIDS instruments are part of an instrument family which is a highly flexible assessment device that can be used to assess patients with any type of chronic medical condition, but which has specific modules for a deeper assessment of some of the most commonly encountered childhood chronic conditions. It is also usable for children between the ages of 4 to 16 years. Compatible proxy and child version are available for the whole age range, which allows greater flexibility where a child may not be able to complete the older age version. There is also greater flexibility in that the instruments are available in all the major European languages. In summary, the DISABKIDS instruments:

- cover a wide range of application possibilities,
- are developmentally appropriate,
- are reliable, valid and sensitive in terms of psychometric criteria,
- are translated into multiple languages, and
- are quick to complete and easy to score as well as to interpret.

### *Cooperation*
The DISABKIDS project is associated with its 'sister' project KIDSCREEN that has developed a generic quality of life questionnaire for children of the general population, for instance to be used in health surveys (Ravens-Sieberer et al., 1991). Both measures, the DISABKIDS and KIDSCREEN measures, have been developed using the same methodology so that it is possible for them to be used in tandem. Information on the instruments involved in both projects are available on a common project website (www.DISABKIDS.org).

# 2   Health-Related Quality of Life Assessment in Children and Adolescents

A paradigm shift in criteria used to evaluate medical outcomes has occurred in the past 20 years. Classical endpoints such as the reduction in symptomatology and increased survival have been supplemented by patient-oriented outcome criteria. A broader definition of health as suggested by the World Health Organisation (WHO, 1948), focusing on the psychological and social dimensions of well-being has contributed to this new look on health. The term HRQoL has been coined to integrate this changed perspective on medical outcomes. The term denotes in psychological terminology a multidimensional construct covering physical, emotional, mental, social, and behavioural components of well-being and function as perceived by patients or proxies (Bullinger 2001). HRQoL is often distinguished from the broader concept of quality of life. In medicine, quality of life clearly relates to health and the subjective well-being of a patient with regard to e.g. a treatment. More specifically, HRQoL is a component of the more general construct of quality of life, which also includes a broader range of aspects such as political freedom and economical issues. In general, HRQoL research has undergone four phases, starting with:

- early considerations of theoretical concepts of the topics (from 1970),
- development of measurement approaches (from 1980),
- the inclusion of measures in different studies (from 1990), and more recently
- examining the clinical impact of HRQoL assessment (from 2000).

While HRQoL research in adults has progressed substantially over recent years, the topic has not yet been systematically investigated in younger populations. Despite the slow development of HRQoL research in children and adolescents, the assessment of well-being and function is considered an important topic especially in paediatric research and practice. One reason for this is the increasing number of children and adolescents suffering from chronic health conditions. Among these are asthma, obesity, and diabetes type 1, but also conditions requiring special care such as arthritis and cerebral palsy as well as those that are requiring continuous management such as diabetes and atopic dermatitis. With regard to the assessment of HRQoL in young populations, researchers have to face a number of challenges. Overall, progress in paediatric HRQoL research was slow due to conceptual and operational difficulties (Drotar 1998). These difficulties refer to age particularities, proxy-report, and cognitive ability of the child. Furthermore, instruments taking into account a cross-national perspective are missing.

In general, HRQoL measures can be divided into generic and condition-specific measures (Guyatt et al. 1995). They can be further categorised into health profiles or preference-based measures. While generic instruments measure HRQoL across health conditions, condition-specific measures do so with regard to a specific disease, treatment or symptom. The disadvantage of generic measures may be that small changes in HRQoL might not be detected. On the other hand, condition-specific instruments may provide more clinically relevant information, but comparison across illnesses is not possible (Bullinger 1997). Moreover, children may have more than one condition and this co-morbidity complicates the development of condition-specific measures. Both types of measures have strengths and weaknesses. The choice of one type of measure depends on the study aims. Sometimes a combined approach is appropriate using bother types of instrument.

Information can be obtained from children or adolescents themselves (self-report) or from significant others, usually the parents (proxy-report). Most instruments are available for different age groups; most of the versions were developed for adolescents from 13-16 years, rarely for school-aged children from 8-13 years, and almost none for the young children. In spite of the availability of different instruments it is unfortunate that only a few instruments are usable for a cross-cultural international research. Although these instruments have been translated into other languages, this procedure reflects the sequential approach, which can be difficult to take into consideration cultural differences between countries. A unique approach for cross-cultural instrument development is the simultaneous approach in which instruments are developed conjointly. In the children's area the DISABKIDS project approached this gap and applied a cross-cultural instrument development procedure.

# 3 The Development of the DISABKIDS Instruments

## 3.1 Rationale for the Development

In view of the necessity to tap at the HRQoL of children with health conditions, especially chronic conditions, the DISABKIDS project was funded by the programme *Quality of Life and Management of Living Resources of the Fifth Framework of the European Union*. A crucial point for this project was to apply an assessment methodology, which gives voice to the children and the adolescents concerns as well as their parents and families. The project proposed a European cooperation to construct an assessment instrument for HRQoL in which the persons concerned play a major role in expressing or structuring the needs for care. The funding of the project by the EU made it possible to construct, develop, test and refine an instrument system, which is now called *The DISABKIDS Questionnaires*. The specific approach, which makes the project unique, is the cross-cultural perspective, the modular system, and the combination of specific and generic aspects, the inclusion of a wide age range and the representation of parent and children's views. This approach was deemed particularly helpful in devising an instrument set that can be applied to a broad range of research in clinical health settings. Different chronic health conditions were selected to contribute to the development of the questionnaire. Concerning the focus of the questionnaire, it was important that it included overall aspects of having a chronic health condition as well as including specific sub-modules. Furthermore, different age ranges are reflected. In summary, the overall objectives of the project were:

- to develop and promote the use of standardised instruments to assess HRQoL in children with chronic health conditions,
- to enhance the possibility of multi-national European studies of HRQoL,
- to assess HRQoL from the patients' perspective by addressing the needs of care, and
- to enhance HRQoL and the independence of children with chronic health conditions.

## 3.2 Conceptual Background

Conceptually the DISABKIDS instruments tools are based on the definition of health-related quality of life assuming mental, social and physical components of quality of life. Furthermore it differentiates between generic and disease-specific quality of life. Concerning the level of operationalisations, the DISABKIDS instrument tool set focusses on the subjective evaluation of symptoms. A developmental approach is taken towards quality of life, which has been elaborated on the literature (Bullinger and Ravens-Sieberer 1995; Eiser and others 1999; Eiser and Morse 2001a).

### 3.3    Description of the DISABKIDS Methodology

The DISABKIDS project is a cooperative effort among experts from different disciplines with experience in HRQoL assessment from different countries (see Figure 3-1). These countries are France, Germany, the Netherlands, Sweden, Austria, and the United Kingdom. The DIS-ABKIDS project has closely cooperated with a cross-cultural epidemiological project, the KIDSCREEN project that employed the same steps in order to develop a survey instrument on quality of life. The HRQoL instruments are applicable in different national and cultural contexts, comply with quality standards in instrument development, and are practical, i.e. short and easy to use and score. The focus of the DISABKIDS project lies on seven chronic health conditions, which are asthma, juvenile rheumatic arthritis, epilepsy, cerebral palsy, diabetes mellitus, atopic dermatitis, and cystic fibrosis.

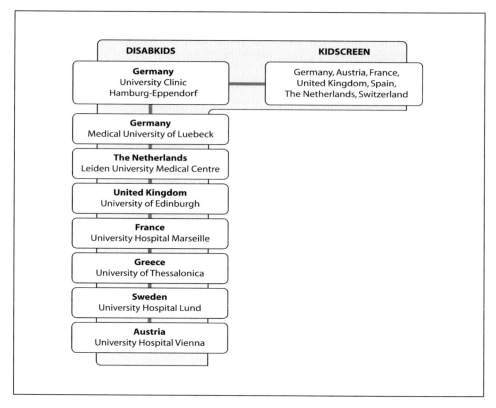

**Figure 3-1 Participating centres and cooperation of the DISABKIDS project**

The DISABKIDS approach followed a methodology, which consists of several work phases (work packages; cf. Table P-1), which reflected a stepwise instrument development procedure. The following paragraphs will give a short overview of the aims and methodology of the different work packages:

### Literature Review

The aim of the process was to review the literature on HRQoL assessment in children and adolescents with a chronic health condition as well as to identify available assessment instruments. Altogether 8233 abstracts were identified in Medline (1985-2000) and reviewed for the purpose to identify dimensions of HRQoL in children and adolescents.

### Focus Groups

The aim of the focus groups was to take the perspective of children and adolescents across Europe into account in the development of the statements in the questionnaire. Focus groups consisted of 3 to 6 children were conducted throughout Europe. In addition, focus groups with parents and professionals were carried out as well as in-depth interviews with some children. The groups were classified according to age, type and severity of disease. Standardised operating procedures ensured the compatibility of the results. The group discussions were content analysed to identify the HRQoL themes relevant to children of different ages and with different conditions.

### Item Development

The results of the focus groups were used to derive items for the generic and condition specific modules. Altogether 3027 statements were formulated as a result of the focus group work. The statements underwent a reduction process involving a redundancy rating performed by three centres, a card sort procedure. Finally, 119 chronic generic and 12-22 disease-specific items for each module were selected to form the draft questionnaire of the pilot test.

### Translation

The pilot questionnaires were forward and backward translated into the languages of the participating centres of the DISABKIDS project. To harmonise translations across countries guidelines were established and each centre followed the standard internationally agreed upon procedure for questionnaire translation. First, two independent translators translated the English pilot draft version into each of the target languages. The two forward translators reviewed the translations for conceptual equivalence and decided upon a reconciled forward translation. A native speaker of the target language or professional translator performed the backward translation into English. Finally, the backward translation was compared with the pilot draft, thus reviewing the respective reconciled forward translation and thereby generating the respective final forward translation. The different languages versions were then harmonised by comparing items across languages.

### Pilot Study

The objectives of the pilot test were to analyse the content of the DISABKIDS draft questionnaires from the respondent's perspective, to collect data for first psychometric analyses, and to simulate the field test. The main psychometric aim of the pilot test analyses was to reduce the number of items and select the best performing items according to predefined criteria. Two methods were chosen to check the appropriateness of the DISABKIDS pilot questionnaires: a quantitative psychometric analysis and a qualitative cognitive debriefing. The questionnaire was administered in each of the project countries during an interview with children drawn from the different conditions. The children completed the questionnaire and were then interviewed using a standard procedure to ascertain the acceptance of the questions, the relevance of the questions to them, their understanding of the questions, and if the wording of the questions could be improved / made more acceptable to children.

Data files were provided by the Hamburg study centre and data entry was done in each country. After data entry, the different data sets were merged and checked in terms of data plausibility. First of all, an analysis of the pilot study was carried out at the international level using classical multi-scaling as well as modern psychometric methods. The criteria applied for the item selection were chosen from a psychometric and clinical perspective. In detail, the results of frequency analyses, cognitive debriefing, exploratory as well as confirmatory factor analysis, item correlations, and Rasch analysis were used to decide upon the inclusion or omission of items. Overall, the item selection process resulted in a 56-item-version of the chronic generic module. The field test version of the chronic generic HRQoL module consists of six domains (independence, emotion, social inclusion, social exclusion, limitation and treatment) and showed a good psychometric performance with reliability coefficients ranging from $\alpha$= .71 to $\alpha$= .90.

With regard to the development of the disease-specific instruments a working group was formed including members of the German, Dutch, and UK team. It was considered important to make use of both a clinical and a statistical perspective during item selection. Data from various sources were first utilised in order to select variables that performed poorly, such as the feasibility and difficulty of the item, its true disease-specific character and it's association with health status variables. The condition specific questionnaires consist of 14-19 items divided over 2-3 domains.

### Field Test

The aim was to analyse the performance of the pilot modules in a representative sample of the target population, to refine the scale structure, and to assess the retest-reliability as well as construct validity of the DISABKIDS modules. The sample was recruited from paediatric hospitals in order to have a homogenous setting. In order to ensure harmony between the DIS-ABKIDS and KIDSCREEN questionnaires the field study instruments included the core items of both questionnaires, and coordinated core determinants, such as sociodemographic items and health status. The field study results provided the reference data reported elsewhere in this manual. Furthermore, core sociodemographic features of the DISABKIDS field study sample are presented (cf. Table 3-1). The DISABKIDS field study was conducted in an overall sample of 1606 cases, about equally distributed across the age groups 4-7 years, 8-12 years, and 13-16 years. Asthma was the only condition tested cross-nationally. In terms of severity of the condition, the sample was primarily in the mild and moderate range (50.7 % respectively 38.7 % of valid cases), however also included children with a more severe impact (10.6 % of valid cases) as indicated by clinical measures on severity assessment

### Implementation: Examples for Application

The DISABKIDS measures were used in different contexts to collect more information about their performance. Implementation studies included clinical feasibility tests and intervention studies. Furthermore, clinical comparative studies on paediatric conditions were conducted, and some countries implemented the DISABKIDS instrument in a survey study.

**Table 3-1 Sociodemographic and clinical characteristics of the sample, crossed for age group\***

| Characteristic | | Total | | Age group I (4-7 years) | | Age group II (8-12 years) | | Age group III (13-16 years) | |
|---|---|---|---|---|---|---|---|---|---|
| N (n$_{total}$ = 1.605) | | 1.556 | 100.00 | 453 | 28.9 | 592 | 37.7 | 525 | 33.4 |
| **Child** | | | | | | | | | |
| Age | Years (M / SD) | 10.44 | 3.75 | 6.04 | 1.57 | 10.06 | 1.52 | 14.69 | 1.52 |
| Gender | Female | 759 | 47.8 | 212 | 47.0 | 274 | 46.5 | 257 | 49.5 |
| | Male | 829 | 52.2 | 239 | 53.0 | 315 | 53.5 | 262 | 50.5 |
| Main diagnosis | Asthma | 609 | 37.9 | 203 | 44.8 | 257 | 43.4 | 135 | 25.7 |
| | Arthritis | 204 | 12.7 | 54 | 11.9 | 75 | 12.7 | 74 | 14.1 |
| | Dermatitis | 111 | 6.9 | 46 | 10.2 | 16 | 2.7 | 46 | 8.8 |
| | Diabetes | 246 | 15.3 | 39 | 8.6 | 98 | 16.6 | 101 | 19.2 |
| | Cerebral Palsy | 147 | 9.2 | 56 | 12.4 | 40 | 6.8 | 46 | 8.8 |
| | Cystic Fibrosis | 58 | 3.6 | 15 | 3.3 | 20 | 3.4 | 20 | 3.8 |
| | Epilepsy | 231 | 14.4 | 40 | 8.8 | 86 | 14.5 | 103 | 19.6 |
| **Parents** | | | | | | | | | |
| Age | Years (M / SD) | 40.16 | 6.54 | 36.94 | 5.76 | 40.23 | 6.31 | 43.08 | 6.02 |
| Respondent | Mother | 1261 | 85.0 | 372 | 86.5 | 484 | 86.3 | 380 | 81.9 |
| | Father | 197 | 13.3 | 46 | 10.7 | 71 | 12.7 | 77 | 16.6 |
| | Other | 25 | 1.7 | 12 | 2.8 | 6 | 1.1 | 7 | 1.5 |
| Marital status | Married | 965 | 78.5 | 297 | 76.9 | 369 | 81.3 | 278 | 77.0 |
| Education | Years (M / SD) | 9.15 | 5.44 | 8.66 | 5.53 | 9.41 | 5.54 | 9.15 | 5.27 |
| Schooling (Other type: .9 %) | No qual. | 95 | 6.9 | 31 | 7.8 | 37 | 7.1 | 23 | 5.3 |
| | Lowest quality | 267 | 19.3 | 78 | 19.5 | 96 | 18.4 | 87 | 20.1 |
| | Above lowest quality | 359 | 26.0 | 114 | 28.5 | 149 | 28.6 | 96 | 22.2 |
| | HSL | 293 | 21.2 | 72 | 18.0 | 111 | 21.3 | 100 | 23.1 |
| | Above HSL | 153 | 11.1 | 48 | 12.0 | 55 | 10.6 | 48 | 11.1 |
| | University | 200 | 14.5 | 57 | 14.3 | 64 | 12.3 | 74 | 17.1 |
| General health | Range 1-5 (M / SD) | 2.66 | .91 | 2.63 | .86 | 2.63 | .95 | 2.73 | .94 |
| **Proxy rating** | | | | | | | | | |
| Childs general health | Range 1-5 (M / SD) | 3.25 | .93 | 3.31 | .91 | 3.29 | .96 | 3.13 | .89 |
| Childs development | Delayed | 229 | 15.6 | 65 | 15.2 | 74 | 13.2 | 88 | 19.3 |
| Child's problems (range: 1-5) | Physical (M / SD) | 1.87 | 1.07 | 1.85 | 1.07 | 1.80 | 1.03 | 1.96 | 1.10 |
| | Emotional (M / SD) | 1.85 | 1.06 | 1.80 | 1.01 | 1.85 | 1.06 | 1.91 | 1.09 |
| | Social (M / SD) | 1.54 | .93 | 1.43 | .81 | 1.51 | .90 | 1.69 | 1.05 |
| **Clinicians rating** | | | | | | | | | |
| Severity | Mild | 524 | 50.7 | 151 | 53.9 | 191 | 49.9 | 170 | 49.3 |
| | Moderate | 400 | 38.7 | 101 | 36.1 | 159 | 41.5 | 129 | 37.4 |
| | Severe | 109 | 10.6 | 28 | 10.0 | 33 | 8.6 | 46 | 13.3 |
| Comorbidity | Yes | 179 | 22.9 | 55 | 23.9 | 64 | 21.8 | 57 | 22.9 |
| Normal cogn. dev. | Yes | 923 | 86.0 | 238 | 84.7 | 355 | 87.4 | 311 | 85.7 |
| Development delay | Yes | 77 | 8.4 | 33 | 13.1 | 12 | 3.4 | 30 | 10.2 |
| Learning difficulty | Yes | 78 | 8.6 | 17 | 6.9 | 32 | 9.1 | 26 | 8.9 |
| Mental retardation | Yes | 47 | 5.2 | 14 | 5.5 | 8 | 2.3 | 29 | 9.7 |

*Note: \* (a) Figures refer to numbers and percent unless otherwise indicated. (b) Absolute frequencies vary as a function of the amount of missing data in each variable.*

# 4 Guidelines for Users - The DISABKIDS measures

The main feature of the DISABKIDS instruments is the modular approach. Table 4-1 gives an overview of the different modules (see also Figure 4-1). In addition, the following pages will describe each module in detail. All modules are available in the six following languages: Dutch, English, French, German, Greek and Swedish.

**Table 4-1 Overview of the DISABKIDS instruments**

| Module | Version | Age | Report | $\sum$ items | Purpose |
|---|---|---|---|---|---|
| *Smileys* | | 4 - 7<br>(8 - 16) | Self/Proxy | 6 | Assessment of Qol in young children, Developmental studies |
| *Chronic*<br>*Generic* | Long Version<br>Short Version | 8 - 16<br>8 - 16 | Self/Proxy | 37<br>12 | Assessment of Qol aspects related to being ill in general; clinical comparative studies; applicable to all chronic conditions |
| *Condition*<br>*Specific* | Arthritis | 8 - 16 | Self/Proxy | 12 | Measurement of Qol that is specific for a particular condition (measuring the impact of the condition); appropriate for condition-specific intervention studies |
| | Asthma | 8 - 16 | Self/Proxy | 11 | |
| | Dermatitis | 8 - 16 | Self/Proxy | 12 | |
| | Diabetes | 8 - 16 | Self/Proxy | 10 | |
| | Cerebral palsy | 8 - 16 | Self/Proxy | 12 | |
| | Cystic fibrosis | 8 - 16 | Self/Proxy | 10 | |
| | Epilepsy | 8 - 16 | Self/Proxy | 10 | |

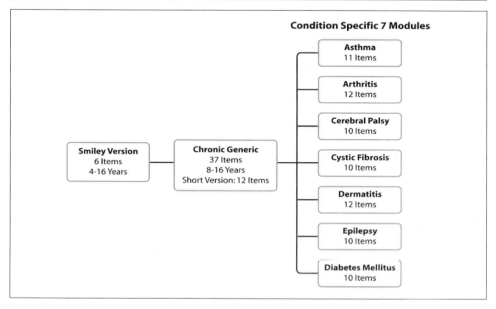

Figure 4-1 Graphical overview on DISABKIDS instruments

## 4.1 The DISABKIDS Chronic Generic Measure - DCGM-37 (long version)

### 4.1.1 Purpose

The DISABKIDS chronic generic module deals with the health-related quality of life (HRQoL) in children and adolescents with different chronic health conditions and addresses HRQoL aspects that pertain not to specific conditions but to chronic conditions in general. The DISABKIDS chronic generic module instrument ought to be applicable in different national and cultural contexts.

### 4.1.2 Development

The proposed DISABKIDS chronic generic module underwent various steps of instrument development in a simultaneous cross-cultural approach (see in detail above, Chapter 3.3). After conducting focus groups and forming an international item pool, only those items were selected that pertain to chronic conditions, while condition specific and generic items were processed separately. Further steps including a translation process following international guidelines (Guillemin and others 1993) and the pilot testing of the instrument (Bullinger and others 2002). The field study analysis of the DISABKIDS chronic generic module comprises additional psychometric evaluations of both the single items and the scale structure. This analyses results in the final version of the DISABKIDS chronic generic module and is reported in detail elsewhere (Debensason and others in press).

### 4.1.3 Description of the instrument

In the following section the scale structure, scoring procedures, reference data for the chronic generic module is described and its convergent and discriminant validity demonstrated. Further reference data is shown in the appendix (T-score, percentiles).

### 4.1.4 Self- and proxy assessment

Two versions of the DISABKIDS chronic generic module are available: the *self-report version (child version)* and a *proxy version (proxy version)*. Both versions of the DISABKIDS chronic generic module are available in six different languages: Dutch, English, French, German, Greek, and Swedish. A *computer-assisted version* of the *paper-and-pencil version* of the DISABKIDS chronic generic module is available as well, in six languages.

### 4.1.5 Scale structure and scoring

The DISABKIDS chronic generic module (DCGM-37) consists of 37 Likert-scaled items assigned to six dimensions: Independence, Emotion, Social inclusion, Social exclusion, Limitation, and Treatment. Pilot test results denoted satisfactory internal consistencies of these scales (Petersen and others 2004), ranging from $\alpha = .79$ (Social inclusion) to $\alpha = .90$ (Emotion). The sub-scales of these six dimensions of the DCGM-37 can be combined to produce a general score for health-related quality of life (HRQoL), denoted as the DCGM-37 total score. The six sub-scales are additionally associated with three domains, denoted as mental, social, and physical. These HRQoL domains have evolved from the mental, social and physical domains of HRQoL, as conceptualised by the WHO. Health-related quality of life is conceived as a second-order factor, underlying the structure of the DCGM-37 (see Figure 4-2).

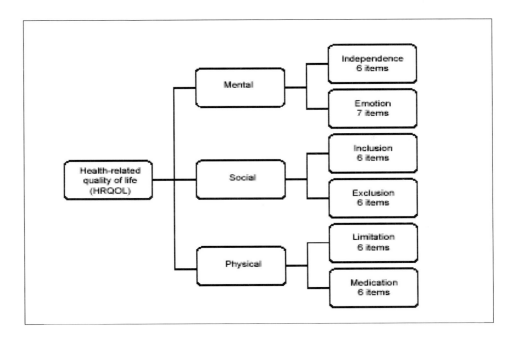

**Figure 4-2 Structure of DISABKIDS chronic generic module**

The 37 items of the DISABKIDS chronic generic module comprise 6 sub-scales each of which has 6 items except for the emotion sub-scale that has 7 items. For 5 of the 6 scales the score can range from 6 to 30, except sub-scale "emotion" with a range from 7 to 35, provided all items of a scale have been completed (see Table 4-2).

**Table 4-2 Items included in the sub-scales of the DISABKIDS chronic generic module**

| | Domain | Facet | $\sum_{items}$ | $\sum_{ranks}$ | Items of sub-scales | Possible range of raw score (Min, Max) |
|---|---|---|---|---|---|---|
| HRQOL | *Mental* | Independence | 6 | 24 | 1+2+3+4+5+6 | 24 (6, 30) |
| | | Emotion | 7 | 28 | 7+8+9+10+11+12+13 | 28 (7, 35) |
| | *Social* | Social inclusion | 6 | 24 | 14+15+16+17+18+19 | 24 (6, 30) |
| | | Social exclusion | 6 | 24 | 20+21+22+23+24+25 | 24 (6, 30) |
| | *Physical* | Physical limitation | 6 | 24 | 26+27+28+29+30+31 | 24 (6, 30) |
| | | Treatment | 6 | 24 | 32+33+34+35+36+37 | 24 (6, 30) |

Table 4-3 describes the main content areas of each of the chronic generic module. The Independence sub-scale describes whether the child is able to live an autonomous life without being impaired by the condition. The Emotional sub-scale assesses emotional reactions caused by the conditions. While the Social inclusion sub-scale describes the perception of positive feedback from friends and family, the Social exclusion sub-scale delineates a very negative impact of the condition that makes the child feel stigmatized and left out. The first Physical sub-scale is related to the limitation experimentally the conditions, while the second Physical sub-scale, the Treatment sub-scale, assesses the impact of taking treatment or receiving any other medical treatment for the condition.

**Table 4-3 Domains and facets of the DISABKIDS chronic generic module**

| | Domain | Facet | Concept/ content |
|---|---|---|---|
| HRQOL | *Mental* | Independence | Confidence about future, living without impairments caused by condition |
| | | Emotion | Emotional worries, concerns, anger, problems because of the condition |
| | *Social* | Social inclusion | Understanding of others, positive social relationships |
| | | Social exclusion | Stigma, feeling left out |
| | *Physical* | Limitation | Functional limitations, perceived health status, difficulties with sleeping |
| | | Treatment | Perceived impact of taking medication, receiving injections, taking insulin, applying cortisone, etc. |

### 4.1.6 Psychometric properties - results of the field study analysis

*Population*

The proposed reference scores for children of the age group 8 to 16 are based on the results of the DISABKIDS field study (n= 1.152, age group 8-16; The DISABKIDS Group Europe, in prep.; see Table 4-4 and Table 4-5). The total sample size differs from the response rates of each survey wave (test or retest) and from the response rates for the study participant (child, proxy). Thus, for some cases there is non-response for the children's test (n = 1.128), although there is a proxy response.

**Table 4-4 Response rates for the DISABKIDS chronic generic module across conditions (age group 8-16; DISABKIDS field study sample)**

| Disease of the child | test | retest | proxy |
|---|---|---|---|
| | *n* | *n* | *n* |
| Asthma | 405 | 146 | 382 |
| Arthritis | 148 | 88 | 141 |
| Atopic dermatitis | 64 | 51 | 41 |
| Diabetes | 204 | 106 | 199 |
| Cerebral palsy | 86 | 38 | 82 |
| Cystic fibrosis | 40 | 6 | 34 |
| Epilepsy | 181 | 32 | 181 |
| Total | 1.128 | 465 | 1.061 |

**Table 4-5 Response rates DISABKIDS chronic generic module across countries (age group 8-16; DISABKIDS field study sample)**

| Disease of the child | test | retest | proxy |
|---|---|---|---|
| | *n* | *n* | *n* |
| Germany | 277 | 184 | 250 |
| Netherlands | 283 | 69 | 271 |
| United Kingdom | 121 | 40 | 108 |
| France | 72 | 24 | 67 |
| Greece | 74 | 30 | 71 |
| Sweden | 200 | 79 | 196 |
| Austria | 101 | 39 | 98 |
| Total | 1.128 | 465 | 1.061 |

The analysis of the data from the DISABKIDS chronic generic module completed by chronically ill children and adolescents and their parents was performed using the SPSS program (version 11.5.1).

### 4.1.7 Descriptive psychometric properties, reliability, and factorial validity

Cronbach's alpha as a measure of internal consistency reached satisfactory values ranging from $\alpha$ =.70 to $\alpha$ =.87 (child version), and $\alpha$ =.77 to $\alpha$ =.90 (proxy version) for the sub-scales, while the overall score displayed a consistency coefficient of $\alpha$ =.93 (child version), respectively $\alpha$ =.95 (proxy version; Table 4-6).

**Table 4-6 Selected descriptive and psychometric properties for the total score and sub-scales of the self-report version (child version) and the proxy-version of the DISABKIDS chronic generic module (DISABKIDS field study sample)**

| | Domain | Facet | M (1-100) | SD | Skewness | $\alpha$ | Split-half | ICC $_{t1,t2}$ |
|---|---|---|---|---|---|---|---|---|
| **HRQOL** | *Mental* | Independence | 76.14 / 76.23 | 18.50 / 17.83 | - 1.02 / - .98 | .78 / .85 | .74 / .84 | .74 / - |
| | | Emotion | 76.24 / 72.04 | 20.98 / 20.78 | - .88 / - .59 | .87 / .90 | .79 / .88 | .83 / - |
| | *Social* | Social inclusion | 74.56 / 73.76 | 18.14 / 18.15 | - .82 / - .81 | .70 / .78 | .75 / .79 | .82 / - |
| | | Social exclusion | 84.41 / 80.67 | 16.24 / 17.17 | - 1.37 / - .90 | .75 / .80 | .79 / .77 | .81 / - |
| | *Physical* | Limitation | 73.96 / 70.63 | 18.92 / 18.57 | - .71 / - .52 | .73 / .77 | .76 / .79 | .79 / - |
| | | Treatment | 72.27 / 69.80 | 22.62 / 22.28 | - .64 / - .64 | .80 / .85 | .70 / .78 | .71 / - |
| | *DCGM-37 total score* | | 76.46 / 73.93 | 14.92 / 15.16 | - .76 / - .62 | .93 / .95 | .86 / .92 | .84 / - |

**Table 4-7 Intercorrelation between total score and sub-scales of the self-report version (child version) and proxy version of the DISABKIDS chronic generic module**

| | Independence | Physical limitation | Social inclusion | Social exclusion | Emotion | Treatment | HRQOL |
|---|---|---|---|---|---|---|---|
| Independence | | | | | | | |
| Emotion | .63 / .63 | | | | | | |
| Social inclusion | .57 / .66 | .44 / .46 | | | | | |
| Social exclusion | .58 / .65 | .67 / .68 | .52 / .61 | | | | |
| Limitation | .62 / .68 | .69 / .70 | .49 / .56 | .62 / .64 | | | |
| Treatment | .33 / .35 | .54 / .56 | .26 / .32 | .40 / .43 | .40 / .40 | | |
| DCGM-37 total score | .79 / .82 | .87 / .87 | .69 / .74 | .80 / .83 | .82 / .83 | .67/ .67 | |

The analyses of the intercorrelation between subscales (see Table 4-7) indicate that all sub-scales show significant correlations with each other suggesting a higher-order quality of life factor. The only exception is the Treatment sub-scale showing lower association ($r = .26-.54$).

### 4.1.8 Concordance between parent and child version

Empirical studies suggested that the degree of convergence between self- and proxy-ratings in HRQoL especially in the field of children and adolescents is different, depending for instance on the health status of the child. Parents of healthy children usually overestimate the quality of life as reported by the children itself, whereas parents of ill children tend to underestimate the child's self-reported quality of life. Furthermore, the divergence seems to be larger in emotional than in physical domains (Eiser and Berrenberg 1995; Eiser and Morse 2001b). The most widely used coefficient for the concordance between different raters is the Pearson correlation coefficient. In addition to this indicator, the concordance between self- and proxy-report was estimated with the intraclass correlation coefficient (ICC). These coefficients are reported for the DISABKIDS scales and indicate a high convergence between parent and child reports of the six domains (see Table 4-8).

**Table 4-8 Intraclass correlation coefficient (ICC) and correlation coefficients (Pearson r) for total score and sub-scales of the self-report version (child version) and the proxy version of the DISABKIDS chronic generic module**

| | Domain | Facet | ICC | r |
|---|---|---|---|---|
| HRQOL | Mental | Independence | .54 | .54 |
| | | Emotion | .60 | .60 |
| | Social | Social inclusion | .55 | .55 |
| | | Social exclusion | .56 | .60 |
| | Physical | Limitation | .62 | .62 |
| | | Treatment | .53 | .53 |
| | DCGM-37 total score | | .65 | .65 |

### 4.1.9 Convergent validity

In terms of convergent validity with other subjective health related measures, the DISAB-KIDS chronic generic module (DCGM-37) sub-scales and the DCGM-37 total score correlated significantly with several self-reported and external reported indicators of subjective health dimensions. Correlations were checked for the CHQ-KINDL-Index (Ellert and others 2001), for the two sub-scales of the Functional Status II (R) measure general health and inter-personal functioning (FSII-R; (Stein and Jessop 1990), the KINDL-R (Ravens-Sieberer 2003), as well as for self and parent reported general health perception (GHP) of the child. It was found that the DCGM-37 total score and sub-scale scores displayed only a moderate correlation with the general health sub-scale of the Functional Status II (R) measure. Altogether, the correlations of the DCGM-37 total score and sub-scale scores with several measures of health status are only moderate. This might reflect the different conceptualisation of the scales. The highest correlation can be found with self-reported general health perception. The correlations for the proxy version of the DISABKIDS chronic generic module are notably higher than for the child version, except for the self-reported general health perception of the child (cf. Table 4-9 to Table 4-10).

**Table 4-9 Correlation coefficients (Pearson r) for total sub-scales of the self-report version (child version) of the DISABKIDS chronic generic module with several health status indicators**

|  | General Health Perception | FS-II-R General health | FS-II-R Interpersonal functioning |
|---|---|---|---|
| Independence | .35 | .34 | .31 |
| Emotion | .40 | .35 | .30 |
| Social inclusion | .24 | .24 | .18 |
| Social exclusion | .30 | .30 | .28 |
| Physical limitation | .41 | .41 | .25 |
| Treatment | .26 | .26 | .21 |
| *Total DCGM-37 score* | .40 | .39 | .30 |

**Table 4-10 Correlation coefficients (Pearson r) for the sub-scales of the self-report version (child version) and the proxy version of the DISABKIDS chronic generic module with the sub-scales of the self-report version (child version) and the proxy version of the KINDL-R**

| | KINDL-R | | | | | | |
|---|---|---|---|---|---|---|---|
| | Physical well-being | Emotional well-being | Self-esteem | Family | Friends | Everyday functioning | Total |
| Independence | .27 / .40 | .39 / .48 | .38 / .49 | .34 / .35 | .42 / .59 | .20 / .25 | .42 / .45 |
| Emotion | .47 / .46 | .53 / .42 | .45 / .36 | .29 / .32 | .41 / .36 | .29 / .11 | .64 / .60 |
| Social inclusion | .23 / .32 | .40 / .45 | .34 / .45 | .27 / .27 | .53 / .68 | .12 / .19 | .35 / .35 |
| Social exclusion | .44 / .43 | .42 / .48 | .35 / .44 | .32 / .33 | .53 / .58 | .22 / .29 | .48 / .42 |
| Physical limitation | .47 / .55 | .42 / .44 | .37 / .39 | .31 / .29 | .45 / .48 | .20 / .14 | .49 / .52 |
| Treatment | .34 / .24 | .32 / .38 | .31 / .32 | .24 / .36 | .31 / .20 | .24 / .31 | .44 / .40 |
| Total DCGM-37 score | .45 / .49 | .53 / .55 | .46 / .51 | .36 / .38 | .58 / .67 | .24 / .25 | .59 / .53 |

## 4.1.10 Discriminant validity

The DISABKIDS chronic generic module for chronically ill children and adolescents, aged 8 to 16 years, discriminates well between chronic conditions as well as between different levels of severity, assessed by clinician's severity assessment measures. It distinguishes between differences in the impairment of health-related quality of life (HRQOL) in children and adolescents with different chronic conditions (asthma, juvenile arthritis, atopic dermatitis, diabetes, cerebral palsy, cystic fibrosis, epilepsy; cf. Table 4-11 % Table 4-12).

**Table 4-11 Transformed raw scores (mean, standard deviation; range 0 - 100) for total score and subscales of the self-report version (child version) and the proxy-version of the DISABKIDS chronic generic module for different chronic conditions**

|  | Asthma | Arthritis | Dermatitis | Diabetes | Cerebral palsy | Cystic fibrosis | Epilepsy |
|---|---|---|---|---|---|---|---|
| *N* | 403 | 148 | 65 | 204 | 84 | 40 | 179 |
| Independence | 79.26 | 77.58 | 72.33 | 78.79 | 64.93 | 71.88 | 71.86 |
| Emotion | 74.47 | 73.02 | 75.49 | 75.09 | 63.23 | 74.33 | 76.91 |
| Social inclusion | 77.59 | 72.86 | 76.54 | 81.29 | 58.95 | 71.78 | 68.24 |
| Social exclusion | 88.97 | 85.79 | 82.09 | 85.20 | 73.74 | 83.50 | 77.98 |
| Physical limitation | 74.47 | 73.02 | 75.49 | 75.09 | 63.23 | 74.33 | 76.91 |
| Treatment | 76.32 | 67.98 | 65.25 | 71.09 | 75.97 | 67.29 | 70.29 |
| *Total DCGM-37 score* | 80.15 | 76.13 | 74.65 | 79.46 | 65.41 | 74.49 | 74.09 |

**Table 4-12 Transformed raw scores (mean, standard deviation; range 0 - 100) for total score and subscales of the proxy version (parent version) of the DISABKIDS chronic generic module for different chronic conditions (DISABKIDS field study sample)**

|  | Asthma | Arthritis | Dermatitis | Diabetes | Cerebral palsy | Cystic fibrosis | Epilepsy |
|---|---|---|---|---|---|---|---|
| *N* | 382 | 141 | 41 | 198 | 82 | 32 | 136 |
| Independence | 80.47 | 79.34 | 75.20 | 78.51 | 57.91 | 73.24 | 68.84 |
| Emotion | 79.18 | 70.24 | 67.00 | 65.55 | 66.74 | 60.30 | 69.63 |
| Social inclusion | 78.42 | 72.59 | 73.52 | 78.53 | 55.29 | 72.99 | 66.49 |
| Social exclusion | 86.35 | 82.69 | 82.72 | 78.04 | 66.73 | 81.09 | 73.18 |
| Physical limitation | 72.49 | 68.54 | 72.38 | 71.56 | 60.39 | 69.35 | 71.54 |
| Treatment | 73.10 | 66.44 | 65.81 | 64.13 | 78.49 | 61.02 | 72.23 |
| *Total DCGM-37 score* | 79.12 | 74.12 | 74.45 | 74.90 | 60.93 | 72.55 | 71.38 |

The DCGM-37 also discriminates well between differences in the impairment of health-related quality of life in children and adolescents with a different clinical severity of condition (cf. Table 4-13 and Table 4-14). The most general finding was that there was a significant difference between conditions with a higher quality of life on all scales, in particular in asthma, and a lower quality of life on all scales, such as cerebral palsy. However, there also appears to be a distinct profile for each condition. For instance, children with Cystic fibrosis had lower scores on Emotion and Treatment, while children with diabetes had particularly low scores on Treatment and children with epilepsy or cerebral palsy on Social exclusion. This good discriminatory performance was observed for both versions of the chronic generic module, the self-report-version (child version) and the proxy version (parent version).

**Table 4-13 Standardized raw scores for total score and sub-scales of the self-report version (child version) and the proxy-version of the DISABKIDS chronic generic module for different groups of clinical severity (DISABKIDS field study sample)**

| Severity | Independence | Physical limitation | Social inclusion | Social exclusion | Emotion | Treatment | Total |
|---|---|---|---|---|---|---|---|
| Mild | 80.44 | 78.94 | 78.44 | 88.18 | 80.25 | 74.44 | 81.15 |
| Moderate | 75.10 | 72.30 | 73.34 | 84.25 | 75.20 | 70.82 | 75.70 |
| Severe | 67.20 | 62.78 | 66.42 | 76.35 | 65.35 | 66.53 | 67.18 |

**Table 4-14 Transformed raw scores (mean, standard deviation; range 0 - 100) for total score and sub-scales of the proxy version (parent version) of the DISABKIDS chronic generic module for different groups of clinical severity (DISABKIDS field study sample)**

| Severity | Independence | Physical limitation | Social inclusion | Social exclusion | Emotion | Treatment | Total |
|---|---|---|---|---|---|---|---|
| Mild | 81.31 | 76.05 | 78.95 | 82.95 | 74.15 | 69.98 | 78.73 |
| Moderate | 75.29 | 69.95 | 72.34 | 80.75 | 72.08 | 69.04 | 73.87 |
| Severe | 64.58 | 56.52 | 63.20 | 72.69 | 62.56 | 66.21 | 64.10 |

## 4.1.11 Interpretation and reference values

The scores achieved on the individual sub-scales of the DISABKIDS chronic generic module and the total score of the DISABKIDS chronic generic module represent an empirical assessment of the child's or adolescent's health-related quality of life (HRQoL) from the respondent's point of view (child/ parents). Until the data from a standard sample is available for the DISABKIDS chronic generic module, the results of the DISABKIDS field study (n = 1152) should be used as a preliminary reference for children and adolescents with chronic conditions. For the following reference values of the DCGM-37 sub-scales and the DCGM-37 total score, the scales have been transformed to a range of 0 to 100 (cf. Table 4-15 to Table 4-16). The scores are shown for males and females and different age groups (8-12 and 13-16).

**Table 4-15 Transformed raw scores (mean, standard deviation; range 0 - 100) for sub-scales and total score of the DISABKIDS chronic generic module (child version), crossed for age group and gender (DISABKIDS field study sample)**

| | Age group I | | | | Age group II | | | | | |
| | Female | | Male | | Female | | Male | | Total | |
| | M | SD | M | SD | M | SD | M | SD | M | SD |
|---|---|---|---|---|---|---|---|---|---|---|
| Independence | 76.31 | 19.12 | 76.79 | 18.77 | 76.93 | 17.38 | 77.76 | 17.83 | 76.90 | 18.34 |
| Emotion | 77.32 | 19.04 | 79.77 | 20.02 | 72.35 | 20.59 | 76.04 | 22.30 | 76.72 | 20.56 |
| Social inclusion | 72.41 | 17.73 | 73.94 | 18.36 | 77.99 | 15.54 | 77.72 | 18.66 | 75.25 | 17.81 |
| Social exclusion | 85.24 | 15.37 | 85.69 | 15.93 | 83.72 | 15.09 | 85.71 | 15.73 | 85.15 | 15.56 |
| Physical limitation | 73.53 | 17.04 | 75.35 | 18.50 | 70.81 | 19.07 | 75.17 | 18.10 | 73.85 | 18.23 |
| Treatment | 72.05 | 20.88 | 76.98 | 21.91 | 66.93 | 23.37 | 71.90 | 23.82 | 72.25 | 22.71 |
| *DCGM-37 total score* | 76.12 | 14.17 | 78.25 | 14.22 | 74.79 | 14.04 | 78.66 | 14.19 | 76.99 | 14.22 |

**Table 4-16 Transformed raw scores (mean, standard deviation; range 0 - 100) for sub-scales and total score of the DISABKIDS chronic generic module (proxy version), crossed for age group and gender (DISABKIDS field study sample)**

| | Age group I | | | | Age group II | | | | | |
| | Female | | Male | | Female | | Male | | Total | |
| | M | SD | M | SD | M | SD | M | SD | M | SD |
|---|---|---|---|---|---|---|---|---|---|---|
| Independence | 78.19 | 16.18 | 77.09 | 17.53 | 75.57 | 16.64 | 75.07 | 18.54 | 76.60 | 17.25 |
| Emotion | 73.10 | 19.18 | 74.81 | 20.31 | 67.36 | 20.04 | 69.56 | 21.81 | 71.61 | 20.49 |
| Social inclusion | 75.81 | 16.39 | 74.10 | 17.54 | 73.87 | 17.34 | 73.17 | 19.47 | 74.28 | 17.65 |
| Social exclusion | 81.87 | 16.00 | 82.11 | 16.55 | 79.02 | 17.26 | 79.98 | 17.46 | 80.91 | 16.79 |
| Physical limitation | 71.36 | 17.66 | 71.97 | 18.62 | 67.51 | 17.56 | 68.97 | 19.10 | 70.19 | 18.32 |
| Treatment | 68.96 | 21.30 | 71.30 | 21.26 | 70.14 | 22.33 | 68.79 | 24.16 | 69.90 | 22.15 |
| *DCGM-37 total score* | 75.82 | 13.62 | 75.93 | 14.49 | 73.28 | 14.25 | 73.97 | 15.83 | 74.90 | 14.55 |

## 4.1.12 Administration - suggested uses

The chronic generic modules can be administered in all clinical, psychosocial and also public health studies. For instance, they can either be used to compare quality of life across different conditions with each other or focus on intervention studies that are conducted across different conditions. In cross-sectional or longitudinal studies on specific conditions, it is suggested to use both the chronic generic modules (in its long or short version) as well as the disease-specific module. When used in a survey approach, it is suggested to use a filter question inquiring about the existence as well as the type of disease. In order to compare data with epidemiological reference data, it is suggested to include the KIDSCREEN measure.

**DISABKIDS Chronic generic measure - DCGM-12 (short version)**

### 4.1.13  Purpose

The short-form of the DISABKIDS condition generic measure (DCGM-37) deals with the same subject as its parental version. It provides a possibility of assessing health-related quality of life (HRQoL) in children and adolescents with different chronic health conditions in a more economic way. This short-form is derived from the same conceptual background as the DCGM-37.

### 4.1.14  Development

The short-form of the DISABKIDS condition generic module was derived from its parental version. In a first pragmatic step, it was decided to transfer the conceptual structure of the DCGM-37 as a framework for short-form development. This approach leads to some restrictions in item selection that is to select the items in a structural representative way. Item selection for short-form development was performed using multivariate methods of test construction. Short-form development and analyses results of the final version of the short-form of the DCGM-37 will be reported (Mühlan et al., in prep.).

### 4.1.15  Description of the instrument

*Self- and proxy assessment*

Two versions of the short-form of the DISABKIDS condition generic module are available: the s*elf-report version (child version)* and a *proxy version (parents` version)*. Both versions of the short-form are available in six different languages: Dutch, English, French, German, Greek, and Swedish. A *computer-assisted version* of the *paper-and-pencil version* of the DISABKIDS chronic generic module is available as well, in six languages.

*Scale structure and scoring*

The short-form of the DISABKIDS chronic generic module consists of 12 Likert-scaled items assigned to the three domains of the parental version: mental, social and physical. The items can be combined to produce a total score.

**Table 4-17 Domains and facets of the DISABKIDS chronic generic module included in the DISABKIDS chronic generic short-form**

| | Domain included | Facet included | Concept/ content |
|---|---|---|---|
| **HRQOL** | *Mental* | Independence | Autonomy, Living without impairments caused by condition |
| | | Emotion | Emotional worries, concerns, anger, problems |
| | *Social* | Social inclusion | Acceptance of others, Positive social relationships |
| | | Social exclusion | Stigma, Feeling left out |
| | *Physical* | Limitation | Functional limitations, Perceived health status |
| | | Treatment | (Emotional) impact of taking medication, Receiving injections, Taking insulin, Applying cortisone, etc. |

Table 4-17 describes the main content areas of the DISABKIDS short-form of the chronic generic measure. The DISABKIDS short-form has been developed in a strictly symmetric representative way. Thus every facet and every domain of its parental version (the DCGM-37) is represented with two items (see Table 4-18). The inclusion of all domains (mental, social, physical) was based on the conceptual model of three higher-order dimensions, following an age adopted and chronic generic diagnostic approach to HRQoL assessment. For a more in-depth view on the concepts included please check the chapter 4.1 "DISABKIDS condition generic measure".

**Table 4-18 Items included in the sub-scales**

| | Domains included | $\sum$ items | Facets included | $\sum$ items | Items | Possible range of raw score (Min, Max) |
|---|---|---|---|---|---|---|
| **HRQOL** | *Mental* | 4 | Independence | 2 | 1+2 | |
| | | | Emotion | 2 | 3+4 | |
| | *Social* | 4 | Social inclusion | 2 | 5+6 | ($\rightarrow$ One score) |
| | | | Social exclusion | 2 | 7+8 | 48 (12, 60) |
| | *Physical* | 4 | Limitation | 2 | 9+10 | |
| | | | Treatment | 2 | 11+12 | |

### 4.1.16 Psychometric properties - results of the field study analysis

*Descriptive psychometric properties, reliability, and factorial validity*

Cronbach's alpha as a measure of internal consistency reached satisfactory values with $\alpha = .84$ (child version) and $\alpha = .86$ (proxy version) for the short-form measure (see Table 4-17), the split-half reliability coefficient reaches values of $=.90$ (child version), respectively .93 (proxy version).

**Table 4-17 Selected psychometric properties for the total score and sub-scales of the self-report version (child version) of the short-form of the DISABKIDS chronic generic module (DISABKIDS field study sample)**

|  | $\Sigma$ items | M (0-100) | SD | Skewness | $\alpha$ | *Split-half* | ICC $_{t1,t2}$ |
|---|---|---|---|---|---|---|---|
| *DCGM-12 score* | 12 | 77.20 / 74.07 | 17.18 / 17.55 | - .79 / - .70 | .84 / .86 | .90 / .93 | .80 / - |

*Concordance between parent and child version*

The concordance between self- and proxy-report was estimated with the Pearson and the intraclass correlation coefficient (ICC). These coefficients indicate a high convergence (ICC = .823; r = .823) between self- and proxy-version of the total score of the DCGM-12 (see Table 4-18).

**Table 4-18 Intraclass correlation coefficient (ICC) and correlation coefficients (Pearson r) for total score and sub-scales of the self-report version (child version) and the proxy version of the short-form of the DISABKIDS chronic generic module**

|  | *ICC* | r |
|---|---|---|
| *DCGM-12 score* | .82 | .82 |

*Convergent validity*

Convergent validity was investigated using other measures of health-related quality of life. The DISABKIDS short-form displays moderate correlations with all subscales of the KINDL-R ($r_{D,K \text{ (self)}} = .317\text{-}.518$; $r_{D,K \text{ (proxy)}} = .370\text{-}.586$) whereas the correlation between the DCGM-12 and the total score of the KINDL-R shows the highest correlation ($r_{D,K \text{ (self)}} = .596$; $r_{D,K \text{ (proxy)}} = .649$). As almost for its parental version, the correlations for the proxy-version of the DISABKIDS short-form are notably higher than for the child version (cf. Table 4-19).

**Table 4-19 Correlation coefficients (Pearson r) for the sub-scales of the self-report version (child version) and the proxy version of the short-form of the DISABKIDS chronic generic module with the sub-scales of the self-report version and the proxy version of the KINDL-R**

| | KINDL-R | | | | | | |
|---|---|---|---|---|---|---|---|
| | *Physical Well-Being* | *Emotional Well-Being* | *Self-esteem* | *Family* | *Friends* | *Everyday functioning* | *Total* |
| *Health-related quality of life* | .44 / .52 | .49 / .53 | .43 / .48 | .32 /.37 | .52 / .59 | .37 /.42 | .60 / .65 |

## Discriminant validity

The DCGM-12 discriminates well between differences in the impairment of health-related quality of life (HRQOL) in children and adolescents with different chronic conditions (asthma, juvenile arthritis, atopic dermatitis, diabetes, cerebral palsy, cystic fibrosis, epilepsy; cf. Table 4-20).

**Table 4-20 Means for total score and sub-scales of the self-report version of the short-form of the DISABKIDS chronic generic module (DCGM-12) for different chronic conditions (DISABKIDS field study sample)**

| | Asthma | Arthritis | Dermatitis | Diabetes | Cerebral Palsy | Cystic Fibrosis | Epilepsy |
|---|---|---|---|---|---|---|---|
| *N* | *382* | *141* | *41* | *198* | *82* | *32* | *136* |
| Independence | 80.47 | 79.34 | 75.20 | 78.51 | 57.91 | 73.24 | 68.84 |
| Emotion | 79.18 | 70.24 | 67.00 | 65.55 | 66.74 | 60.30 | 69.63 |
| Social inclusion | 78.42 | 72.59 | 73.52 | 78.53 | 55.29 | 72.99 | 66.49 |
| Social exclusion | 86.35 | 82.69 | 82.72 | 78.04 | 66.73 | 81.09 | 73.18 |
| Physical limitation | 72.49 | 68.54 | 72.38 | 71.56 | 60.39 | 69.35 | 71.54 |
| Treatment | 73.10 | 66.44 | 65.81 | 64.13 | 78.49 | 61.02 | 72.23 |
| *Total DCGM-37 score* | 79.12 | 74.12 | 74.45 | 74.90 | 60.93 | 72.55 | 71.38 |

It also discriminates between differences in the impairment of health-related quality of life in children and adolescents with a different clinical severity of condition (cf. Table 4-21 and Table 4-22). Discriminant validity are observable for the self-report as well as for the proxy-version.

**Table 4-21 Means for total score and sub-scales of the self-report version (child version) and the proxy-version of the short-form of the DISABKIDS chronic generic module for different chronic conditions**

|  | Asthma | Arthritis | Dermatitis | Diabetes | Cerebral palsy | Cystic fibrosis | Epilepsy | Total |
|---|---|---|---|---|---|---|---|---|
| *N* | 356 | 115 | 52 | 196 | 22 | 32 | 157 | 930 |
| Total (self) | 80.76 | 71.96 | 72.44 | 77.90 | 63.07 | 75.33 | 74.20 | 76.89 |
| *N* | 348 | 110 | 38 | 195 | 29 | 23 | 120 | 863 |
| Total (proxy) | 78.79 | 69.83 | 73.63 | 71.83 | 59.84 | 67.30 | 71.46 | 73.88 |

**Table 4-22 Means for total score and sub-scales of the self-report version (child version) and the proxy-version of the short-form of the DISABKIDS chronic generic module for different groups of clinical severity (DISABKIDS field study sample)**

| *Severity* | Total (self) | | Total (proxy) | |
|---|---|---|---|---|
|  | *M (SD)* | *N* | *M (SD)* | *N* |
| *Mild* | 81.37 (15.82) | 362 | 77.93 (16.29) | 334 |
| *Moderate* | 75.92 (15.73) | 287 | 73.76 (15.87) | 260 |
| *Severe* | 66.59 (17.92) | 77 | 61.37 (17.97) | 66 |
| Overall | 77.65  (16.64) | 726 | 74.63  (16.98) | 660 |

## 4.1.17 Interpretation and reference values

The scores achieved on the DISABKIDS short-form represent a global screening assessment of the child's or adolescent's HRQoL from the respondent's point of view (child/ proxy). Until the data from a standard sample is available for the DISABKIDS short-form, the results of the DISABKIDS field study (n = 1152; see above) should be used as a preliminary reference for children and adolescents with chronic conditions. For the reference values (see chapter 6), the raw scores have been also transformed to a range of 0 to 100. The scores are shown for males and females, different age groups (8-12 and 13-16) and conditions.

## 4.1.18 Administration - suggested uses

The DISABKIDS short-form should be used whenever a short version is needed for economic reasons, e.g. in survey studies on quality of life in children with chronic conditions, in survey studies on the general child population with a filter asking for a chronic condition, or in studies where different modules (generic measures, chronic generic measure, conditions-specific measure, smileys) need to be combined so that comparisons can be made to children of a specific age.

## 4.2    The DISABKIDS-Smileys

### 4.2.1    Purpose

The purpose of the DISABKIDS-Smiley measure is to assess general quality of life and the level of distress caused by a chronic disease. The questionnaire is simple and fast to complete and is aimed at cognitive levels of children between 4 to 7 developmental years. It should also be used for children above 7 years who have not reached the level of reading ability necessary for the completion of the generic DISABKIDS questionnaire. It can also be used in older children if comparisons between younger and older children are intended.

### 4.2.2    Development

The items for the questionnaire were derived from focus groups with parents of children bet-ween 4 and 7 years. Research on the use of smileys has guided the graphical layout of the questionnaire. The questionnaire was pilot tested and refined not only by using psychometric approaches but also by results of the 'cognitive applicability'.

### 4.2.3    Population

The DISABKIDS-Smiley measure is designed for children aged 4-7 years and completed, in particular for younger children, with the help of the interviewer/nurse or parent. Children and adolescent can also complete this short questionnaire.

### 4.2.4    Score

A single summary score is produced which is compared to the scores on a reference table of children in 7 countries with various chronic medical conditions.

### 4.2.5    Time

The questionnaire should take no more than 5 minutes to administer to the child.

### 4.2.6    Description of the instrument

The DISABKIDS-Smiley measure includes a separate paediatric scale designed for children aged 4-7 years and a proxy/parent response form. Responses are in the form of "smiley" faces, and the paediatric questionnaire is completed, at least for younger children, with the help of the interviewer/nurse or parent. The paediatric version is read aloud to the child who is encou-raged to point to the appropriate answer category. The interviewer records the first answer of the child. The parental version is completed without reference to the paediatric version.

### 4.2.7 Scoring and scale structure

A 5-point scale of smiley faces response scale is used. The children respond by indicating one of 5 smiley faces representing a scale between very happy and very sad. The happiest face (on the right of the scale) scores the highest number and the unhappiest face receives the lowest score. The DISABKIDS-Smiley measure consists of 6 Likert-scaled items. Pilot test results denoted satisfactory internal consistency of the original 12-item-scale.

### 4.2.8 Self- and proxy assessment

Two versions of the DISABKIDS-Smiley measure are available: the *self-report version (child version)* and a *proxy version*. Both versions of the DISABKIDS smiley module are available in six different languages: Dutch, English, French, German, Greek, and Swedish. A *computer-assisted version* of the *paper-and-pencil version* of the DISABKIDS-Smiley measure is available as well, in six languages.

### 4.2.9 Descriptive psychometric properties, reliability, and factorial validity

Cronbach's alpha as a measure of internal consistency reached moderate values ranging from $\alpha = .67$ (child version) to $\alpha = .71$ (proxy-report) for the smiley total score (see Table 4-23), while the split-half reliability displayed a coefficient of .72 (child version), respectively .71 (proxy version).

Table 4-23 Selected psychometric properties for the total score of the DISABKIDS-Smiley measure (DISABKIDS field study sample), for self- report (test) and parent version (proxy version)

| | Version / module | N | M (0-100) | SD | Skewness | $\alpha$ | Split-half | ICC $_{t1,t2}$ |
|---|---|---|---|---|---|---|---|---|
| 1 | Self-report version (test) | 1.444 | 68.97 | 95.83 | -.29 | .69 | .72 | .69 |
| 3 | Proxy-report version (parent version) | 402 | 70.66 | 70.83 | -.28 | .71 | .71 | - |

### 4.2.10 Convergent validity

The convergent validity of the child and parent version of DISBAKIDS-Smiley with all KINDL-dimensions is shown in Table 4-26.

**Table 4-26 Correlation coefficients (Pearson r) for total score of the self-report version (child version) of the DISABKIDS smiley measure with different indicators of health status and health-related quality of life**

| Smileys | KINDL-R | | | | | | |
|---|---|---|---|---|---|---|---|
| | Physical well-being | Emotional well-being | Self-esteem | Family | Friends | Everyday functioning | Total |
| Child version | .41 | .43 | .55 | .34 | .40 | .44 | .60 |
| Proxy version | .11 | .41 | .52 | .23 | .38 | .28 | .47 |

| | GHP | CHQ-KINDL-Index | KIDSCREEN |
|---|---|---|---|
| Child version | .45 | .53 | .72 |
| Proxy version | .30 | .52 | .82 |

## 4.2.11 Interpretation and reference values

The scores achieved on the DISABKIDS-Smiley measure represent an empirical assessment of the child's or adolescent's health-related quality of life from the respondent's point of view (child/parent's). Until the data from a standard sample is available for the DISABKIDS Smiley version, the results of the DISABKIDS field study (n = 1563) should be used as a preliminary reference for children and adolescents with chronic conditions. For the following reference values the scales has been transformed to a range of 0 to 100 (see Table 4-27 to Table 4-8).

**Table 4-27 Transformed raw scores (mean, standard deviation; range 0 - 100) for the DISABKIDS-Smiley measure (child version), crossed for age group and gender (DISABKIDS field study sample)**

| Age group | Female | | | Male | | | Total | | |
|---|---|---|---|---|---|---|---|---|---|
| | M | SD | N | M | SD | N | M | SD | N |
| Age group I | 73.63 | 14.74 | 203 | 69.34 | 16.22 | 232 | 71.34 | 15.67 | 435 |
| Age group II | 67.78 | 15.12 | 260 | 70.67 | 15.42 | 300 | 69.33 | 15.34 | 560 |
| Age group III | 64.57 | 14.82 | 243 | 68.11 | 15.41 | 242 | 66.34 | 15.20 | 485 |

**Table 4-28 Transformed raw scores (mean, standard deviation; range 0 - 100) for the DISABKIDS-Smiley measure (child version), crossed type of chronic condition and gender (DISABKIDS field study sample)**

| | Female | | | Male | | | Total | | |
|---|---|---|---|---|---|---|---|---|---|
| Condition | M | SD | N | M | SD | N | M | SD | N |
| Asthma | 70.79 | 15.28 | 247 | 71.34 | 14.69 | 355 | 71.11 | 14.92 | 602 |
| Arthritis | 66.01 | 14.74 | 127 | 63.53 | 16.30 | 73 | 65.10 | 15.33 | 200 |
| Atopic dermatitis | 61.72 | 16.57 | 62 | 62.59 | 17.05 | 48 | 62.10 | 16.71 | 110 |
| Diabetes | 69.57 | 14.90 | 119 | 70.17 | 15.90 | 122 | 69.88 | 15.39 | 241 |
| Cerebral palsy | 69.61 | 12.07 | 55 | 68.56 | 16.63 | 82 | 68.98 | 14.93 | 137 |
| Cystic fibrosis | 69.39 | 14.69 | 19 | 71.14 | 11.31 | 27 | 70.42 | 12.69 | 46 |
| Epilepsy | 66.89 | 16.26 | 87 | 70.34 | 17.17 | 79 | 68.53 | 16.73 | 166 |

The DISABKIDS-Smiley measure discriminates well between different degrees of severity. Children with more severe conditions show lower quality of life scores on the DISABKIDS-Smiley dimensions (see Table 4-9).

**Table 4-29 Transformed raw scores (mean, standard deviation; range 0 - 100) for the DISABKIDS-Smiley measure (child version), crossed for clinical severity scoring and gender (DISABKIDS field study sample)**

| | Female | | | Male | | | Total | | |
|---|---|---|---|---|---|---|---|---|---|
| Severity | M | SD | N | M | SD | N | M | SD | N |
| Mild | 69.67 | 14.23 | 249 | 71.94 | 15.06 | 265 | 70.84 | 14.70 | 514 |
| Moderate | 69.19 | 16.12 | 192 | 67.97 | 15.23 | 195 | 68.58 | 15.67 | 387 |
| Severe | 62.73 | 13.16 | 57 | 65.14 | 19.96 | 49 | 63.84 | 16.61 | 106 |

## 4.2.12 Administration - suggested uses

Used for all children between 4 and 7 years with a chronic medical condition. It is also useful for children above 7 years whose reading abilities or cognitive level do not allow the administration of the generic DISABKIDS questionnaire.

## 4.3    The DISABKIDS Condition specific measures

### *General Introduction*

The different DISABKIDS condition specific modules deal with the health-related quality of life (HRQoL) in children and adolescents with different chronic health conditions by developing European instruments for HRQoL assessment from the perspective of children and adolescents, as well as their parents. A common conceptual and empirical approach was applied to the development of each of the condition-specific modules. The aim was to have short and economic disease – specific versions at hand that can be used for intervention studies. The DISABKIDS condition specific modules ought to be applicable in different national and cultural contexts. The DISABKIDS questionnaire set contains seven disease-specific modules for the following conditions: asthma bronchiale, arthritis, dermatitis, diabetes mellitus, cerebral palsy, cystic fibrosis and epilepsy.

### *Severity Assessment*

In addition to the condition-specific quality of life modules, there are three questions for each of the modules to self-report on the perceived severity of symptoms, e.g.: the frequency of having asthma attacks from the child perspective. The items on perceived severity are displayed in the appendix.

### *Clinical severity assessment*

The clinical severity was assessed by paediatricians. For each of the conditions, clinical severity measures were adopted from international measures of severity assessment and are described for each of the conditions. Additionally parental measures for severity assessment were included. The aim of both assessment types was to have a mild - moderate - severe – categorization on the severity for the condition.

In the following sections the background and content of each of the condition specific modules is described. All modules were developed according to a common approach, all scoring instructions and reference values are shown in chapter 4.4.1.10 pp.

### 4.3.1 The DISABKIDS Asthma Module (AsM)

#### *Background*

Asthma is a chronic inflammatory disorder of the airways. It is the most common chronic dis-ease among children, however the prevalence varies greatly between countries (ISAAC 1998). A diagnosis of asthma is based mainly upon clinical observations of symptoms (US Depart-ment of Health and Human Services 1997). Airway inflammation and airway narrowing are the cause of the symptoms, which consist of recurrent episodes of wheezing, breathlessness, chest tightness and coughing (nocturnal or exercise related, US Department of Health and Hu-man Services 1997, 2003). Acute asthma exacerbations symptoms can be more severe and in some cases even life threatening (Silverstein and others 1994). The symptoms can arise spontaneously or can be triggered by allergens such as pollen, cigarette smoke, house dust mite and chemicals or factors as respiratory infections, physical activity, emotional stress and weather changes (US Department of Health and Human Services 1997, 2003). The majority of children develop their asthma during their preschool years (Silverstein and others 1994) (Croner and Kjellman 1992) Management of patients with asthma consists of monitoring the course of the disease, pharmacological therapy, non-pharmacological management (identifying and avoiding asthma triggers in order to prevent asthma exacerbations) and educating patients (Ross and others 2003) Pharmacological medication is focussed on suppressing inflammation and reversing airway narrowing. Initial treatment usually includes inhaled bronchodilators as intermittent reliever and, if this is insufficient, inhaled anti-inflam-matory agents like corticosteroids as protector in a daily doses (Anderson and others 1996; Ross and others 2003).

#### *Severity assessment in asthma*

In daily practice asthma severity is frequently based on a combination of several parameters, including symptom frequency and severity, use of treatment, physical limitations and pulmo-nary function tests (US Department of Health and Human Services 1997; Williams and others 2003). Several classifications have been developed for asthma severity in recent years (US Department of Health and Human Services 1997; Rosier and others 1994; Gautier and others 1996; Redier and others 1995). Information can be collected from the parents, the child or the clinician. However, as asthma symptoms are subject to change on a daily basis, are influenced by physical activity and exposure to triggers, there is no simple or standard way to score seve-rity.

Severity was evaluated in several ways in the DISABKIDS project. There were single items, for children and parents, assessing general health (*In general, how would you say your health is?*) and disease severity (*How severe was your asthma during the last year?*). Parents were also asked to complete a symptom checklist for asthma severity, based on a scale by Rosier and others (1994). Clinicians were also asked to rate the asthma severity. There was a single item assessing severity (*How would you rate this child's asthma severity?*) and a short questionnaire which was used as the assessment measure for clinicians (Hargreave and others 1990). The calculated score was based on questions including symptoms, medication and lung function.

### *Impact of asthma on quality of life*

Asthma impacts a child's life in several areas. Children need to cope with taking their medication (daily). Some may be concerned about the adverse effects of the asthma medication. The symptoms they experience can lead to physical limitations, for example during sport or play. Nocturnal symptoms may disturb their sleep (US Department of Health and Human Services, 1997). Children might miss school days or experience poor school performance (Hilton et al., 1994). Their social activities may be limited for instance due to the necessity of avoiding potential trigger factors (eg. tobacco smoke, allergens) or due to physical limitations. The above factors can also add to the fear of being rejected by peers due to being "different" (French et al., 1994). Teenagers with complaints of asthma experience more physical and emotional problems, lower perceived well being, more activity restrictions and more negative behaviours that threaten social development (Forrest et al., 1997). A meta-analysis by McQuaid et al. (2001) shows that children with asthma have more adjustment difficulties and behavioural problems, which are also related to the severity of their asthma (McQuaid et al., 2001). Asthma can also disrupt the family routines and cause an increase in family stress (Schulz et al., 1994). Parents may overprotect a child with asthma, creating the possibility of limiting them in their normal daily activities (Hilton et al., 1994). Due to these aspects it is important for clinicians to become aware of the impact of asthma on a child and his/her family. Quality of Life questionnaires for children are therefore becoming increasingly important for the future of paediatric health care and research.

### *Content of the DISABKIDS Asthma Module*

The condition specific asthma questionnaire can be used in addition to the chronic generic module. It focuses more on the specific physical and emotional aspects of asthma. The module consists of two domains: the impact domain (6 items) concerns limitations and symptoms and the worry domain (5 items) concerning fears related to asthma. The internal reliability of the impact domain is α =.83, for the domain worry the α =.84. There is a parent proxy version that consists of similar questions, but asks the parent to answer how they think their child feels. The condition specific modules will be explained in more detail in chapter 4.4.9 pp.

### 4.3.2 The DISABKIDS Arthritis Module (ArM)

*Background*

Chronic arthritis in childhood is a heterogeneous group of disorders characterized by joint inflammation, onset before 16 years of age and disease duration of a minimum of 6 weeks. The prevalence is approximately 30-150 per 100,000, the incidence 5-18 per 100,00 children, girls being two to three times more often affected than boys (Gare 1999).

Classification of juvenile arthritis has been complicated by differences between the classification of juvenile chronic arthritis (JCA) by the European League Against Rheumatism (EULAR), and the classification of juvenile rheumatoid arthritis (JRA) by the American College of Rheumatology (ACR). A unifying classification, juvenile idiopathic arthritis (JIA), encompasses JCA and JRA, with reactive arthritis classifying as 'other arthritis' (Petty and Cassidy 2001). In this study, we used the ILAR classification and additionally included children and adolescents with reactive arthritis in the analysis.

There is neither a known aetiology nor any known cure for juvenile idiopathic arthritis. Subgroups are diagnosed using clinical symptoms 6 months after onset of the disease. Oligoarthritis (less than 5 joints affected) is the most common form of JIA. The prognosis is good for most children, although they are at risk for uveitis and damage of a critical joint may threaten function. Systemic arthritis (fever at onset) and polyarthritis (5 ore more joints affected) are the most severe forms, often treated with steroids and immune-suppressive drugs. Other important subgroups are enthesitis-related arthritis and psoriatic arthritis, which show a wide range of symptoms. Apart from idiopathic arthritis reactive arthritis due to viral or bacterial infections is a common form of arthritis in childhood.

*Severity assessment in arthritis*

To monitor clinical change, the Pediatric Rheumatology International Trials Organization (PRINTO) has developed a set of core outcome variables and defined improvement, which has been used in this study. The core outcome variables include patient or parent global assessment of disease impact, physician's global assessment of activity, number of active and limited joints, an index of inflammation (ESR or CRP) and a functional assessment by parents (usually the CHAQ) (Giannini and others 1994; Giannini and others 1997). However, there is yet no published index to calculate overall clinical severity of juvenile idiopathic arthritis from clinical parameters. To assess the clinical severity of the child's chronic arthritis, we used a global assessment by the rheumatologist (mild, moderate, severe) as well as an assessment of the severity in the last year by the child and a parent (not at all, a little bit, moderately, quite a bit, extremely). Disease impact on the child according to the PRINTO core set was assessed by a parent on a VAS-Scale with a range from 1 to 10 for all age groups.

### *Impact of arthritis on quality of life*

Chronic arthritis can produce serious limitations in functioning and well-being. Typical symptoms include swollen joints, acute and chronic pain, stiffness, fatigue, limited mobility and functional impairment. Symptoms may change from day to day even from morning to afternoon. Young people often report that others fail to understand the fluctuation of complaints and the unpredictability of the disease. In addition to pain and physical limitations, children may suffer from altered body image and anxieties around stigmatisation and social acceptance as well as fears about independence and uncertainty about the future. Disease management is often complex, involving medication, using medical aids such as splints and doing exercises. Regularly visits to specialised medical services such as rheumatologists, ophthalmologists and physiotherapy may be time consuming and place further limitations on social and leisure time activities. While most disease burdens are supposed to increase when the condition is more severe, children who are not using any visible medical aids or do not suffer very severe symptoms also tend to feel discriminated and marginalized. In these children, lack of understanding from peers and especially in school and from teachers may have an impact on their HRQOL (Barlow and others 1999; Sällfors and others 2002).

### Content of the DISABKIDS Arthritis Module (ArM)

*The arthritis module* has been developed as a supplement to the chronic-generic module with a focus on arthritis–specific physical symptoms and limitations. It comprises two main scales, *Impact* and *Understanding* (see Table 4-31). As in the chronic-generic measure, the scale scores have been transformed to a range of 0 to 100, higher values indicating better arthritis-specific HRQOL. The *Impact* scale is related to physical symptoms and disease-specific impacts on activities of daily living, well-being and social relations. For clinical interpretation, the impact scale may also be divided into two sub-domains, *Pain* (3 items, $\alpha = .79$) and *Limitations* (6 items, $\alpha = .82$). The P*ain* subscale refers to general adaptation to pain and pain-related impact on activities, the *Limitation* subscale addresses other arthritis-related functional and social limitations due to joint problems and exhaustion. Children with more active or severe arthritis are expected to report lower HRQOL in this domain. The *Impact* scale is also supposed to be sensitive to treatment changes or improvement of the condition. The *Understanding* scale has been developed to address feelings of social exclusion and lack of empathy by peers and teachers. This arthritis-specific burden is related to the invisibility of the condition and the fluctuation of symptoms and is assumed to have a greater impact on HRQOL in children with a moderate disease severity. Low HRQOL of the patient in this domain may indicate an unmet need for comprehensive care like health education or cooperation with school based services or other health services.

### 4.3.3   The DISABKIDS Atopic Dermatitis Module (ADM)

*Background*

Atopic dermatitis is very common in all parts of the world. It affects about 10% of infants and 3% of the total population. The word "atopic" means there is a tendency for excess inflammation of the skin and linings of the nose and lungs. This often runs in families with allergies such as hay fever and asthma, sensitive skin, or a history of atopic dermatitis. Although most people with atopic dermatitis have family members with similar problems, 20% of them are the only ones in their family with the condition.

It can occur at any age but is most common in infants young adults. The skin rash is very itchy and can be widespread, or limited to a few areas. The condition frequently improves with adolescence, but many patients are affected throughout life, although not as severely as in early childhood.

*Impact of atopic dermatitis on quality of life*

Quality of life has increasingly become an integral part in outcome measurement in dermatology, with the majority of quality of life measures developed for adults with a variety of skin conditions such as psoriasis and Atopic dermatitis (Ben-Gashir 2003; Herd and others 1997). There are many characteristics of atopic dermatitis that may affect quality of life in children with atopic dermatitis such a symptoms of itching, and its impact on sleep and social activities, or the perceived impact of the appearance of the condition. Since atopic dermatitis is a widespread condition that begins in infancy in more than 60% of cases (Hanifin 1991), the need has been recognised to develop quality of life instruments for children, either as self-report (Lewis-Jones and Finlay 1995) or but primary as proxy-versions (Lewis-Jones and others 2001; von Rüden and others 1999).

### *Severity assessment in atopic dermatitis*

For clinical severity assessment, the SCORAD (cf. European-Task-Force-on-Atopic-Dermatitis 1993) was used. The SCORAD Assessment results in a 0 – 100 score, with higher scores indicating higher severity. The parental severity assessment instrument was the Nottingham Eczema Severity Scoring (Emerson and others 2000). Parents rate the extent of symptoms, the intensity of itching as well as the amount of sleep problems.

### Content of the DISABKIDS Atopic Dermatitis Module (ADM)

The Impact scale describes symptoms (e.g. of itching) and emotional and functional limitations; the Stigma scale describes feeling of being stigmatised, when others look at the skin condition. The scales are measured on a 0-100 range. Cronbach's alpha values were .79 for the Impact scale and .69 for the Stigma scale.

### 4.3.4    The DISABKIDS Diabetes Module (DM)

### *Background*

Diabetes mellitus type 1 is a chronic condition that is characterised by an abnormal glucose metabolism. The onset of the disease mostly occurs in childhood, adolescence or early adulthood. The clinical features of a young and slim patient with high blood glucose may give a hint in the differential diagnosis between type 1 and type 2 diabetes. Acute manifestations include hypoglycaemic attacks and diabetic coma.

The therapy consists of lifelong substitution of insulin by several daily injections or by insulin pump therapy. The therapeutic aim is to achieve a near to normal metabolic situation while avoiding hypoglycaemic attacks (IDF 2003; Rosenbloom and Hanas 1996).

After several years signs of tissue damage due to the hyperglycaemic metabolism may become apparent. Typical signs are visual impairment due to retinal damage, renal function impairment, vascular diseases of the peripheral arteries, the heart and the brain, and neurological symptoms due to damaged peripheral nerves.

The prevalence of diabetes mellitus type I is about 0,19% in Europe and about 0,25% in the USA (IDF 2003).

*Severity assessment in diabetes*

Diabetes is a condition that causes only mild or even no symptoms in many cases. Therefore it is difficult to determine severity. Metabolic control may be assessed by measuring the HbA1c level and the occurrence of severe hypoglycaemias, hyperglycaemic exacerbations and long-term sequelae of diabetes.

*Impact of diabetes on quality of life*

For adequate management of the glucose level it is necessary that the patient measures his/ her blood glucose levels and injects adequate amounts of insulin. In younger children these tasks may have to be accomplished by a parent. Numerous needle pricks per day are necessary.

The therapy of diabetes mellitus type 1 amounts to a serious impact on the everyday life. The patient has to plan his daily routine according to the necessity of measuring the blood glucose level and injecting insulin several times a day. Therefore the testing and injecting equipment must be carried with him/ her at any time.

Minor changes in the daily routine can have a serious impact on the diabetic metabolism and may lead to acute complications such as hypoglycaemic attacks or diabetic coma. The quality of life may be influenced seriously by the procedures that are necessary to control the blood glucose levels, but also by fear of high blood glucose levels, acute complications or long-term sequelae. These issues may affect not only the patient but also his/ her family and friends.

**Content of the DISABKIDS Diabetes Module (DM)**

The Diabetes Module has two scales, an Impact and a Treatment scale. The Impact scale describes emotional reactions of needing to control every day life, and to restrict one's diet; the Treatment scale refers to carrying equipment and planning treatment. Cronbach's alpha values were .84 for the Impact scale and .85 for the Treatment scale.

**4.3.5   The DISABKIDS Cystic Fibrosis Module (CFM)**

*Background*

Cystic Fibrosis is a chronic, multi-system genetic disease with wide variability in clinical severity (Lissauer and Clayden 2001; Nelson 2000; Taussig and Landau 1999). As the disease progresses, respiratory infection causes symptoms such as coughing, breathlessness, weight loss and decreased exercise tolerance. These impair patient's QoL and eventually result in premature death. Cystic Fibrosis (CF) is the commonest cause of chronic suppurative lung disease in Caucasians. In the past, CF led to death in early childhood from progressive bronchiectasis and respiratory failure, but with improved antibiotic and nutritional therapy, survival into mid-adult life can now be expected for most patients. CF is an autosomal recessive disease. In Caucasians the carrier rate is 1 in 25, with 1 in 2500 affected births. The disease is much less common in other ethnic groups (Lissauer and Clayden 2001; Nelson 2000; Taussig and Landau 1999). In CF there is an abnormal ion transport across the epithelial cells of the exocrine glands of the respiratory tract and pancreas; this results in increased viscosity of secretions. Abnormal function of the sweat glands results in excessive concentrations of sodium and chloride in the sweat. This forms the basis of the essential diagnostic procedure, the sweat test. Most children with CF present with malabsorption and failure to thrive from birth, accompanied by recurrent or persistent chest infection. The child has a persistent, loose cough productive of purulent sputum.

The effective management of CF requires a multi- disciplinary team approach, including paediatricians, physiotherapists, dieticians nursing staff and most importantly, the child and parents. The condition cannot be cured. The principal aims of therapy are to prevent progression of the lung disease and to maintain adequate nutrition and growth. Children should have physiotherapy at least twice a day. Persistent bacterial chest infection is the major problem. Most centres recommend prompt and vigorous intravenous therapy for acute exacerbations. Nebulised antibiotics are used in patients colonized with Pseudomonas. Up to one-third of children have reversible airways obstruction and may benefit from bronchodilators and inhaled steroids. Dietary status should be assessed regularly. Pancreatic insufficiency is treated with oral pancreatic supplements. A high-calorie diet is essential and fat- soluble vitamin supplements are routinely given.

### *Impact of cystic fibrosis on quality of life*

Most CF sufferers now survive into adult life. The improved survival rate has been accompanied by a change in the range of problems seen. The psychological repercussions on the affected child and family of a chronic and ultimately fatal illness that requires regular physiotherapy and drugs, frequent hospital admissions and absences from school are considerable. The team should provide psychological and emotional support. Adolescents have particular needs, which must receive special consideration.

Cystic fibrosis (CF) is the most common inherited disease with a fatal outcome in industrialized countries. Today the majority of patients with CF will grow into adulthood. However, despite improvement in survival, the disease is progressive, especially with respect to the decline in pulmonary function and growth, which in turn may have an impact on a patient's quality of life (QoL).

### Severity assessment in cystic fibrosis

There are several clinical scoring systems for CF, over the past 40 years. Shwachman and Kulczycki introduced in 1958 the most widely used method of evaluation the health status in CF (Shwachman and Kulczycki 1958). This continues to be popular for classifying patients into various categories of disease severity. Its disadvantage is that it doesn't include pulmonary function tests, and serious pulmonary complications, which affect patient's life. The "National Institute of Health" (NIH) scoring system was introduced in 1973 by Taussing et al. (1973). The criteria for several items were poorly defined. These were composed of several elements or had point ranges for scoring, not clearly graduated and it did not include scoring for respiratory failure. Huang et al in 1981 introduced a scoring system for the short-term evaluation of patients with CF as a means for assessing the efficacy of antibiotic treatment for acute exacerbation. As the pulmonary complications account over 90% of morbidity and associated mortality CF, we measure the severity level as the severity of lung disease. (Defined by values of the highest recorded forced expiratory volume in 1 sec (FEV1) In our study, we used a simplified combination of Shwachman and Huang scores, in order to assess the severity of Cystic Fibrosis Patients.

$FEV_1$, % ideal body weight, frequency of IV treatment and the respiratory combined score (respiratory rate/ breathing pattern/ cardiac frequency) were used as predictors of disease severity.

### Content of the DISABKIDS Cystic Fibrosis Module

The DISABKIDS Cystic Fibrosis Module has two scales, named Impact and Treatment. The Impact scale describes feeling tired and exhausted as well as out of breath, needing rest, impact on sports' activities. The Treatment scale denotes emotional reaction about taking enzymes, and having a special diet, having physiotherapies and time spent on treatment. The scale is measured between 0-100; higher values indicate better adjustment to cystic fibrosis.

Internal consistency values were α =.82 for the Impact scale and α =.88 for the Treatment scale.

### 4.3.6   The DISABKIDS Cerebral Palsy Module (CPM)

*Background*

Cerebral Palsy is a term covering a group of disorders involving motor function, movement, tone and posture that is due to non-progressive defects or lesions of the immature brain (Aicardi 1998; McKinlay 2004). Most studies in developed countries show an incidence of around 2 per 1000.

Cerebral Palsy has many aetiologies. Historically, it was attributed mainly to birth trauma and asphyxia, although this has been questioned more recently. A more useful approach is to divide causes into pre-natal, peri-natal and post-natal. Prenatal factors include genetic and chromosome abnormalities, congenital infections and cerebral maldevelopment. Peri-natal factors refer to those factors operative from the onset of labour to the end of the first week of life. They include brain haemorrhage, infection and asphyxia. Post-natal factors (responsible for less than 10% of cases) are often due to post-convulsive or vascular aetiologies. Two major risk factors in general are pre-term birth and intra-uterine growth retardation (Aicardi 1998; McKinlay 2004). As aetiology is often unclear, a system based on the muscle/limb groups affected is most suitable. The commonly used classification system is as follows:

- Hemiplegia - Unilateral motor disability
- Spastic diplegia - Affects four limbs with lower limbs affected more than upper limbs
- Tetraplegia - Severe form affecting all limbs with upper limbs affected more, usually involves muscles, associated with feeding and swallowing.
- Dyskinetic/Dystonic - Inability to execute co-ordinated movements and to maintain posture
- Ataxic - Poorly co-ordinated movement with intentional tremor
  *(Note: Wide variation in severity of motor disabilities.)*

*Impact of cerebral palsy on quality of life*

Few, if any, quantitative studies are available though anecdotal qualitative reports have been published. Major determinants of quality of life are the severity of the motor disability, cognitive abilities and the presence of behavioural problems. Recently, Goodman and colleagues

(Goodman 1998) have shown that over 50% of children with hemiplegia have significant behavioural problems.

A major issue in quality of life research for children with cerebral palsy is that physical limitations preclude many children from self-completion of a questionnaire. In addition to the motor disability, additional disabilities that have a major determinant on long-term adjustment are common. These include feeding difficulties, epilepsy, communication disorders, cognitive and learning disorders, and behavioural problems.

### Severity assessment in cerebral palsy

This is based on the Lifestyle Assessment Questionnaire (LAQ-CP) developed by Mackie and colleagues (Mackie and others 1998). It assesses the child's ability to perform activities of daily living including mobility and independence, the clinical and social burden and schooling. The classification of severity used was mild, moderate or severe, depending on the LAQ-CP score. This classification was used in the clinical as well as parental severity assessment.

### Content of DISABKIDS Cerebral Palsy Module

The 14 disease specific questions are focussed around one domain of the impact of the condition, as well as 2 further items on communications about the conditions. Higher scores indicate betters quality of life. The scale is measured between 1-100, higher values indicate better adjustment to the cerebral palsy. Internal consistency values were α =. 80 for the Impact scale, and α =. 72 for the Communication scale.

### 4.3.7   The DISABKIDS Epilepsy Module (EM)

### Background

Epilepsy is a condition of the brain characterised by recurring seizures. Epilepsy is a group of disorders with different origins, manifestations, courses and prognoses. The prevalence of the condition is approximately 0.4% in all countries. In about 70% of cases the seizures can be fully controlled with anti-convulsant therapy. However, epilepsy has considerable impact on HRQoL in children relating to the severity, controllability, medication, age at onset and social and family acceptance. Epilepsy can affect the cognitive ability of the child thought brain damage or side-effects of medication, the social and personally development and family life of the child through over-protection, restricted social exposure, disrupted education and stigmatisation. The HRQoL consequences of epilepsy have been widely recognised and researched over the past 60 years however the effects on quality of life are sometimes underestimated by professionals and by the individuals themselves must cope with the consequences of recurrent seizures. HRQoL instruments for adults have been in development in recent years to try to identify the HRQoL effects of epilepsy however instruments designed for children have been lacking. Proxy instruments have been the first to be developed but it is widely recognised that instruments designed for children themselves to complete is the goal for quality of life measurement. DISABKIDS is the first multi-language European Questionnaire designed especially for completion by children based on the qualitative reality of the lives of children with epilepsy.

### Severity assessment in epilepsy

The determination of severity in epilepsy is complicated by the range of types of epilepsy, frequency and types of seizures, combination of different types of seizures, presence of a warning (aura) before the seizure, the reliability of this warning, behaviour before, after and during the seizure, number of medications, side-effects from medication, social, emotional and educational (cognitive) problems related to the epilepsy and the combination of multiple problems. Several schemes have been developed to determine severity, which vary in specificity. For example: the Seizure Severity Questionnaire developed by J.A.Cramer (Cramer 2003; Cramer and others 2002) has eleven questions which concern aura, behaviour during a seizure, alterations in consciousness, recovery time after a seizure, cognitive, emotional and physical effects and an overall assessment. Carpey and colleagues (Carpey and Arts 1996; Carpey and others 1996) from the Netherlands has scales for the parents to complete. However the Epilepsy Foundation of America uses a simpler category system based on presence or absence of seizures and presence or absence of 'problems' or multiple problems, giving three categories:

- Uncomplicated - those whose condition is uncomplicated because the seizures are controlled with medication;
- Compromised - those whose condition is compromised because of social, emotional and educational (cognitive) problems; and
- Devastated - those whose condition is devastated by virtue of multiple problems.

Another measure of severity can be based on the type of epilepsy alone. Dunn et al (Dunn and others 2004) has, using a Delphi technique categorised different epileptic syndromes on a ten point scale of severity.

There is however, no internationally agreed index to measure epilepsy severity and due to the inclusion of social and psychological variables as in the Epilepsy Foundation categorisation the judgement must lie with the patient's physician. Smith and colleagues (Smith and others 1995; Smith and others 1993) have investigated the issue of severity in relation to quality of life measurement and concluded that the judgement from the physician is the most suitable method of measuring severity in this context. Therefore, to assess the clinical severity of the child's epilepsy in DISABKIDS, we collected data concerning syndromes, seizure type and frequency; injuries; auras; automatisms; medication and side effects from the neurological hospital records as background to the overall clinical assessment made by the clinician. An assessment within the last year was also made by the child (mild, moderate severe) and by a parent (mild, moderate, sever). We therefore, have three measures of severity, clinical (based on the medical records and assessment of the paediatrician, judgement from the child and from the parent.

**Content of the DISABKIDS Epilepsy Module (EM)**

The epilepsy module has been developed as a supplement to the chronic generic module and comprises of two scales - Impact which includes anxiety about having seizures and the potential public stigma (5 items) and Social which self-esteem and comparison to others (5 items), in both child and parent versions for the 8-16 year olds and a proxy/parent version for the 4-7 year olds. The scale is measured between 0-100; higher values indicate better adjustment to the epilepsy. Internal consistency values are $\alpha$ =.90 for the Impact scale, and .83 for the Social scale.

### 4.3.8  Scale structure of condition specific modules

The DISABKIDS condition-specific modules consists of varying number of Likert-scaled items (10-12), for each module assigned to two dimensions (see Table 4 3). The content of the two dimensions of each of the condition – specific modules is shown in Table 4-31. First of the dimensions for all DISABKIDS condition specific modules refers to the (emotional or physical) "impact" of the condition, the second dimension refers to a topic that is specific for each condition (e.g. "stigma" for dermatitis, "treatment" in diabetes).

**Table 4-30 Structure and design of the different DISABKIDS condition specific modules**

| Module | $\sum_{items}$ | $\sum_{dimensions}$ | Dimension I | $\sum_{item}(I)$ | Dimension II | $\sum_{item}(II)$ |
|---|---|---|---|---|---|---|
| Asthma | 11 | 2 | Impact | 6 items | Worry | 5 items |
| Arthritis | 12 | 2 | Impact | 9 items | Understanding | 3 items |
| Dermatitis | 12 | 2 | Impact | 8 items | Stigma | 4 items |
| Diabetes | 10 | 2 | Impact | 6 items | Treatment | 4 items |
| Cerebral palsy | 12 | 2 | Impact | 10 items | Communication | 2 items |
| Cystic fibrosis | 10 | 2 | Impact | 4 items | Treatment | 6 items |
| Epilepsy | 10 | 2 | Impact | 5 items | Social | 5 items |

### 4.3.9 Structure of (sub-)scales and classification of items

The content of each of the condition-specific dimension is shown in Table 4-31.

**Table 4-31 Dimensions of the different DISABKIDS condition specific modules**

| Module | No. | Dimension | Concept/ content |
|---|---|---|---|
| Asthma | I | Impact | Experience of limitations and symptoms during sports and activities |
| | II | Worry | Worries about having asthma (asthma attack, night time, emergency room) |
| Arthritis | I | Impact | Impact of pain, feeling exhausted and stiff or restricted in movement |
| | II | Understanding | Reaction from teachers, parents and friends in terms of understanding symptoms |
| Dermatitis | I | Impact | Impact of symptoms (e. g. itching) and emotional and functional limitations |
| | II | Stigma | Feeling of being stigmatised, when others look at the skin condition |
| Diabetes | I | Impact | Emotional and functional impact of Diabetes to control every day life, restrictions on diet |
| | II | Treatment | Carrying equipment and planning treatment |
| Cerebral palsy | I | Impact | Problems with walking and other physical activities (c.f. swimming, getting dressed, sports, moving, climbing stairs) |
| | II | Communication | Impact of condition on communicating with others |
| Cystic fibrosis | I | Impact | Feeling tired and exhausted as well as out of breadth, needing rest, impact on sports' activities |
| | II | Treatment | Emotional reaction about taking enzymes, and having a special diet, having physiotherapies time spent on treatment |
| Epilepsy | I | Impact | Anxieties about having seizures (feeling hurt, being recognised in public) |
| | II | Social | Feeling ashamed of having seizures, loosing control in respect to others |

### 4.3.10 Scoring

The scoring instructions for the condition-specific dimension are shown in
Table 4-32. The number of items for sub-scales ranges from 2 to10, corresponding to that, the
possible range of raw scores varies between 8 (minimum raw score: 2, maximum raw score:
10) and 40 (minimum raw score: 10, maximum raw score: 50).

**Table 4-32 Items included in the modules and dimensions of the different condition specific modules**

| Module | No. | Dimension | $\sum$ items | $\sum$ ranks | Items of dimensions | Possible range of raw score (Min, Max) |
|--------|-----|-----------|--------------|--------------|---------------------|-----------------------------------------|
| *Asthma* | I | Impact | 6 | 24 | 1+2+3+9+10+11 | 24 (6,30) |
| | II | Worry | 5 | 20 | 4+5+6+7+8 | 20 (5,25) |
| *Arthritis* | I | Impact | 9 | 36 | 1+2+3+4+5+6+7+8+9 | 36 (9,45) |
| | II | Understanding | 3 | 12 | 10+11+12 | 12 (3,15) |
| *Dermatitis* | I | Impact | 8 | 32 | 1+2+3+4+5+6+7+8 | 32 (8,40) |
| | II | Stigma | 4 | 16 | 9+10+11+12 | 16 (4,20) |
| *Diabetes* | I | Impact | 6 | 24 | 3+4+5+6+7+8 | 24 (6,30) |
| | II | Treatment | 4 | 16 | 1+2+9+10 | 16 (4,20) |
| *Cerebral palsy* | I | Impact | 10 | 40 | 1+2+3+4+5+6+7+8+9+10 | 40 (10,50) |
| | II | Communication | 2 | 8 | 11+12 | 8 (2,10) |
| *Cystic fibrosis* | I | Impact | 4 | 16 | 1+2+3+4 | 16 (4,20) |
| | II | Treatment | 6 | 24 | 6+7+8+9+10 | 24 (6,30) |
| *Epilepsy* | I | Impact | 5 | 20 | 1+2+3+4+5 | 20 (5,25) |
| | II | Social | 5 | 20 | 6+7+8+9+10 | 20 (5,25) |

### 4.3.11 Psychometric properties - results of the field study analysis

The proposed reference scores are based on the results of the DISABKIDS field study (n= 1152; Schmidt et al., 2006). The analysis of the data from the DISABKIDS condition specific modules completed by chronically ill children and adolescents and their parents was performed using the SPSS program (version 11.5.1). Response rates for different groups of chronic conditions are reported in Table 4-243.

**Table 4-243 Response rates for the DISABKIDS condition specific modules (DISABKIDS field study sample)**

| Module | test | retest | proxy |
|---|---|---|---|
| | *n* | *n* | *n* |
| Asthma | 405 | 146 | 382 |
| Arthritis | 148 | 88 | 141 |
| Atopic dermatitis | 64 | 51 | 41 |
| Diabetes | 204 | 106 | 199 |
| Cerebral palsy | 86 | 38 | 83 |
| Cystic fibrosis | 40 | 4 | 34 |
| Epilepsy | 181 | 32 | 181 |
| *Total* | *1.128* | *465* | *1.061* |

## 4.3.12 Descriptive psychometric properties, reliability, and factorial validity

Descriptive characteristics of the condition-specific measures are reported in Table 4-254, including means and standard deviations for the transformed raw scores (range 0-100) as well as floor and ceiling effects (as indicated by the percentage of answering frequency for the lowest and highest possible raw score).

**Table 4-254 Selected descriptive characteristics for the sub-scales of the self-report version (child version) of the different DISABKIDS condition specific modules (DISABKIDS field study sample)**

| Module | No. | Dimension | N | M (0-100) | SD | Floor | Ceiling |
|--------|-----|-----------|---|-----------|-----|-------|---------|
| *Asthma* | I | Impact | 375 | 65.40 | 22.72 | 0.3 % | 5.8 % |
| | II | Worry | 397 | 79.42 | 21.10 | 0.0 % | 22.8 % |
| *Arthritis* | I | Impact | 143 | 63.37 | 22.61 | 0.0 % | 4.1 % |
| | II | Understanding | 140 | 67.80 | 26.55 | 2.8 % | 21.4 % |
| *Dermatitis* | I | Impact | 64 | 41.13 | 18.06 | 6.3 % | 1.6 % |
| | II | Stigma | 63 | 71.92 | 20.54 | 1.6 % | 46.0 % |
| *Diabetes* | I | Impact | 205 | 62.73 | 22.22 | 0.0 % | 3.0 % |
| | II | Treatment | 205 | 58.94 | 23.41 | 2.5 % | 8.6 % |
| *Cerebral palsy* | I | Impact | 82 | 60.06 | 20.52 | 0.0 % | 2.4 % |
| | II | Communication | 83 | 81.33 | 26.22 | 4.9 % | 22.0 % |
| *Cystic fibrosis* | I | Impact | 26 | 66.83 | 20.14 | 0.0 % | 3.2 % |
| | II | Treatment | 28 | 54.38 | 24.13 | 3.2 % | 12.9 % |
| *Epilepsy* | I | Impact | 180 | 68.37 | 27.65 | 3.9 % | 21.7 % |
| | II | Social | 179 | 75.72 | 24.24 | 0.6 % | 28.3 % |

**Table 4-265 Selected psychometric properties for the sub-scales of the self-report version (child version) of the different DISABKIDS condition specific modules (DISABKIDS field study sample)**

| Module | No. | Dimension | $N_{valid}$ | $\alpha$ | $ICC_{t1,t2}$ | $r_{I,II}$ |
|--------|-----|-----------|-------------|----------|---------------|------------|
| *Asthma* | I | Impact | 375 | .83 | .77 | .56 |
| | II | Worry | 397 | .84 | .76 | |
| *Arthritis* | I | Impact | 143 | .87 | .78 | .11 |
| | II | Understanding | 140 | .74 | .45 | |
| *Dermatitis* | I | Impact | 64 | .71 | .74 | .83 |
| | II | Stigma | 63 | .69 | .74 | |
| *Diabetes* | I | Impact | 205 | .84 | .85 | .66 |
| | II | Treatment | 205 | .85 | .85 | |
| *Cerebral palsy* | I | Impact | 82 | .80 | .79 | .40 |
| | II | Communication | 83 | .72 | - | |
| *Cystic fibrosis* | I | Impact | 26 | .82 | - | .34 |
| | II | Treatment | 28 | .88 | - | |
| *Epilepsy* | I | Impact | 180 | .90 | .74 | .69 |
| | II | Social | 179 | .83 | .41 | |

### 4.3.13 Concordance between child and proxy version

The concordance between the child and the proxy version (parent report) of the condition-specific modules is displayed in Table 4-36. The concordance is in general high except for perceived stigma in children with atopic dermatitis where parents have lower Quality of life values.

**Table 4-36 Intraclass correlation coefficient (ICC) and correlation coefficients (Pearson r) for total score and sub-scales of the self-report version (child version) and the proxy version of the DISABKIDS condition specific modules**

| Module | No. | Dimension | ICC | r |
|--------|-----|-----------|-----|---|
| Asthma | I | Impact | .67 | .67 |
| | II | Worry | .52 | .53 |
| Arthritis | I | Impact | .72 | .72 |
| | II | Understanding | .44 | .444 |
| Dermatitis | I | Impact | .77 | .77 |
| | II | Stigma | .67 | .68 |
| Diabetes | I | Impact | .49 | .50 |
| | II | Treatment | .49 | .50 |
| Cerebral palsy | I | Impact | .79 | .79 |
| | II | Communication | .77 | .77 |
| Cystic fibrosis | I | Impact | .62 | .62 |
| | II | Treatment | .69 | .69 |
| Epilepsy | I | Impact | .60 | .60 |
| | II | Social | .67 | .67 |

### 4.3.14 Convergent validity

Convergent validity was assessed by implementing widely used measures of quality of life in children in the DISABKIDS field study. Correlations between the sub-scales of the different DISABKIDS condition specific measures and the multifactorial KINDL-R displayed a wide range of covariation between the sub-scales, however, with conceptually associated subscales displaying higher associations. For example, at the average the "impact" sub-scales of the DCGM`s showing a sufficient correlation with the "physical well-being" sub-scale of the KINDL-R, but this tendency is not consistent over all "impact" sub-scales. For the "impact" sub-scale of the DISABKIDS dermatitis module, the correlation is very low (r = .178).

Table 4-37 Correlation coefficients (Pearson r) for the sub-scales of the self-report version (child version) of the DISABKIDS chronic generic module with the sub-scales of the self-report version (child version) and the proxy version of the KINDL

| Module | No. | Dimension | Physical Well-Being | Emotional Well-Being | Self-esteem | Family | Friends | Everyday functioning | Total |
|---|---|---|---|---|---|---|---|---|---|
| Asthma | I | Impact | .57 | .28 | .45 | .13 | .42 | .33 | .51 |
| | II | Worry | .37 | .22 | .32 | .17 | .37 | .25 | .37 |
| Arthritis | I | Impact | .62 | .25 | .32 | .10 | .13 | .17 | .38 |
| | II | Understanding | .22 | .22 | .26 | .27 | .36 | .35 | .37 |
| Dermatitis | I | Impact | .18 | .49 | .35 | .15 | .37 | .01 | .34 |
| | II | Stigma | .06 | .40 | .38 | .21 | .43 | .22 | .37 |
| Diabetes | I | Impact | .32 | .22 | .29 | .32 | .38 | .48 | .45 |
| | II | Treatment | .28 | .22 | .26 | .26 | .31 | .46 | .40 |
| Cerebral palsy | I | Impact | .59 | .24 | .62 | .58 | .18 | .49 | .66 |
| | II | Communication | .15 | .21 | -.07 | .37 | .20 | .27 | .27 |
| Cystic fibrosis | I | Impact | .56 | .17 | .32 | .39 | .29 | .41 | .45 |
| | II | Treatment | .21 | .32 | .52 | .31 | .20 | .65 | .46 |

### 4.3.15 Discriminant validity

For each condition, a severity assessment was obtained by both the clinician and parents. These severity assessments were obtained from international research groups. Table 4-278 shows the condition-specific scale scores for different levels (mild, moderate, severe) of clinical severity, categorized by physicians.

**Table 4-278 Means of transformed raw scores (range 0-100) for the sub-scales of the self-report versions (child version) of the DISABKIDS condition specific modules for different groups of clinical severity (DISABKIDS field study sample)**

| Module | No. | Dimension | Mild | | Moderate | | Severe | | Overall | |
|--------|-----|-----------|------|------|----------|------|--------|------|---------|------|
| Asthma | I | Impact | 70.37 | 21.87 | 65.20 | 23.42 | 56.67 | 23.24 | *66.83* | *22.96* |
| | II | Worry | 82.65 | 19.94 | 76.81 | 21.23 | 73.33 | 25.89 | *79.05* | *21.17* |
| Arthritis | I | Impact | 68.77 | 20.37 | 56.70 | 23.20 | 54.22 | 23.28 | *62.83* | *22.53* |
| | II | Understanding | 69.33 | 27.47 | 61.32 | 28.45 | 73.26 | 19.50 | *67.75* | *26.73* |
| Dermatitis | I | Impact | 43.33 | 17.19 | 49.22 | 17.98 | 52.13 | 14.67 | 47.57 | 17.19 |
| | II | Stigma | 75.99 | 17.95 | 73.44 | 17.31 | 68.06 | 19.38 | 73.44 | 17.76 |
| Diabetes | I | Impact | 64.07 | 21.53 | 59.08 | 21.09 | 38.33 | 20.07 | *61.67* | *21.81* |
| | II | Treatment | 59.15 | 22.98 | 54.74 | 23.25 | 34.00 | 20.12 | *56.94* | *23.34* |
| Cerebral palsy | I | Impact | 73.38 | 24.61 | 66.41 | 16.62 | 41.85 | 20.21 | 61.40 | 23.00 |
| | II | Communication | 93.75 | 12.15 | 88.82 | 18.58 | 51.14 | 35.56 | 79.69 | 28.96 |
| Cystic fibrosis | I | Impact | 81.25 | 18.54 | 51.56 | 20.65 | 55.56 | 17.35 | *65.16* | *20.98* |
| | II | Treatment | 47.92 | 7.22 | 41.7 | 17.68 | 45.84 | 11.79 | *49.78* | *27.02* |
| Epilepsy | I | Impact | 76.93 | 25.84 | 71.08 | 24.19 | 63.84 | 26.01 | *73.96* | *25.34* |
| | II | Social | 80.72 | 21.83 | 71.09 | 30.58 | 80.95 | 20.11 | *77.46* | *25.21* |

### 4.3.16 Reference values

References values for the different condition specific modules are reported in the appendix.

### 4.3.17 Administration - suggested uses

The DISABKIDS condition-specific measure should be used in intervention studies and clinical studies on specific conditions.

## 4.4 Background of the DISABKIDS Computer Version

### 4.4.1 Summary

To improve health-related quality of life (HRQoL) assessment of children and adolescents with chronic diseases and disabilities is a major goal of the DISABKIDS project. In recent years the notion of quality of life (QoL) and how to measure it has become a core feature of healthcare. When measuring QoL, consultation with patients and their families concerning the physical and psychosocial consequences of treatment is useful and desirable. In children, computer-aided measurement of HRQoL enables the healthcare professional to form an opinion of the QoL experienced by the child and the thoughts of the parents concerning their child's situation. The measurement of HRQoL can supplement outpatient and paramedical treatment, supplying better insight into the kind of support needed by the child or the parents. With the help of standardized data the care of the chronically ill child and the support the parents are receiving can be improved. Data obtained from small numbers of patients at several hospitals can be combined and reference values developed, leading to easily accessible and comparable information concerning the child, obtained from the child and his/her parents. Measurement of HRQoL can be integrated into the care of a child with a chronic illness as a standard part of healthcare practice. The physician, nurse or other healthcare professional can obtain data on the HRQoL experienced by the child and his/her parents relatively simply and at any time.

### 4.4.2 The development of the DISABKIDS computer program RUNQUEST

Initially, computer programs focused primarily on the level of direct clinical care. Using a computer in regular (outpatient) clinical practice enables several advantages to be realized. The quality of care for the child and his/her parents can be improved by means of broader, deeper and standardized patient contact. Furthermore, the course of the individual rating of the (chronic) illness by the child and his/her parents can be more easily monitored. By combining individual data, computer-aided HRQoL research can eventually lead to the establishment of age- and gender-specific reference values for specific chronic conditions.

Three stages can be distinguished in the development of the DISABKIDS computer program.

*Stage 1: Design*

The first stage of development involves the design of the computer program RUNQUEST and computer versions of the DISABKIDS questionnaires. The main criteria for the design are an appealing layout and ease of use by the child, parents and physician. Individual data from the child and parents can be linked to (secure) databases for a specific chronic conditions and repeated use of the DISABKIDS questionnaires is possible. Individual results from children and parents can be shown on screen or in print in several formats, and the results can be used instantly as a resource for deciding upon further diagnosis and treatment. Additionally, a feature is available for expanding the (modular build) test battery with condition-specific DISABKIDS questionnaires and longitudinal data analyses.

### Stage 2: Testing

The feasibility and effectiveness of the periodic, systematic general registration and feedback of data from computer-aided DISABKIDS questionnaires to physicians, parents and children is researched (suitability in several patient populations, user friendliness) and evaluated (measurement of satisfaction, etc.). The DISABKIDS computer program is tested in terms of transparency, simplicity, user-friendliness and stability. Adjustments are made on the basis of the test results obtained and the experiences of the child, parents and physicians.

### Stage 3: Implementation

In the future (public relation) meetings and interactive workshops with patient groups, physicians and other healthcare workers have to be organized. The advantages for the healthcare workers of using the computer program RUNQUEST and the DISABKIDS questionnaires can be illustrated. Publicity is given to the existence and possibilities of the DISABKIDS instruments by means of correspondence and consultation with patient groups. Users can be consulted about the DISABKIDS program and software. User satisfaction can be monitored and the need for possible enhancements noted. If needed, new and improved versions of the DISABKIDS computer programs can be developed and distributed. In this way, reliable, instantly usable products are realized, based on soundly structured (normalized, valid, reliable) DISABKIDS measurement instruments.

### 4.4.3   The DISABKIDS computer program RUNQUEST

The RUNQUEST computer program on the Internet (Link to the DISABKIDS computer version website: http://www.capiqol.nl) consists of:

- Install and uninstall programs
- A program with which the DISABKIDS questionnaires (child and proxy versions) can be completed and the results displayed

- A program with which the DISABKIDS database can be constructed to aid the treatment of individual patients and facilitate research by patient groups.

The central features of the DISABKIDS program are flexibility for the user and an allowance for future developments. The computer screens are visually attractive and completely adjustable. The layout is automatically adjusted to the screen resolution.

Completion of the DISABKIDS questionnaires is possible using either a keyboard or mouse. A training module is provided. The client data and the DISABKIDS questionnaires are stored in a database and can be related to averages of norm populations. Data from the constructed files are easily exported to other applications (e.g. SPSS PC and DBASE). Both current and future DISABKIDS questionnaires can be installed in several languages. There is an extensive user-friendly manual. The questionnaires are protected against interruptions and application changes during completion. Only a co-operator can close down the program after all the results have been imported. All programs can be used on a stand-alone PC; single and multiple use is also possible on a network. Built-in scripting language gives maximum control of the flow of administration. The graphical user interface conforms to Microsoft Windows 95/98 and later versions. The applications have been developed using a 32-bit version of Delphi 5. The minimum configuration necessary for the correct functioning of the program is as follows: 133 MHz Intel Pentium processor; 32 MB of RAM; 600 by 800 graphic resolution screen; and 20 MB of free space on the hard disk. The program automatically puts the data into a database and checks the data range. Immediately after completing the questionnaire the data can be processed and analyzed. Within a few seconds the desired output (possibly including available reference values for the general population and a specific population) can be obtained. Condition-specific databases normalized for gender, age and background can be constructed. DISABKIDS data address those facets of children's and parents' well being which are not often addressed in a routine medical consultation.

For different countries in Europe several DISABKIDS modules have been developed, normalized and validated. The pediatricians and other healthcare professionals involved are learning to use these questionnaires via repeated use of the questionnaires and via feedback on DISABKIDS data that they receive. An additional advantage for the patient is the fact that, using DISABKIDS data, pediatricians can improve communication with family practitioners and school doctors. Enhancement of mutual communication leads to better (adjustment of) care and better opportunities for standardization and continuity of care. The computer can show separate reference values for boys and girls in cases where there are significant differences within the standard database. Likewise, reference values can be presented for every period of life, so that the maturational changes that every child experiences can be taken into account. Some of the disadvantages of a DISABKIDS computer program include:

- Absence of sufficient and/or adequate hardware
- Patient consultations may be less flexible (e.g. they may take more time or require a different patient order) because the completion of the DISABKIDS questionnaires by the child and the parents has to be taken into account
- The presence of a research assistant is often desirable to facilitate the work on the computer, especially for the parents (support for the children is often not found to be necessary).
- In addition, possible advantages (namely the broadening and deepening of client information) can be added to the list of disadvantages, and can give rise to the following questions:
- What do you do with the information received from the children and parents?
- How should one take into account or adjust for the experiences and perceptions reported by the children or parents?
- How much time does it take to be able to use a computer program?
- How can DISABKIDS profiles be interpreted?
- What problems surface when completing the program?

The DISABKIDS allows one to form a systematic, reliable and valid opinion of the child's and parents' (or proxy) effective appreciation of the child's daily functioning. On average, children with a chronic condition report a lower HRQoL than healthy children in the reference group. In addition, the DISABKIDS HRQoL domains enable a distinction to be made between the consequences of the different chronic conditions on the children.

### 4.4.4 Structural embedding of the DISABKIDS computer program in healthcare

To improve healthcare for both children and parents it is necessary to distribute the available DISABKIDS computer program and the matching software as openly and as broadly to the workers in the field as possible. Other aims are to achieve the highest possible user-friendliness and the lowest cost, and to keep the program relevant.

The DISABKIDS software is distributed via the DISABKIDS Web page. This page consists of general information and a user section where it is possible to download the necessary software and new developments (adapted norm data, improvements to the program or new software) using a password.

Frequently asked questions can be clarified and user requests can be registered to support the work of the Help Desk. Furthermore, there is the possibility of creating a user forum. Individual users can receive guidance in the use of the DISABKIDS computer program in groups or through occupational societies. A manual containing a description of the DISABKIDS program and software is distributed via the Web page.

### 4.4.5 Advantages and disadvantages of the DISABKIDS computer program

Advantages of a DISABKIDS computer program include: acquisition of more detailed and extensive information from the child and the parents, acquisition of a greater depth of information concerning the impact of a chronic condition experienced by the child and the parents, comparisons over long periods of time by means of the standardization of patient consultations (individual trend analyses), possibility of comparing DISABKIDS HRQoL results with normalized data from healthy children.

The building of a database for a specific group of patients is also considered an advantage because it facilitates the comparison of HRQoL within the same chronic patient group.

The DISABKIDS computer program makes it easier for healthcare professionals to obtain information from the child, as well as saving time and money. Time savings are greatest if the questionnaire is completed on a computer.

To avoid unnecessary strain on the child and parents the pediatrician/physician must be disciplined in the outpatient clinic. The healthcare worker is stimulated to supply more continuity of care by giving precise feedback on the well being experienced in relation to medication given, advice or treatment.

### 4.4.6 Conclusions

The medical and psychosocial care of the child with a chronic illness and his/her parents can be improved with the aid of computer-aided DISABKIDS instrument or questionnaires.

HRQoL data collection can be carried out on almost a routine basis and used in the care of patients. In this way the possibility is created for the child and the parents to share their thoughts and visions with their physician. The DISABKIDS computer version directly enables the healthcare worker to obtain more insight into how the child experiences his/her QoL and how parents think of their child's situation. Data collected in this manner can contribute to the clinical and medical treatment of the patient and his/her ongoing care. Better insight can be obtained into the kind of support or guidance required by the child and parents. With the help of these data, obtained in a standardized way, the care of children with a chronic condition and their parents in Europe can be supplied more adequately. Data can be made easily accessible and comparable. Information on the often-small numbers of patients in different hospitals and healthcare centres can be combined. When taking into account the time saved in terms of data collection, data input, correction, scoring and summarizing, the use of the DISABKIDS computer program can lead to substantial cost savings. The start-up phase may bring extra expenses with regard to software and computer infrastructure; however, many institutes already have such an infrastructure.

Use of this new technology can lead to lower costs when measurement of DISABKIDS is included in clinical trials, enable a better assessment of care, create a more transparent view of the thoughts of the patient for the physician, possibly improve the quality of care and support the direct care of the patient in Europe. The implementation of the DISABKIDS computer project is not only an important contribution towards the care of the child with a chronic condition and his/her parents, but also strengthens cooperation on a national or international level Figure 4-3 to Figure 4-6 give examples from our DISABKIDS computer program RUNQUEST.

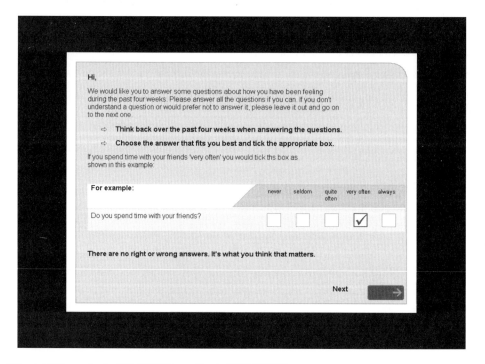

**Figure 4-3 Example of a DISABKIDS question in RUNQUEST**

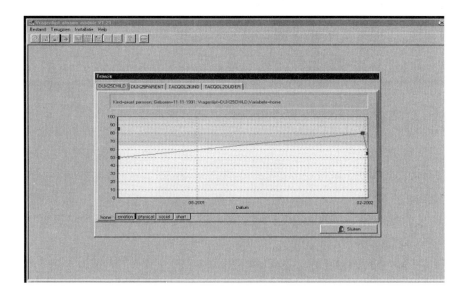

**Figure 4-4 Example of a trend analysis in RUNQUEST for a child who is doing better physically after intervention.**

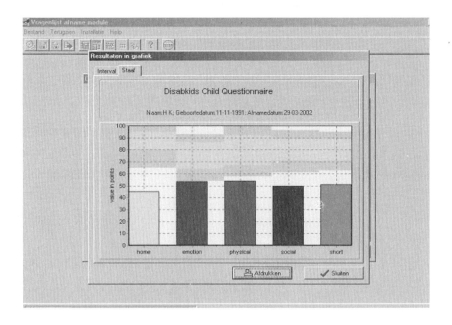

**Figure 4-5 A DISABKIDS profile of a child obtained using RUNQUEST**

| | home | emotion | physical | social | short | V01 | V02 | V03 | V04 | V05 | V06 | |
|---|---|---|---|---|---|---|---|---|---|---|---|---|
| 1 | 85.00 | 39.29 | 20.83 | 60.71 | 50.00 | a bit sad | normal | a bit happy | a bit happy | a bit happy | normal | |
| 2 | 35.00 | 60.71 | 54.17 | 50.00 | 51.00 | a bit happy | normal | a bit sad | normal | a bit happy | normal | |
| 3 | 90.00 | 82.14 | 95.83 | 92.86 | 90.00 | very happy | very happy | very happy | a bit sad | very happy | very happy | |
| 4 | 40.00 | 57.14 | 54.17 | 60.71 | 54.00 | a bit happy | normal | very happy | very sad | normal | a bit happy | |
| 5 | 40.00 | 57.14 | 62.50 | 50.00 | 53.00 | normal | normal | a bit happy | very happy | very happy | a bit sad | |
| 6 | 30.00 | 28.57 | 29.17 | 25.00 | 28.00 | normal | a bit sad | very sad | a bit sad | normal | a bit sad | |
| 7 | 50.00 | 50.00 | 50.00 | 50.00 | 50.00 | normal | normal | normal | normal | normal | normal | |
| 8 | 65.00 | 53.57 | 45.83 | 60.71 | 56.00 | normal | normal | a bit happy | a bit happy | very happy | very happy | |
| 9 | 75.00 | 67.86 | 75.00 | 75.00 | 73.00 | normal | normal | a bit happy | a bit happy | a bit happy | a bit happy | |
| 10 | 45.00 | 53.57 | 54.17 | 50.00 | 51.00 | normal | a bit happy | a bit sad | normal | a bit happy | normal | |

**Figure 4-6 DISABKIDS database in RUNQUEST and the export feature.**

## 4.5 Use of the DISABKIDS measures in individual patients

The DISABKIDS measure can be used both on a group and an individual level. Individual diagnostics includes application of the questionnaire to single children for diagnostic, predictive, or evaluative purposes. Whenever a child fills in a questionnaire and the clinician is interested in the results immediately in order to act upon, it is important that easy scoring and interpretation with regard to reference groups is possible. To accomplish this following information is necessary on the questionnaire level:

1. Each item belongs to a scale and is depicted in a template version of the questionnaire, indicating a scoring direction between one and five (with five representing the highest possible level of health-related quality of life accommodating of reversed items). Scales can be identified by the heading under which the items are grouped. Positively worded items will be scored 1, 2, 3, 4, 5 and negatively worded items will be scored 5, 4, 3, 2, 1 already in the template version of the questionnaire.

2. The items are then added per subscale to a raw score per subscale. They can also on a sub-scale level be transformed to a zero to hundred score. Both raw score and transformed raw score can be used for comparison with the reference data tables in the end of the manual. The total raw score can be identified be adding up the individual raw scores of each sub-scale, or by adding up all item scores. Again, this total raw score could be transformed in a zero to hundred score.

3. In order to interpret the scores, a description on a sub-scale level is necessary. In general, higher values on sub-scales or general scores indicate better quality of life for each of the DISABKIDS modules. For example, a raw score of 20 on the sub-scale "social inclusion", of the DISABKIDS chronic generic module (long version), with a range of possible raw scores from 6 to 30, indicates a higher quality of life in terms of feelings of social integration and acceptance by others, than a raw score of 15 does. A raw score of 6 represents the lowest value reachable on this measurement, thus indicating a worse quality of life with respect to aspects of social inclusion. Individual scorings down to 6 are highly associated with social isolation and feelings of loneliness. On the other side, a raw score of 30 as the highest possible value reachable at this measurement indicates a very high quality of life with respect to aspects social inclusion Children scoring up to 30 are thought to have stable

and satisfying social interactions and relationships. In addition the raw scores of the individual child can be compared to the tables in the back of the manual (0-100 transformed raw scores, percentile scores, t-scores), indicating the relative location of the patient with regard to his health-related quality of life to his/ her reference groups. In addition it is recommended that a profile template is used in which the physician can fill in either raw or percentile scale scores to see in which scale the patient is within the average range or beyond or below. For easy scoring, the template questionnaire is depicted so that it can be copied on an overhead, which can be put on top of the patient questionnaire for easy scoring.

4. In the reference score part at the end of the manual (see Chapter 6) every observable category of the raw scores for each subscale score and total score of the DISABKIDS measures is represented for different reference groups (crossed for gender and age group). The raw score tables are added by the transformation of this raw scores into zero to hundred scores, percentile scores and for t-scores. Ideally, the scores should be shaded so that the position of the person within the shades indicates their relative position in the reference group, indicates of high health-related quality of life, average health-related quality of life, low health-related quality of life. In order to understand how the manual tables work an individual example is given (see below).

5. An Example: Child X has filled in the DISABKIDS condition generic measure. The first scale is independence scale, the individual score can be calculated by putting the overhead with the answer scale values on the child's questionnaire and adding up the numbers which can range for each item between 1 and 5. The first scale, independence, contains six items, for six items therefore the scale range can vary between 6 and 30, with 24 different possible raw scores. In this case, the child is a boy, about 10 years old and has a raw score of 15. This means that his transformed raw score (zero to hundred) is 37.50, his percentile score is 2.5 and his t-score is 28.42. A percentile score of 2.5 means that 97.5% of boys in the same age group of 8 to 12 years have a higher score than him, basically then this child's health-related quality of life is very low. With regard to the t-score 28.42 (the average t-score is 50 and the standard deviation is 10) a value of 28.42 means that the child is more than two standard deviations below the average of its reference group, again indicating a very low health-related quality of life. With the help of the transformed raw score, which is also included in the reference tables, individual cases can also be identified by searching their individual cases zero to hundred values on the reference tables and then comparing it

with the percentile score. For use of the DISABKIDS measure in research and on a group level, a scoring disk is included which describes an SPSS program for calculating subscales and total scores.

6. **Profile sheet (for the DISABKIDS Chronic Generic Module DCGM-37)**.

   *(Next page)*

## DISABKIDS CHRONIC GENERIC MODULE (DCGM-37) – PROFILE SHEET

| Date | .................................................................... |
|---|---|
| **Code/ Name** | .................................................................... |
| **Age** | .................................................................... |
| **Gender** | ☐ male    ☐ female |

| Reference data | ≤ 4 | ≤ 11 | ≤ 23 | ≤ 40 | ≤ 60 | ≤ 77 | ≤ 89 | ≤ 96 | ≤ 100 | *PR* |
|---|---|---|---|---|---|---|---|---|---|---|
| (DISABKIDS Group | 4 | 7 | 12 | 17 | 20 | 17 | 12 | 7 | 4 | *%* |
| field study sample) | 1 | 2 | 3 | 4 | 5 | 6 | 7 | 8 | 9 | *Stanine* |

|  | *(low)* | | | *Health-related Quality of Life* | | | | *(high)* | | **Score** |
|---|---|---|---|---|---|---|---|---|---|---|
| **1. INDEPENDENCE** | • | • | • | • | • | • | • | • | • | ... |
| **2. EMOTION** | • | • | • | • | • | • | • | • | • | ... |
| **3. INCLUSION** | • | • | • | • | • | • | • | • | • | ... |
| **4. EXCLUSION** | • | • | • | • | • | • | • | • | • | ... |
| **5. LIMITATION** | • | • | • | • | • | • | • | • | • | ... |
| **6. TREATMENT** | • | • | • | • | • | • | • | • | • | ... |
|  | | | | ← 54 % → | | | | | | |
| **• TOTAL SCORE** | • | • | • | • | • | • | • | • | • | ... |

| **Comments** | ...................................................................... |
|---|---|
| | ...................................................................... |
| | ...................................................................... |

# 5 Future Directions

In addition to the DISABKIDS quality of life questionnaires, the following assessment tools have been developed by the group:

- CHC-SUN: **C**hild **H**ealth **C**are Questionnaire on **S**atisfaction, **U**tilisation and **N**eeds (Schmidt et al., 2006)
- CODI: **Co**ping with Chronic **Di**sease Inventory (Petersen et al., 2004)
- Clinical and Parental Severity Assessment (The DISABKIDS Group, 2006)

Information on these measures can be obtained at the Hamburg Centre. For information on the CODI- Coping Inventory please contact Dr. Corinna Petersen (copeters@uke.uni-hamburg.de). For information on the CHC-SUN (Child Health Care Questionnaire on Satisfaction, Utilisation and Needs) please contact Dr. Silke Schmidt (sischmid@uke.uni-hamburg.de).

# 6 Final remarks on the project: Experiences of the DISABKIDS group

The preceding part of this book was devoted to the description of aims, methods, results and conclusions from the European DISABKIDS project "Quality of Life in children with chronic conditions and disabilities". While the previous chapters described the scientific part of the study, the final chapter will address some aspects of conducting collaborative European research projects in terms of the organisational and human aspects of working together.

Within the European project, a total of eight countries worked together to develop the study protocol, consent on the methods, recruit the subjects, collect the data and do the statistic analysis. In wise foresight of potential problems to be solved during such a collaborative process, the grant proposals to the European Union requested a description of the organisational structure of the project as well as of the nature of the collaboration in the DISABKIDS project. This already helped to clarify some of the issues, which are related not only to regulatory and financial matters, but also to the actual conduct of the project in the respective responsibilities. Basically, the nature of the collaboration is a network of partners (principal investigators) with special expertise in specific areas of research or clinical knowledge as well as of a central institution coordinating the work in the project. As for the DISABKIDS project, the study centre was located in Hamburg, and had both scientific as well as organisational tasks in terms of planning and monitoring the programme while conducting the project. The principal investigators originally had, in the formation phases of the study protocol, indicated their interest in specific activities within the project and helped shaping the project protocol. Therefore it was clear and also described in the project proposal which centre would be active in the eleven work phases in the DISABKIDS project. While the general progress of the project was planned ahead in the consent of all members, specific work steps and decisions to be made during the process could not be anticipated. Therefore it was necessary convene as much as possible in person, via telephone and email for the group of researchers to identify the state of the work and to plan further activities. Although the role of the study centres was important in terms of time lines, pace-making and management as well as scientific input, it was well understood by all participants that this was a group of partners and that decisions had to be made in consensus.

In addition, the DISABKIDS and KIDSCREEN projects shared similar aims and methodology, so that DISABKIDS and KIDSCREEN meetings were held together. Plenary sessions were held together, but study related sessions held apart. This made it possible to include the views of all project partners, from both projects and on different levels of cooperation.

A special challenge during the group process was the decisions at the milestones and deliverables of the study. For example, as regards the literature research, the search strategies had to be streamlined in order to employ the relevant keywords. The literature search was conducted with great care, used different approaches and yielded at a total of 8.000 articles relevant for the topic in the DISABKIDS project and a comparable number in the KIDSCREEN project. How to conduct the literature search and how to analyse it, was one of the first discussions within the project. Another discussion was related to the ideal properties of the instruments to be developed, the type and number of domains, types of questions, time frames and sources of information for items were intensely debated and led to the publication of the paper describing ideal properties of quality of life instruments in children, derived from an expert Delphi exercise (Herdman et al. 2002).

On the level of focus groups, the question was how best to address children's views and values, the writing of focus group manuals and the standardisation of the item eliciting procedure proved to be very helpful for both projects. Some dissent arose over the question how to sort the statements and how to write them up. One problem here was how to agree on the nature of item (generic versus the disease specific) and whether to reformulate the items. Here questions of framing (1-week recalls, 4-week recalls, present tense/ past tense questions) were intensely debated. The wording and framing issue was one of the few questions/statements in which both studies of KIDSCREEN and DISABKIDS diverged and came up with different solutions. KIDSCREEN used a 1-week recall, while in DISBAKIDS; statements were assessed within a 4-weeks time frame in order to tap more rare experiences with conditions.

The translation procedure as the next work step went smoothly with regard to the employment of expert services, although some of the translations had to be reviewed critically and changed, especially after pilot-testing. In the pilot-test, the two projects diverged, the DISABKIDS project used a comparatively small proportion of parents and children of three age groups to conduct the pilot testing and the sites involved contributed in different fashion to the recruitment process. This was not due to motivational problems, but mainly to organisational problems in terms of difficulties with patient's recruitment, especially during the summer months. Nevertheless, an appropriate sample size could be obtained.

Different persons, however, performed analysis of the pilot data within the DISABKIDS project, consenting on the analysis strategy which itself was a matter of much discussion and debate. However, the strategy employed proved to be useful: consensus on the data analysis was reached and data were published adequately. Revision to be done according to the questions as well as modifications of the questionnaire were discussed within the meetings and consented upon, so that the field study phase within the DISABKIDS project could begin. Here, the recruitment also was different across sites, however, sites being not so strong in the pilot test proved to be strong in the field test and vice versa. With an extension of the project duration of 6 months, which was due to problems in ethical approval as well as patient recruitment, the field test phase was completed.

With regard to the final analysis, again analysis groups were assembled to discuss procedures and methods used for data analysis. This included both descriptive statistics as well as complex procedures using IRT as new psychometric methods. Three subgroups addressed the psychometric analysis and came up in the end with comparable solutions, so that consensus on the final version of the questionnaire was possible. Decision points here were the number of items to be extracted, the identification of a short form, which was finally agreed upon, and a small children's version. A problem within the process was the parallel development of a computer-assisted form due to the many languages involved in the different forms. It was especially the magnitude of factors - such as the construction of generic and disease specific modules, different language modules, modules for different conditions, different respondents and different age groups - that made it difficult to reconcile the whole tool set in the development process.

At the end, KIDSCREEN and DISABKIDS projects reunited after completion of the respective field studies. Their work came together in a common website which includes both information about the generic instrument KIDSCREEN as well as the condition-generic and condition-specific (disease-specific) instruments of the DISABKIDS questionnaire family. Together with manuals and information how to use the site, this is a helpful resource both in terms of documentation of accomplishment as well as comprehensive information about the methods developed, their psychometric properties and their implementation so far.

As regards organisation matters, telephone conferences and workshops were of utmost importance as were emails contacts between members of the group. One critical issue was the question whether people helping along the project but not being original members of the group should be included in the work process and especially the publications. To take care of this problem, publication rules were formulated both within the DISABKIDS and KID-SCREEN groups and exchanged, so that a common approach to publication policy was possible. However, rather than following rules, having the publications finished is of major importance, so that the publication rules were thought of as a general outline of strategies how to publish and how to assure the quality of the publication.

In general, group processes such as multinational collaborative groups go through different phases that are well known from social psychology. This includes the introductory phase, the conflict phase, the resolution phase, the working phase and the departure phase. These phases could also easily be discerned in the DISABKIDS project. Controversial phases necessary for groups to move on with their tasks, and if settled in a consensual way can be very fruitful, as it was the case with the DISABKIDS process. Sometimes the organisational work took a lot of time with special regard to relating to the European commission in preparing short reports, cost statements and the administration in a way that is helpful for the projects. This rather time-consuming and for scientists novel aspect of working also administratively together in the European project could have been helped by professional support with the administrative part of this relatively huge endeavour.

In terms of personal relations forming within partners in a project, the European DISABKIDS project was a very positive experience. People who had known and valued each other work before, got together to reach a common goal and this was done with effort and fervour and with fun. For example, a DISABKIDS and KIDSCREEN songbook was put together because the group tended after a long days work to relax together and sing songs from the different nations involved. This "songbook" became rather a sportive activity for all of the meetings and fostered group cohesion.

As is often the case with such projects, much of the work still needs to be done when the project is over, especially as concerns the publications emanating from many different scientific topics researched in the project. This is the phase that the DISABKIDS project will be in for some time as well as KIDSCREEN. In terms of the product, it is hoped that the DISABKIDS as well as the KIDSCREEN will well used in the European Community, so that the group effort which was put into the conduct of the study will be implemented further for the benefit of the patients.

All in all, all members at the last meeting expressed their gratitude for having had the experience of working together. There was also sadness of having to depart, especially as concerns the many possibilities of further ongoing studies that were applied for, but on the European level were not funded. It is important to keep such a network of motivated researchers alive and active. One possibility would be to reapply for another EU study, emanating from the current efforts, and researching more intensely about the application of the measures developed in the DISABKIDS and KIDSCREEN.

# 7 References

Abott J, Webb K, Dodd M. 1997. Quality of life in cystic fibrosis. Journal of the Royal Society of Medicine; 90 (Suppl 31): 37-42.

Aicardi J. 1998. Diseases of the Nervous System in Childhood. London: MacKeith Press.

Anderson RT, McFarlane M, Naughton MJ, A SS. 1996. Conceptual issues and considerations in cross-cultural validation of generic health-related quality of life instruments. In: Spilker B, editor. Quality of life and pharmacoeconomics in clinical trials. Philadelphia: Lippincott-Raven Publishers. p 605-612.

Barlow JH, Shaw KL, Harrison K. 1999. Consulting the 'experts': Children's and parents' perceptions of psycho-educational interventions in the context of juvenile chronic arthritis. Health Education Research 14 (5):597-610.

Ben-Gashir MA. 2003. Relationship between quality of life and disease severity in atopic dermatitis/eczema syndrome during childhood. Current Opinion in Allergy & Clinical Immunology. p 369-373.

Beryl J.Rosenstein, MD, and Carry R. Cutting, MD, for Cystic Fibrosis Foundation Concensus Panel 1998. The Journal of Pediatrics; 132: 589-95.

Bullinger M. 1997. Health related quality of life and subjective health. Literature review. PPmP 3(4):76-91.

Bullinger M, Ravens-Sieberer U. 1995. Health-related quality of life assessment in children: A review of the literature. Euro Rev Appl Psychol 45:245-254.

Bullinger M, Schmidt S, Petersen C, The-DISABKIDS-Group. 2002. Assessing quality of life of children with chronic health conditions and disabilities: A European approach. International Journal of Rehabilitation Research 25:197-206.

Carpey HA, Arts WFM. 1996. Outcome assessment in epilepsy: available rating scales for adults and methodological issues pertaining to the development of scales for childhood epilepsy. Epilepsy Research. p 127-136.

Carpey HA, Arts WFM, Vermeulen J, Stronik H, Brouwer OF, Boudewn Peters AC, Conselaar van CA, Aldenkamp AP. 1996. Parent-completed scales for measuring seizure severity and severity of side-effects of anticpileptic drugs in childhood epilepsy: development and psychometric analysis. Epilepsy Research. p 173-181.

Congleron J, Hodson M, Duncan- Skingle F. 1996. Quality of life in adults with cystic fibrosis. Thorax; 51: 936-940.

Cooperman E, park M, McKee J, et al. 1971. A simplified cystic fibrosis scoring system. Can Med Assoc J; 105:580-582.

Cramer JA. 2003. Seizure Severity Questionnaire.

Cramer JA, Baker GA, Jacoby A. 2002. Development of a new seizure severity questionnaire: initial reliability and validity testing. Epilepsy Research. p 187-197.

Croner S, Kjellman NI. 1992. Natural history of bronchial asthma in childhood. A prospective study from birth up to 12-14 years of age. Allergy 47:150-157.

Drotar D. 1998. Measuring Health-Related Quality of Life in Children and Adolescents. Mahwah, NJ: Erlbaum.

Dunn DW, Buelow JM, Austin JK, Shinnar S, Perkins SM. 2004. Development of syndrome severity scores for pediatric epilepsy. Epilepsia. p 661-666.

Eiser C, Berrenberg JL. 1995. Assessing the impact of chronic disease on the relationship between parents and their adolescents. J Psychosom Res 39(2):109-14.

Eiser C, Cotter I, Oades P, Seamark D, Smith R. 1999. Health-related quality-of-life measures for children. International Journal of Cancer Supplement. p 87-90.

Eiser C, Morse R. 2001a. The measurement of quality of life in children: past and future perspectives. Journal of Developmental & Behavioral Pediatrics. p 248-56.

Eiser C, Morse R. 2001b. Quality-of-life measures in chronic diseases of childhood. Health Technol Assess 5(4):1-157.

Elborn JS, Shale DJ, Britton JR. Cystic fibrosis: current survival and population estimates to the year 2000. Thorax. 1991; 46: 81-5.

Ellert U, Thomas C, Ravens-Sieberer U, Kosinski M, Björner JB, Dewey J, Ware JE. 2001. Using item response theory to improve QoL measures for children - first results from the child dynamic health assessment project. Abstract Issue 8th Annual Conference of the International Society for Quality of Life Research. Quality of Life Research 10(3):203.

Emerson RM, Charman CR, Williams HC. 2000. The Nottingham Eczema Severity Score: preliminary refinement of the Rajka and Langeland grading. British Journal of Dermatology 142(2):288.

European-Task-Force-on-Atopic-Dermatitis. 1993. Severity scoring of atopic dermatitis: the SCORAD index. Dermatology 186(1):23-31.

Fitz-Simmons SC, The changing epidemiology of cystic fibrosis. J. Pediatr. 1993; 122:1-8.

French D. Quality of life in cystic fibrosis. Thorax 1998; 53:721-722.

Gare BA. 1999. Juvenile arthritis- who gets it, where and when? A review of current data on incidence and prevalence. Clin Exp Rheumatol. p 367-374.

Gautier V, Redier H, Pujol JL, Bousquet J, Proudhon H, Michel C, Daures JP, Michel FB, Godard P. 1996. Comparison of an expert system with other clinical scores for the evaluation of severity of asthma. European Respiratory Journal 9:58-64.

Gee L, Abbott J, Conway SP, et al. Development of a disease specific health related quality of life measure for adults and adolescents with cystic fibrosis. Thorax 2000; 55:946-954

Giannini EH, Lovell DJ, Felson DT, Goldsmith CH. 1994. Preliminary core set of outcome variables for use in juvenile rheumatoid arthritis clinical trials. Arthritis & Rheumatism. p 428.

Giannini EH, Ruperto N, Ravelli A, Lovell DJ, Felson DT, Martini A. 1997. Preliminary definition of improvement in juvenile arthritis. Arthritis & Rheumatism. p 1202-1209.

Goodman R. 1998. The Longitudinal Stability of Psychiatric Problems in Children with Hemiplegia. Journal of Child Psychology and Psychiatry 39:347-354.

Guillemin F, Bombardier C, Beaton D. 1993. Cross-cultural adaption of health-related quality of life measures: Literature review and proposed guidelines. Journal of Clinical Epidemiology 46(12):1417-1432.

Guyatt G, Jaeschke R, Heddle N, Cook D, Shannon H, Walter S. 1995. Basic statistics for clinicians: 1. Hypothesis testing. p 27-32.

Hanifin JM. 1991. Atopic dermatitis in infants and children. Pediatr Clin North Am 38:763-789.

Hargreave FE, Dolovich J, Newhouse MT. 1990. The Assessment and Treatment of Asthma: a Conference Report. Journal of Allergy and Clinical Immunology 85:1098-1111.

Herd RM, Tidman MJ, Ruta DA, Hunter JAA. 1997. Measurement of quality of life in atopic dermatitis: Correlation and validation of two different methods. British Journal of Dermatology 136:502-507.

Hodson ME and Geddes DM. Cystic Fibrosis. Arnold Ed. 2000.p: 13-27, 203-218.

International Diabetes Federation (IDF). 2003. The Diabetes Atlas. Brussels.

ISAAC. 1998. Worldwide Variations in the Prevalence of Asthma Symptoms. European Respiratory Journal 12:315-335.

Jong W, Kaptein A, Ceens van der Schans, et al. 1997 Quality of life in Patients with cystic fibrosis. Pediatric Pulmonology; 23:95-100.

Lewis-Jones MS, Finlay AY. 1995. The Children's Dermatology Life Quality Index (CDLQI): initial validation and practical use. British Journal of Dermatology 132(6):942-949.

Lewis-Jones MS, Finlay AY, Dykes PJ. 2001. The Infants' Dermatitis Quality of Life Index. British Journal of Dermatology 144(1):104-110.

Lissauer T, Clayden G. 2001. Illustrated Textbook of Paediatrics. Mosby.

Mackie P, E J, Jarvis S. 1998. The Lifestyle Assessment Questionnaire: An Instrument to Measure the Impact of Disability on the Lives of Children with Cerebral Palsy and Their Families. Child: Care, Health and Development 24:473-486.

Marshall BC, Pathophysiology of pulmonary disease in cystic fibrosis. Semin Respir Crit Care Med. 1994; 15:364-74.

Matouk E, Ghezzo R, Gruber R, et al. Internal consistency and predictive validity of a modified N. huang clinical scoring system in adult cystic fibrosis patients. Eur Respir J 1997 ; 10 : 2004-2013.

McKinlay I. 2004. Cerebral Palsy. London: Churchill Livingstone.

Mühlan, H., Schmidt, S., Debensaason, D. Simeoni, M .C. and the DISABKIDS Group. (in prep.) Developing a Short form of the DISABKIDS CGM.

Nelson. 2000. Textbook of Pediatrics. 17, editor: Saunders Company.

Orenstein DM. In: Cystic Fibrosis. A guide for patient and family. Lippincott- Raven Edition. 1997.p: 13-75

Orestaein D, Nixon P, Ross E, Kaplan R. The quality of weel-being scale in cystic fibrosis. Chst 1989; 95:344-347.

Petersen C, Schmidt S, Bullinger M. 2004. Gesundheitsbezogene Lebensqualität von Kindern und Jugendlichen mit einer chronischen Erkrankung - ein internationaler Ansatz zur Entwicklung eines Fragebogens. In: Bullinger M, editor. Lebensqualität: Nützlichkeit und Psychometrie des Short Form 12/36 in der medizinischen Rehabilitation.

Petty RE, Cassidy JT. 2001. The juvenile idiopathic arthritides. In: Petty RE, editor. Textbook of Rheumatology. 4 ed. Philadelphia, London, New York, St. Louis, Sidney, Toronto: Saunders. p 214-217.

Quittner Al. Measurement of quality of life in cystic fibrosis. Current Opinion in Pulmonary Medicine 1998; 4:326-331.

Quittner Al, Buu A. Effects of Tobramycin solution for inhalation on global ratings of quality of life in patients with cystic fibrosis and pseudomonas aeruginosa Infection. Pediatric Pulmonology 2002; 33: 269-276.

Ravens-Sieberer U. 2003. Der Kindl-R Fragebogen zur Erfassung der gesundheitsbezogenen Lebensqualität bei Kindern und Jugendlichen - Revidierte Form. In: Schumacher J, Klaiberg A, Brähler E, editors. Diagnostische Verfahren zu Lebensqualität und Wohlbefinden. Göttingen: Hogrefe. p 184-188.

Redier H, Daures JP, Michel C, Proudhon H, Vervloet D, Charpin D, Marsac J, Dusser D, Brambilla C, Wallaert B. 1995. Assessment of the severity of asthma by an expert system. Description and evaluation. American Journal of Respiratory and Critical Care Medicine 151:345-352.

Robinson P. Cystic fibrosis. Thorax 2001;56:237–241.

Rosenbloom A, Hanas R. 1996. Diabetic Ketoacidosis (DKA): Treatment Guidelines. Clinical Pediatrics 35:261-266.

Rosenstein BJ, Langbaum TS. Diagnosis. In: Taussing LM, ed. Cystic fibrosis. New York, NY: Thieme: 1984:p85-114.

Rosier MJ, Bishop J, Nolan T, Robertson CF, Carlin JB, Phelan PD. 1994. Measurement of functional severity of asthma in children. American Journal of Respiratory and Critical Care Medicine 149:1434-1441.

Ross MH, Mjaanes CM, Lemanske R. 2003. Rudolph CD, Rudolph AM, eds., Rudolph's Pediatrics. Asthma. New York: McGraw-Hill.

Sällfors C, Fasth A, Hallberg LR. 2002. Oscillating between hope and despair- a qualitative study. Child: Care, Health and Development. p 495-505.

Saiman L, Cacalano G, Gruenert D, et al. Comparison of adherence of Pseudomonas aeruginosa to respiratory epithelial cells from cystic fibrosis patients and healthy subjects. Infect Immun. 1992; 60:2808-14.

Schidlow DV, Taussing LM, Knowles MR. Cystic fibrosis foundation consensus conference report on pulmonary complications of cystic fibrosis. Pediatr Pulmonol. 1993; 15:187-98.

Schmidt S, Thyen U, Chaplin J, Mueller-Godeffroy E, The-European-DISABKIDS-Group. in press. Development of a child health care questionnaire on satisfaction, utilization and needs (CHC-SUN): Results from a European pilot study. Ambulatory Pediatrics

Schmidt, S., Bullinger, M. (2003). Current issues in cross-cultural quality of life instrument development. *Archives of Physical Medicine and Rehabilitation, 84 (4), 29-35.*

Schmidt, S., Morfeld, M., Petersen, C., Bullinger, M. (2003). Die Bedeutung subjektiver Indikatoren bei der Ermittlung des Gesundheitsversorgungsbedarfs. *Praxis Klinische Verhaltensmedizin und Rehabilitation, 63, 278-284.*

Shwachman H, Kulczycki LL. Long term study of one-hundred-five patients with cystic fibrosis. Am .J. Dis. Child 1958; 96:6-15.

Silverstein MD, Reed CE, O'Connell EJ, Melton LJ, O'Fallon WM, Yunginger J. 1994. Long-term survival of a cohort of community residents with asthma. The New England Journal of Medicine 331:1537-41.

Smith D, Baker GA, Jacoby A, Chadwick DW. 1995. The contribution of the measurement of seizure severity to quality of life research. Quality of Life Research. p 143-158.

Smith D, Chadwick D, Baker G, Davis G, Dewey M. 1993. Seizure severity and the quality of life. Epilepsia. p s31-s35.

Staab D, Wenninger K, Gebert N, et al. Quality of life in patients with cystic fibrosis and their parents: what is important besides disease severity? Thorax 1998; 53: 727-731.

Stein RE, Jessop DJ. 1990. Functional status II(R). A measure of child health status. Med Care 28(11):1041-1055.

Taussig L, Landau L. 1999. Textbook of paediatric respiratory medicine. Mosby, St Luis.

Tomashefski JF, Jr., Abramowsky CR, Dahms BB. The pathology of cystic fibrosis in: Davis PB, ed. Cystic fibrosis. New York, NY: Marcel Dekker; 1993:435-89.

Tullis E, Gordon G. Quality of life in cystic fibrosis. Pharmacoeconomics 1995; 8(1): 23-33.

US Department of Health and Human Services NIoH. 1997. Expert Panel Report 2: guidelines for the diagnosis and management of asthma. National Heart, Lung and Blood Institute National Asthma Education and Prevention Program. Bethesda MD: US Department of Health and Human Services, National Institutes of Health. Report nr 97-4051.

von Rüden U, Staab D, Kehrt R, Wahn U. 1999. Entwicklung und Validierung eines krankheitsspezifischen Fragebogens zur Erfassung der Lebensqualität von Eltern neurodermitiskranker Kinder. Zeitschrift für Gesundheitswissenschaft 7(H.4):335-350.

Williams SG, Schmidt DK, Redd SC, Storms W. 2003. Key clinical activities for quality asthma care. Recommendations of the National Asthma Education and Prevention Program. The MMWR Recommendations and Reports 52:1-8.

Wood RE. Treatment of CF lung disease in the first two years. Pediatr Pulmonol Suppl. 1989; 4:68-70. Abstract.

Wolter J, Bowler S, Nolan P, McCormack J. Home intravenous therapy in cystic fibrosis: a prospective randomized trial examining clinical Quality of life and cost aspects. Eur Respir J 1997; 10:896-900.

# 8 List of DISABKIDS Publications

*Published*

Baars, R., Atherton, C., Koopmann, H., Bullinger, M., Power, M., and the DISABKIDS group (2005). The European DISABKIDS project: development of seven condition-specific modules to measure health related quality of life in children and adolescents. *Health and Quality of Life Outcomes* 2005, 3: 70-79.

Baars, R.M., van der Pal, S.M., Koopman, H.M., Wit, J.M (2004). Clinicians' perspective on quality of life assessment in paediatric clinical practice. Acta-Paediatr.; 93(10): 1356-62.

Bullinger, M. & the DISABKIDS group. (2002). Assessing Quality of Life with Chronic Health Conditions and Disabilities – a European Approach. *International Journal of Rehabilitation Research, 25,* 197-206.

Bullinger, M., Petersen, C., Schmidt, S. & DISABKIDS group (2002). European Paediatric Health-Related Quality of Life Assessment. *Quality of Life Newsletter*, 29, 4-5.

Hatziagorou, E., Karagianni, P., Vidalis, A., Bullinger, M., Tsanakas, I. (2002). Association of Clinical Variables in Children with Cystic Fibrosis and Health-Related Quality of Life. *Hippokratia, 6(1),* 75-78.

Hatziagorou, E., Karagianni, P., Vidalis, A., Bullinger, M., Tsanakas, I. (2002). Association of Asthma Severity and Health-Related Quality of Life in Children. *Hippokratia, 6(1), 88-90.*

Hatziagorou, E., Karagianni, P., Vidalis, A., Bullinger, M., Tsanakas, I. (2002). Quality of Life in Children with Cystic Fibrosis and Asthma. *Hippokratia, 6(1),*12-14.

Hatziagorou, E., Karagianni, P., Vidalis, A., Bullinger, M., Tsanakas, I. (2002). Quality of Life in Cystic Fibrosis. *Hippokratia, 6(1),* 67-71.

Herdman, M., Rajmil, L., Ravens-Sieberer, U., Bullinger, M., Power, M., Alonso, J. & the European KIDSCREEN and DISABKIDS Group (2002). Expert consensus on the development of a European health related quality of life measure for children and adolescents: A Delphi study. *Acta Paediatrica, 91*, 1385-1390.

Petersen, C. (2003). Development and pilot-testing of a health related quality of life and coping inventory for children and adolescents with chronic health conditions. Dissertation. *Universität Hamburg.* http://www.sub.uni-hamburg.de/disse/1087/dissertation.pdf.

Petersen, C., Schmidt, S., Bullinger, M. and the DISABKIDS Group (2004). Brief Report: Development and Pilot Testing of a Coping Questionnaire for Children and Adolescents With Chronic Health Conditions *Journal of Pediatric Psychology, 29*, 635-640.

Petersen, C., Schmidt, S., Power, M. and the-DISABKIDS group (2005). Developing and pilot testing a chronic generic quality of life questionnaire for children with chronic conditions. *Quality of Life Research, 73 (2), 1065-75.*

Petersen, C., Schmidt, S., Bullinger, M. and the DISABKIDS Group (2006). Coping with a chronic pediatric health condition and Health-Related Quality of Life. European Psychologist, 11 (1), 50-57.

Petersen, C., Schmidt, S. & Bullinger, M. (2003). Erfassung der gesundheitsbezogenen Lebensqualität von Kindern und Jugendlichen mit einer chronischen Erkrankung, submitted: Lebensqualität: Nützlichkeit und Psychometrie des Short Form 12/ 36 in der medizinischen Rehabilitation. In: C. Maurischat, M. Morfeld, Th. Kohlmann & M. Bullinger (Hrsg.), Lebensqualität: Nützlichkeit und Psychometrie des Health Survey SF-36/ SF-12 in der medizinischen Rehabilitation. Lengerich, Pabst Verlag, 227-238.

Schmidt, S., Thyen, U., Petersen C., Bullinger, M. and the European DISABKIDS group. The performance of the screener to identify children with special health care needs in a European sample of children with chronic conditions. *European Journal of Pediatrics*, 2004, 9, 517-21.

*In press*

Schmidt, S., Debensason, D., Petersen, C., Mühlan, H., Simeoni, M.C., Bullinger, M. and the DISABKIDS group (2005). Cross-cultural performance of the DISABKIDS condition generic measure. *Journal of Clinical Epidemiology* (in press).

Schmidt S, Thyen U, Chaplin J, Mueller-Godeffroy E, The-European-DISABKIDS-Group. in press. Development of a child health care questionnaire on satisfaction, utilization and needs (CHC-SUN): Results from a European pilot study. Ambulatory Pediatrics

Schmidt, S., Thyen, U., Chaplin, J., Mueller-Godeffroy, E., Bullinger, M. and the DISABKIDS group. Health Care Needs and Health Care Satisfaction of families of children with chronic conditions: The DISABKIDS approach (in press).

*In preparation*

Baars, R.M., Koopman, H.M. & the DISABKIDS group. Focus Groups in Children with Asthma.

Baars, R.M., Koopman, H.M. & the DISABKIDS group. Item Development within the DIS-ABKIDS Project.

Baars, R.M., Koopman, H.M. & the DISABKIDS group. Questionnaire Development after Focus Group Research: the Reduction Process.

Baars, R., Hatziagorou, E. The Development of the DISABKIDS Asthma module.

Chaplin, J., Simeoni, MC. Development of a DISABKIDS Epilepsy Module.

Debensasson, D., Schmidt, S., Simeoni, M, Petersen, C. and the DISABKIDS group. Development of a proxy version of the European DISABKIDS instrument.

Debensasson, D., Schmidt, S., Simeoni, M, Petersen, C. and the DISABKIDS group. Field test results on the proxy version.

Hatziagorou, E., Vidales, T., Tsanakas, A. and the DISABKIDS group. Development of a DISABKIDS Cystic Fibrosis module.

Hoare, P., Atherton, C. and the DISABKIDS Group. Development of ´the DISABKIDS Cerebral Palsy module.

Koopman, H. and the DISABKIDS Group. Development of a DISABKIDS Computer Version.

Mueller-Godeffroy, E., Petersen, C. and the DISABKIDS Group, Development of a DISABKIDS arthritis module.

Mühlan, H., Schmidt, S., Debensasson, D. Simeoni, M .C. and the DISABKIDS Group. Developing a Short form of the DISABKIDS CGM. (Submitted 2006)

Schmidt, S., Thyen, U., Chaplin, J., Mueller-Godeffroy, E., Bullinger, M. and the DISABKIDS group. Development and testing of a child health care questionnaire on satisfaction, utilisation and needs (CHC-SUN). *Submitted.*

Schmidt, S., Simeoni, M. and the DISABKIDS group. Developing a quality of life module for children with atopic dermatitis. *Dermatology  and Psychomatics*

Schuhfried, O., Quittan, U.,  Field test results on the Diabetes Module (comparison proxy/child)

Simeoni, M., Schmidt, S., Muehlan, H., Debensasson, D. and the DISABKIDS group. Testing and improving the chronic generic module: The DISABKIDS field test experience.

Thyen, U., Schmidt, S., Mueller-Godeffroy, E., Chaplin, J. and the DISABKIDS group. Health care needs in children with chronic conditions. (Submitted to Ambulatory Pediatrics)

Thyen, U., Schmidt, S., Mueller-Godeffroy, E., Chaplin, J. Development of a Clinical Severity Assessment System for the DISABKIDS Group. Technical Report, University of Hamburg, Campus Schleswig-Holstein, 2006.

*Abstracts are not listed. A list of abstracts as well as presentations and posters can be obtained separately.*

# 9    Contact

***Central coordination centre:***

*Prof. Dr. Monika Bullinger*

bullinger@uke.uni-hamburg.de

Institute and Policlinic of Medical Psychology

Centre of Psychosocial Medicine

*Dr. Silke Schmidt*

University Hospital of Hamburg-Eppendorf

sischmid@uke.uni-hamburg.de

Martinistr. 52, S 35

20246 Hamburg

*Dr. Corinna Petersen*

Germany

copeters@uke.uni-hamburg.de

*Holger Muehlan*

hmuehlan@uke.uni-hamburg.de

***German Clinical Centre***

Department of Paediatrics

Medical University of Lübeck

Ratzeburger Allee 160

23538 Lübeck

Germany

*PD Dr. Ute Thyen*

thyen@paedia.ukl.mu-luebeck.de

*Dr. Esther Mueller-Goddefroy*

mueller-g@paedia.ukl.mu-luebeck.de

*National contact partners:*

**Austria**

Department of Physical Medicine and Rehabilitation

University of Vienna

Währinger Gürtel 18-20

1090 Wien

Austria

*Prof. Dr. Michael Quittan*

Michael.quittan@akh-wien.ac.at

*Dr. Othmar Schuhfried*

Othmar.Schuhfried@univie.ac.at

*Bettina Bandur*

disabkids.phys-med-rehab@univie.ac.at

**France**

Department of Public Health

University Hospital of Marseille

27 BD. J. Moulin

13885 Marseille cedex 5

France

*Dr. Marie Claude Siméoni*

lsp@medecine.univ-mrs.fr

*Dr. Audrey Clement*

lsp@medecine.univ-mrs.fr

*Delphine Orbicini*

Delphine.Orbicini@medecine.univ-mrs.fr

*David Debensasson*

lsp@medecine.univ-mrs.fr

**Greece**

Department of Paediatrics Respiratory Unit

Hippocratio Hospital

Konstantinoupoleos 49

Thessaloniki T.K. 54642

Greece

*Prof. John Tsanakas*

tsanakas@spark.net.gr

*Dr. Elpis Hatziagorou*

elpcon@otenet.gr

*Dr. Voula Paraskevi Karagianni*

*Prof. Dr. Athanasios Vidalis, PhD*

vidalis@med.auth.gr

Psychiatric Department

Hippokratio General Hospital

Konstantinoupoleos 49

Thessaloniki T.K. 54642

Greece

**Netherlands**

Department of Paediatrics
Leiden University Medical Centre
PO Box 9600
Albinusdreef 2
2300 RC Leiden
Netherlands

*Dr. Henrik M. Koopman*
H.M.Koopman@lumc.nl

*Dr. Rolanda M. Baars*
R.M.Baars@lumc.nl

**Sweden**

*Dr. John Eric Chaplin PhD Leg.psyk.*
Göteborg Pediatric Growth Research Center
The Sahlgrenska Academy at Göteborg University
Institute of Clinical Sciences
Department of Pediatrics
The Queen Silvia Children's Hospital
Växthuset
SE-41685 Göteborg, Sweden
Tel.: 0046 (0) 31 343 57 88
Fax: 0046 (0) 31 84 89 52
Epost: john.chaplin@vgregion.se

**United Kingdom**

Child & Family Mental Health Service
RHSC
3 Rillbank Terrace
Edinburgh EH9 1LL
United Kingdom

*Dr. Peter Hoare*
P.Hoare@ed.ac.uk

Section of Clinical and Health Psychology
University of Edinburgh
Royal Edinburgh Hospital
Morningside Park
Edinburgh EH 10 5HF
United Kingdom

*Prof. Dr. Mick Power*
mj@srvl.med.ed.ac.uk

*Dr. Clare Atherton*
C.Atherton@ed.ac.uk

# 10    Summary Sheet of the DISABKIDS Instruments

**Authors:** The DISABKIDS Group (2006).

**Publisher:** Pabst Publisher.

**Purpose:** Designed to assess health-related quality of life (HRQoL) in children and adolescents with chronic health conditions.

**Description:** The DISABKIDS instruments were designed to address quality of life with chronic conditions. They are based on a comprehensive process of development across different countries. The instruments are designed to assess health-related quality of life in a standardized format as reported by children/ adolescents or parents. A paper and pencil as well as a computer version are available.

**Population:** The DISABKIDS instruments are applicable to chronically ill children and adolesecents from 4 to16 years. Additionally, proxy versions for parents or other caregivers are available.

**Scoring:** The DISABKIDS instruments can be self-administered or administered. Depending on the module, the instruments consist of 10 to 37 items, which are scored on a 5-point scale ranging from never to always. The time frame refers to the last four weeks. Scores can be calculated for each dimension of the different DISABKIDS instruments. Reference data (percentages and t-values) are reported for different conditions, age groups and gender (only for DISABKIDS-Smileys and DISABKIDS Chronic Generic Measures).

**Time required:** DISABKIDS-Smileys approx. 5 minutes; DISABKIDS Chronic Generic Measures: approx. 10-30 minutes; DISABKIDS Condition-Specific Measures: approx. 10-20 minutes.

**Reliability:** DISABKIDS-Smileys: Internal consistency values (Cronbach`s Alpha) reaches .69 for the self-report version; test-retest reliability at a 2-4 week interval reaches .46. Item intraclass correlation (ICC) between self-reported scores and scores from parents filling out the DISABKIDS-Smileys proxy-version reaches .69.

DISABKIDS Chronic Generic Measures: Internal consistency values (Cronbach`s Alpha) varied between .70 ("Social Inclusion") and .87 ("Emotion") for the different dimensions of the self-report versions, test-retest reliability at a 2-4 week interval varies between .71 and .83. Item intraclass correlations (ICC) between self-reported scores and scores from parents filling out the DISABKIDS proxy-versions ranging from .53 ("Treatment") to .62 ("Limitation").

DISABKIDS Condition-Specific Measures: Internal consistency values (Cronbach`s Alpha) varied between .69 (Dermatitis - "Stigma") and .90 (Epilepsy - "Impact") for the different dimensions of the conditions-specific self-report versions, test-retest reliability at a 2-4 week interval varies between .45 (Arthritis - "Understanding") and .85. (Diabetes - "Impact"). Item intraclass correlations (ICC) between self-reported scores and scores from parents filling out the DISABKIDS proxy-versions ranging from .44 (Arthritis - "Understanding") to .79 (Cerebral Palsy - "Impact").

**Validity:** Validity could be assumed for all DISABKIDS modules, as indicated by association with different other measures of HRQoL and general health (KINDL, CHQ; convergent validity) and by discrimination of different levels of clinical severity (discriminatory validity).

**Administration/ Suggested Uses:** All types of paediatric studies: Clinical comparative studies on different conditions, intervention studies on specific conditions and across conditions, integrated outcome measurement, developmental studies, psychosocial studies, economic studies. Administration is recommended for health and medical professionals in different fields (medicine, epidemiology, public health) and institutions (schools, hospitals, research labs, medical establishment) of the health care system.

**Selected bibliographical information:**

Baars, R., Atherton, C., Koopmann, H., Koopmann1, Bullinger, M., Power, M., and the DISABKIDS group (2005). The European DISABKIDS project: development of seven condition-specific modules to measure health related quality of life in children and adolescents. Health and Quality of Life Outcomes 2005, 3: 70-79.

Bullinger, M. & the DISABKIDS group. (2002). Assessing Quality of Life with Chronic Health Conditions and Disabilities – a European Approach. *International Journal of Rehabilitation Research, 25,* 197-206.

Herdman, M., Rajmil, L., Ravens-Sieberer, U., Bullinger, M., Power, M., Alonso, J. & the European KIDSCREEN and DISABKIDS Group (2002). Expert consensus on the development of a European health related quality of life measure for children and adolescents: A Delphi study. *Acta Paediatrica, 91,* 1385-1390.

Petersen, C., Schmidt, S., Power, M., Bullinger, M. & the DISABKIDS Group (2003). Development and pilot-testing of a health-related quality of life chronic generic module for children and adolescents with chronic health conditions – A European perspective, submitted: *QUALITY OF LIFE RESEARCH, 73 (2), 1065-75.*

Schmidt, S., Debensason, D., Petersen, C., Mühlan, H., Simeoni, M.C., Bullinger, M. and the DISABKIDS Group (2005). Cross-cultural performance of the DISABKIDS disease-generic measure. *Journal of Clinical Epidemiology* (in press)

Schmidt, S., Thyen, U., Petersen, C., Bullinger, M. and the European DISABKIDS Group (2004). The performance of the screener to identify children with special health care needs in a European sample of children with chronic conditions. *European Journal of Pediatrics* 163:517-523, 517-523.

**Internet Site**: http://www.disabkids.org

# Appendix

## Content

## A-I      The DISABKIDS questionnaires

On the following pages, the DISABKIDS questionnaires are demonstrated using the English version. All other language versions will be available on the CD-ROM that is included in this book.

The questionnaires are presented in the following sequence:

**Child version**

- DISABKIDS Chronic Generic Measure – long form (DCGM-37)
- DISABKIDS Chronic Generic Measure – short form (DCGM-12)
- DISABKIDS Smiley Measure
- Condition-specific modules for asthma, arthritis, cerebral palsy, cystic fibrosis, dermatitis, diabetes, and epilepsy.

**Parent version**

- DISABKIDS Chronic Generic Measure – long form (DCGM-37)
- DISABKIDS Chronic Generic Measure – short form (DCGM-12)
- DISABKIDS Smiley Measure
- Condition-specific modules for asthma, arthritis, cerebral palsy, cystic fibrosis, dermatitis, diabetes, and epilepsy.

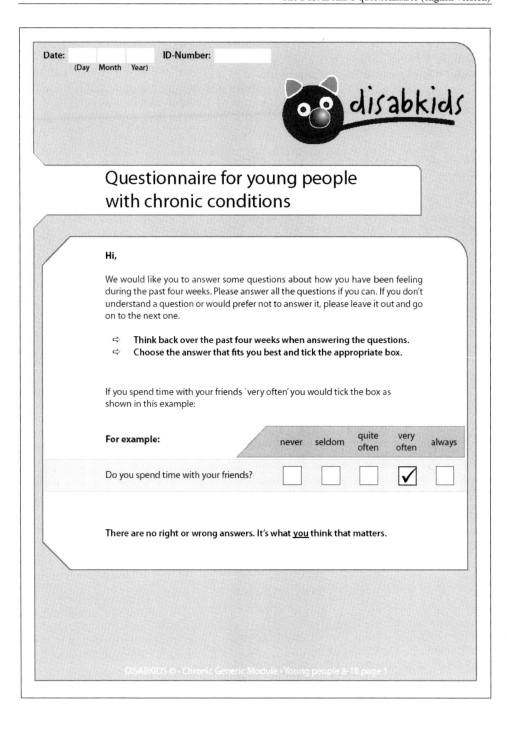

Date: _____   ID-Number: _____

(Day   Month   Year)

# disabkids

## Questionnaire for young people with chronic conditions

**Hi,**

We would like you to answer some questions about how you have been feeling during the past four weeks. Please answer all the questions if you can. If you don't understand a question or would prefer not to answer it, please leave it out and go on to the next one.

⇨  **Think back over the past four weeks when answering the questions.**
⇨  **Choose the answer that fits you best and tick the appropriate box.**

If you spend time with your friends 'very often' you would tick the box as shown in this example:

| **For example:** | never | seldom | quite often | very often | always |
|---|---|---|---|---|---|
| Do you spend time with your friends? | ☐ | ☐ | ☐ | ✓ | ☐ |

There are no right or wrong answers. It's what <u>you</u> think that matters.

## Some questions about you

| A. | Are you male or female? | ☐ female | ☐ male |

| B. | How old are you? | ☐ years |

C. Which condition do you have?

☐ asthma          ☐ arthritis          ☐ dermatitis

☐ cerebral palsy  ☐ diabetes           ☐ cystic fibrosis

☐ epilepsy        ☐ other  ⟶  Which? [                    ]

In some questions we use the word „condition". When you see condition, please think about what you filled in above.

## About your life

**Think about the past four weeks!**

| | | never | seldom | quite often | very often | always |
|---|---|---|---|---|---|---|
| 1. | Are you confident about your future? | ☐ | ☐ | ☐ | ☐ | ☐ |
| 2. | Do you enjoy your life? | ☐ | ☐ | ☐ | ☐ | ☐ |
| 3. | Are you able to do everything you want to do even though you have your condition? | ☐ | ☐ | ☐ | ☐ | ☐ |
| 4. | Do you feel like everyone else even though you have your condition? | ☐ | ☐ | ☐ | ☐ | ☐ |
| 5. | Are you free to lead the life you want even though you have your condition? | ☐ | ☐ | ☐ | ☐ | ☐ |
| 6. | Are you able to do things without your parents? | ☐ | ☐ | ☐ | ☐ | ☐ |

DISABKIDS © · Chronic Generic Module · Young people 8-18 page 2

## About your typical day

**Think about the past four weeks!**

| | | never | seldom | quite often | very often | always |
|---|---|---|---|---|---|---|
| 7. | Are you able to run and move as you like? | ☐ | ☐ | ☐ | ☐ | ☐ |
| 8. | Do you feel tired because of your condition? | ☐ | ☐ | ☐ | ☐ | ☐ |
| 9. | Is your life ruled by your condition? | ☐ | ☐ | ☐ | ☐ | ☐ |
| 10. | Does it bother you that you have to explain to others what you can and can't do? | ☐ | ☐ | ☐ | ☐ | ☐ |
| 11. | Is it difficult to sleep because of your condition? | ☐ | ☐ | ☐ | ☐ | ☐ |
| 12. | Does your condition bother you when you play or do other things? | ☐ | ☐ | ☐ | ☐ | ☐ |

## About your feelings

**Think about the past four weeks!**

| | | never | seldom | quite often | very often | always |
|---|---|---|---|---|---|---|
| 13. | Does your condition make you feel bad about yourself? | ☐ | ☐ | ☐ | ☐ | ☐ |
| 14. | Are you unhappy because of your condition? | ☐ | ☐ | ☐ | ☐ | ☐ |
| 15. | Do you worry about your condition? | ☐ | ☐ | ☐ | ☐ | ☐ |
| 16. | Does your condition make you angry? | ☐ | ☐ | ☐ | ☐ | ☐ |
| 17. | Do you have fears about the future because of your condition? | ☐ | ☐ | ☐ | ☐ | ☐ |
| 18. | Does your condition get you down? | ☐ | ☐ | ☐ | ☐ | ☐ |
| 19. | Does it bother you that your life has to be planned? | ☐ | ☐ | ☐ | ☐ | ☐ |

DISABKIDS © · Chronic Generic Module · Young people 8-18 page 3

## About you and other people

**Think about the past four weeks!**

| | never | seldom | quite often | very often | always |
|---|---|---|---|---|---|
| 20. Do you feel lonely because of your condition? | ☐ | ☐ | ☐ | ☐ | ☐ |
| 21. Do your teachers behave differently towards you than towards others? | ☐ | ☐ | ☐ | ☐ | ☐ |
| 22. Do you have problems concentrating at school because of your condition? | ☐ | ☐ | ☐ | ☐ | ☐ |
| 23. Do you feel that others have something against you? | ☐ | ☐ | ☐ | ☐ | ☐ |
| 24. Do you think that others stare at you? | ☐ | ☐ | ☐ | ☐ | ☐ |
| 25. Do you feel different from other children/adolescents? | ☐ | ☐ | ☐ | ☐ | ☐ |

## About your friendships

**Think about the past four weeks!**

| | never | seldom | quite often | very often | always |
|---|---|---|---|---|---|
| 26. Do other children/adolescents understand your condition? | ☐ | ☐ | ☐ | ☐ | ☐ |
| 27. Do you go out with your friends? | ☐ | ☐ | ☐ | ☐ | ☐ |
| 28. Are you able to play or do things with other children/adolescents (like sports)? | ☐ | ☐ | ☐ | ☐ | ☐ |
| 29. Do you think that you can do most things as well as other children/adolescents? | ☐ | ☐ | ☐ | ☐ | ☐ |
| 30. Do your friends enjoy being with you? | ☐ | ☐ | ☐ | ☐ | ☐ |
| 31. Do you find it easy to talk about your condition to other people? | ☐ | ☐ | ☐ | ☐ | ☐ |

DISABKIDS © • Chronic Generic Module • Young people 8-18 page 4

## About your medical treatment

Do you take any medicine for your condition? (by medicine we mean tablets, cream, spray, insulin or any other medicine)   yes ☐   no ☐

**Think about the past four weeks!**

| If yes, please fill in the following questions, if no, please skip this section. | never | seldom | quite often | very often | always |
|---|---|---|---|---|---|
| 32. Does having to get help with medication from others bother you? | ☐ | ☐ | ☐ | ☐ | ☐ |
| 33. Is it annoying for you to have to remember your medication? | ☐ | ☐ | ☐ | ☐ | ☐ |
| 34. Are you worried about your medication? | ☐ | ☐ | ☐ | ☐ | ☐ |
| 35. Does taking medication bother you? | ☐ | ☐ | ☐ | ☐ | ☐ |
| 36. Do you hate taking your medicine? | ☐ | ☐ | ☐ | ☐ | ☐ |
| 37. Does taking medication disrupt everyday life? | ☐ | ☐ | ☐ | ☐ | ☐ |

**Thank you for your assistance!**

DISABKIDS © · Chronic Generic Module · Young people 8-18 page 5

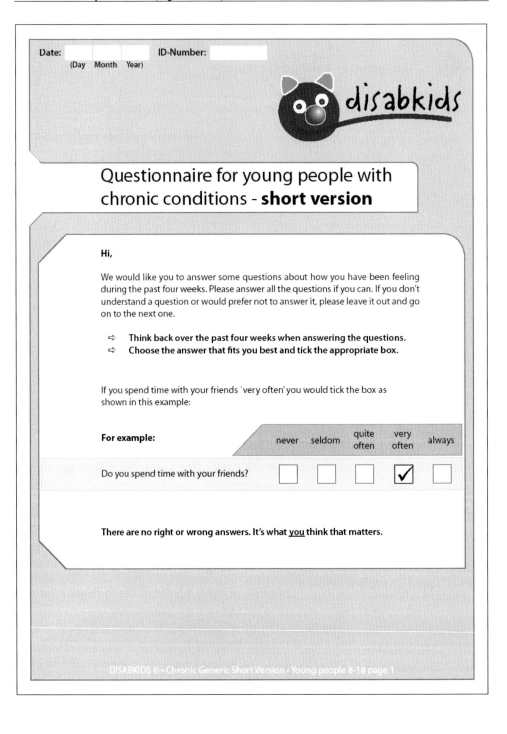

Date: _____ ID-Number: _____
(Day Month Year)

**disabkids**

## Questionnaire for young people with chronic conditions - **short version**

**Hi,**

We would like you to answer some questions about how you have been feeling during the past four weeks. Please answer all the questions if you can. If you don't understand a question or would prefer not to answer it, please leave it out and go on to the next one.

⇨ Think back over the past four weeks when answering the questions.
⇨ Choose the answer that fits you best and tick the appropriate box.

If you spend time with your friends `very often' you would tick the box as shown in this example:

| For example: | never | seldom | quite often | very often | always |
|---|---|---|---|---|---|
| Do you spend time with your friends? | ☐ | ☐ | ☐ | ✔ | ☐ |

**There are no right or wrong answers. It's what <u>you</u> think that matters.**

DISABKIDS © - Chronic Generic Short Version - Young people 8-18 page 1

## Some questions about you

A.   Are you male or female?   ☐ female   ☐ male

B.   How old are you?   ☐ years

C.   Which condition do you have?

☐ asthma   ☐ arthritis   ☐ dermatitis

☐ cerebral palsy   ☐ diabetes   ☐ cystic fibrosis

☐ epilepsy   ☐ other   ⟶   Which? ☐

In some questions we use the word „condition". When you see
condition, please think about what you filled in above.

## About your life

**Think about the past four weeks!**

| | never | seldom | quite often | very often | always |
|---|---|---|---|---|---|
| 1. Do you feel like everyone else even though you have your condition? | ☐ | ☐ | ☐ | ☐ | ☐ |
| 2. Are you free to lead the life you want even though you have your condition? | ☐ | ☐ | ☐ | ☐ | ☐ |
| 3. Is your life ruled by your condition? | ☐ | ☐ | ☐ | ☐ | ☐ |
| 4. Does your condition bother you when you play or do other things? | ☐ | ☐ | ☐ | ☐ | ☐ |
| 5. Are you unhappy because of your condition? | ☐ | ☐ | ☐ | ☐ | ☐ |
| 6. Does your condition get you down? | ☐ | ☐ | ☐ | ☐ | ☐ |
| 7. Do you feel lonely because of your condition? | ☐ | ☐ | ☐ | ☐ | ☐ |

DISABKIDS © · Chronic Generic Short Version · Young people 8-18 page 2

## About your life

**Think about the past four weeks!**

| | never | seldom | quite often | very often | always |
|---|---|---|---|---|---|
| 8. Do you feel different from other children/adolescents? | ☐ | ☐ | ☐ | ☐ | ☐ |
| 9. Do you think that you can do most things as well as other children/adolescents? | ☐ | ☐ | ☐ | ☐ | ☐ |
| 10. Do your friends enjoy being with you? | ☐ | ☐ | ☐ | ☐ | ☐ |

## About your medical treatment

Do you take any medicine for your condition? (by medicine we mean tablets, cream, spray, insulin or any other medicine)  yes ☐  no ☐

**Think about the past four weeks!**

| If yes, please fill in the following questions, if no, please skip this section. | never | seldom | quite often | very often | always |
|---|---|---|---|---|---|
| 11. Does taking medication bother you? | ☐ | ☐ | ☐ | ☐ | ☐ |
| 12. Do you hate taking your medicine? | ☐ | ☐ | ☐ | ☐ | ☐ |

**Thank you for your assistance!**

DISABKIDS © · Chronic Generic Short Version · Young people 8-18 page 3

Date: ___ (Day Month Year)    ID-Number: ___    Condition: ___

**disabkids**

# Questionnaire for children with chronic conditions

**Hi,**

We want to know how you felt lately. On every question, can you tell us how that feeling was? Put a circle around the face that fits best. With every question you can choose one of the five faces.

**This is an example.**

When I play with my friends I feel:

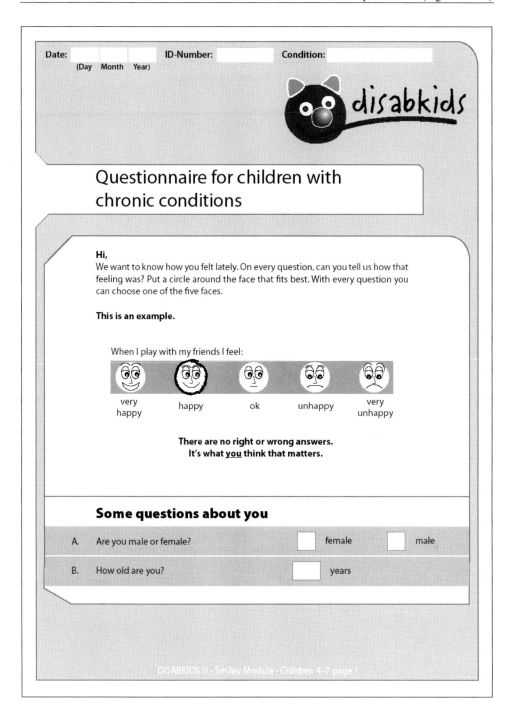

| very happy | happy | ok | unhappy | very unhappy |

**There are no right or wrong answers.**
**It's what _you_ think that matters.**

## Some questions about you

| A. | Are you male or female? | ☐ female | ☐ male |
| B. | How old are you? | ☐ years | |

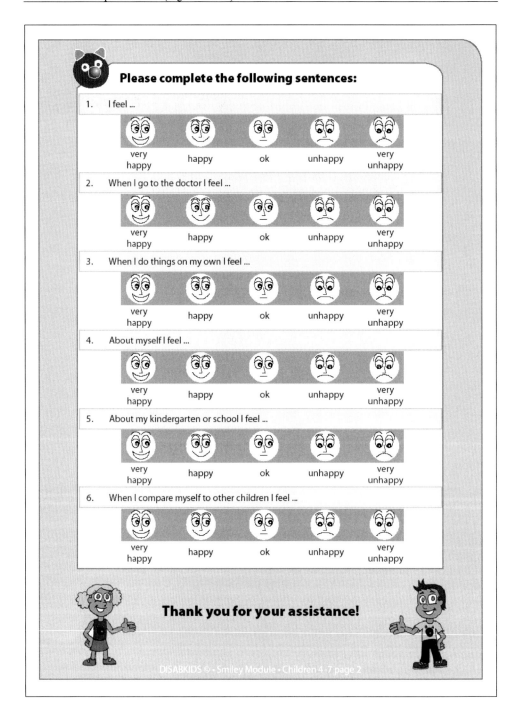

**Please complete the following sentences:**

1. I feel ...

   very happy · happy · ok · unhappy · very unhappy

2. When I go to the doctor I feel ...

   very happy · happy · ok · unhappy · very unhappy

3. When I do things on my own I feel ...

   very happy · happy · ok · unhappy · very unhappy

4. About myself I feel ...

   very happy · happy · ok · unhappy · very unhappy

5. About my kindergarten or school I feel ...

   very happy · happy · ok · unhappy · very unhappy

6. When I compare myself to other children I feel ...

   very happy · happy · ok · unhappy · very unhappy

**Thank you for your assistance!**

DISABKIDS © · Smiley Module · Children 4 -7 page 2

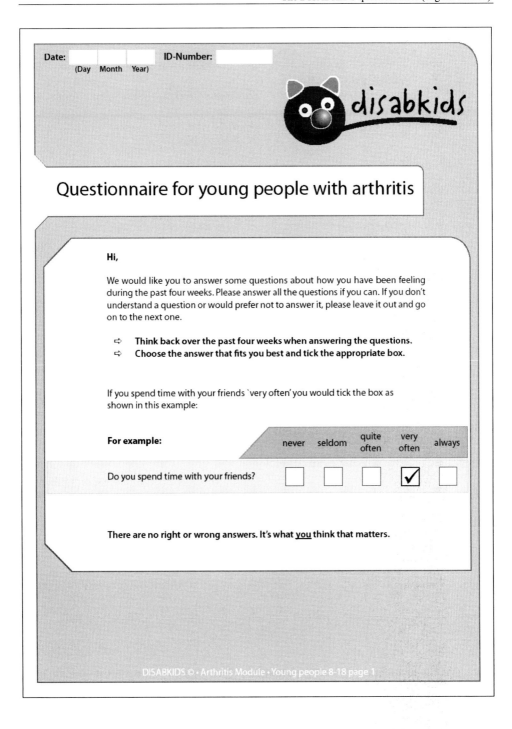

Date: _____ ID-Number: _____
(Day   Month   Year)

disabkids

# Questionnaire for young people with arthritis

**Hi,**

We would like you to answer some questions about how you have been feeling during the past four weeks. Please answer all the questions if you can. If you don't understand a question or would prefer not to answer it, please leave it out and go on to the next one.

⇨ **Think back over the past four weeks when answering the questions.**
⇨ **Choose the answer that fits you best and tick the appropriate box.**

If you spend time with your friends ˋvery often' you would tick the box as shown in this example:

| For example: | never | seldom | quite often | very often | always |
|---|---|---|---|---|---|
| Do you spend time with your friends? | ☐ | ☐ | ☐ | ☑ | ☐ |

**There are no right or wrong answers. It's what <u>you</u> think that matters.**

DISABKIDS © · Arthritis Module · Young people 8-18 page 1

## About your arthritis

**Think about the last four weeks!**

| | | never | seldom | quite often | very often | always |
|---|---|---|---|---|---|---|
| 1. | Do you feel stiff in the mornings (like an old grandma/granddad)? | ☐ | ☐ | ☐ | ☐ | ☐ |
| 2. | Do you get exhausted easily? | ☐ | ☐ | ☐ | ☐ | ☐ |
| 3. | Does arthritis make you feel too exhausted to be with friends? | ☐ | ☐ | ☐ | ☐ | ☐ |
| 4. | Do you hate being in pain? | ☐ | ☐ | ☐ | ☐ | ☐ |
| 5. | Does it annoy you that the pain sometimes comes on so suddenly? | ☐ | ☐ | ☐ | ☐ | ☐ |
| 6. | Does pain stop you from doing what you want? | ☐ | ☐ | ☐ | ☐ | ☐ |
| 7. | Does it bother you that you can't do all sports/hobbies because of your arthritis? | ☐ | ☐ | ☐ | ☐ | ☐ |
| 8. | Do you hate being restricted in movement? | ☐ | ☐ | ☐ | ☐ | ☐ |
| 9. | Does it bother you that you have trouble writing/ drawing? | ☐ | ☐ | ☐ | ☐ | ☐ |

## About your arthritis

**Think about the last four weeks!**

| | | never | seldom | quite often | very often | always |
|---|---|---|---|---|---|---|
| 10. | Do others understand that your symptoms may change suddenly? | ☐ | ☐ | ☐ | ☐ | ☐ |
| 11. | Do your friends understand that you may feel poorly quite suddenly? | ☐ | ☐ | ☐ | ☐ | ☐ |
| 12. | Do teachers understand that you sometimes can't join in? | ☐ | ☐ | ☐ | ☐ | ☐ |

The last three questions are about how much trouble you have had **with** your arthritis **in the last year.**

## About symptoms

| | Think about the last year | | | | |
|---|---|---|---|---|---|
| | never | few times | every month | every week | daily |
| a. How often did you have problems with your arthritis during the last year? | ☐ | ☐ | ☐ | ☐ | ☐ |

| | not at all | a little bit | mode-rately | quite a bit | ex-tremely |
|---|---|---|---|---|---|
| b. How severe was your arthritis during the last year? | ☐ | ☐ | ☐ | ☐ | ☐ |

| | never | seldom | quite often | very often | always |
|---|---|---|---|---|---|
| c. How often did you have pain in your joints or muscles during the last year? | ☐ | ☐ | ☐ | ☐ | ☐ |

**Thank you for your assistance!**

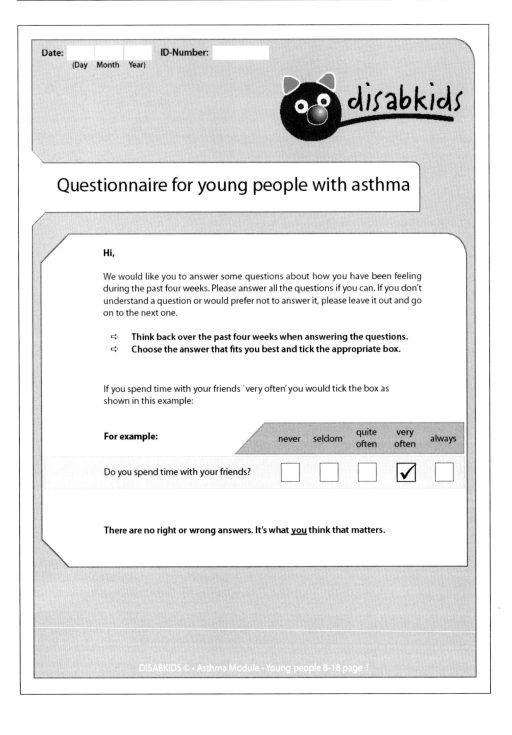

**Date:** ⬚⬚  **ID-Number:** ⬚⬚⬚

(Day  Month  Year)

# disabkids

## Questionnaire for young people with asthma

**Hi,**

We would like you to answer some questions about how you have been feeling during the past four weeks. Please answer all the questions if you can. If you don't understand a question or would prefer not to answer it, please leave it out and go on to the next one.

⇨  **Think back over the past four weeks when answering the questions.**
⇨  **Choose the answer that fits you best and tick the appropriate box.**

If you spend time with your friends ´very often´ you would tick the box as shown in this example:

| **For example:** | never | seldom | quite often | very often | always |
|---|---|---|---|---|---|
| Do you spend time with your friends? | ☐ | ☐ | ☐ | ☑ | ☐ |

**There are no right or wrong answers. It's what <u>you</u> think that matters.**

DISABKIDS © · Asthma Module · Young people 8-18 page 1

## About your asthma

**Think about the last four weeks!**

| | never | seldom | quite often | very often | always |
|---|---|---|---|---|---|
| 1. Do you feel that you get easily exhausted? | ☐ | ☐ | ☐ | ☐ | ☐ |
| 2. Does asthma bother you if you want to go out? | ☐ | ☐ | ☐ | ☐ | ☐ |
| 3. Are you unable to take part in certain sports (like long-distance running)? | ☐ | ☐ | ☐ | ☐ | ☐ |
| 4. Do you feel short of breath when you do sports? | ☐ | ☐ | ☐ | ☐ | ☐ |
| 5. Are you bothered by the amount of time you spend wheezing? | ☐ | ☐ | ☐ | ☐ | ☐ |
| 6. Do you feel terrible when you are out of breath? | ☐ | ☐ | ☐ | ☐ | ☐ |

## About your asthma

**Think about the last four weeks!**

| | never | seldom | quite often | very often | always |
|---|---|---|---|---|---|
| 7. Are you worried that you might have an asthma attack? | ☐ | ☐ | ☐ | ☐ | ☐ |
| 8. Do you worry that others do not know what to do if you have an attack? | ☐ | ☐ | ☐ | ☐ | ☐ |
| 9. Do you feel scared that you might have difficulty breathing? | ☐ | ☐ | ☐ | ☐ | ☐ |
| 10. Are you scared that you might have to go to the emergency ward? | ☐ | ☐ | ☐ | ☐ | ☐ |
| 11. Are you scared at night because of your asthma? | ☐ | ☐ | ☐ | ☐ | ☐ |

DISABKIDS © · Asthma Module · Young people 8-18 page 2

123

The last three questions are about how much trouble you have had with your asthma **in the last year.**

## About symptoms

Think about the last year

| | never | in the last year | last 6 months | last month | last week |
|---|---|---|---|---|---|
| a. When was the last time you had an asthma attack? | ☐ | ☐ | ☐ | ☐ | ☐ |

| | never | 1 time | 2 times | 3 times | more than 3 times |
|---|---|---|---|---|---|
| b. How many asthma attacks did you have during the last year? | ☐ | ☐ | ☐ | ☐ | ☐ |

| | not at all | a little bit | mode-rately | quite a bit | extre-mely |
|---|---|---|---|---|---|
| c. How severe was your asthma during the last year? | ☐ | ☐ | ☐ | ☐ | ☐ |

**Thank you for your assistance!**

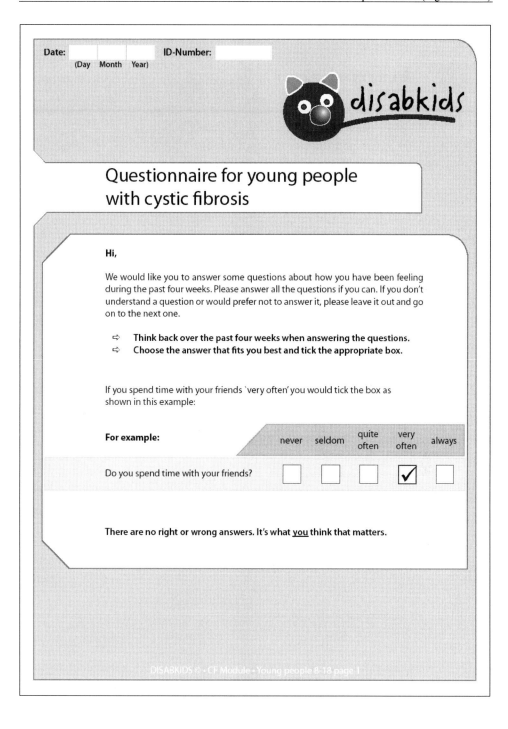

Date: _____ ID-Number: _____

(Day   Month   Year)

disabkids

# Questionnaire for young people with cystic fibrosis

**Hi,**

We would like you to answer some questions about how you have been feeling during the past four weeks. Please answer all the questions if you can. If you don't understand a question or would prefer not to answer it, please leave it out and go on to the next one.

➪   **Think back over the past four weeks when answering the questions.**
➪   **Choose the answer that fits you best and tick the appropriate box.**

If you spend time with your friends `very often' you would tick the box as shown in this example:

| For example: | never | seldom | quite often | very often | always |
|---|---|---|---|---|---|
| Do you spend time with your friends? | ☐ | ☐ | ☐ | ✔ | ☐ |

**There are no right or wrong answers. It's what _you_ think that matters.**

DISABKIDS © · CF Module · Young people 8-18 page 1

## About your cystic fibrosis

**Think about the last four weeks!**

| | | never | seldom | quite often | very often | always |
|---|---|---|---|---|---|---|
| 1. | Do you get exhausted when you do sports? | ☐ | ☐ | ☐ | ☐ | ☐ |
| 2. | Do you feel tired during the day? | ☐ | ☐ | ☐ | ☐ | ☐ |
| 3. | Do you get out of breath? | ☐ | ☐ | ☐ | ☐ | ☐ |
| 4. | Do you need to rest more than others? | ☐ | ☐ | ☐ | ☐ | ☐ |

## About your cystic fibrosis

**Think about the last four weeks!**

| | | never | seldom | quite often | very often | always |
|---|---|---|---|---|---|---|
| 5. | Does it bother you that you must take your enzymes before every meal? | ☐ | ☐ | ☐ | ☐ | ☐ |
| 6. | Does it bother you that you have to eat a special diet to keep you healthy? | ☐ | ☐ | ☐ | ☐ | ☐ |
| 7. | Does it bother you that you have to spend a lot of time having treatment? | ☐ | ☐ | ☐ | ☐ | ☐ |
| 8. | Are you bothered because you have to do physiotherapy everyday? | ☐ | ☐ | ☐ | ☐ | ☐ |
| 9. | Have you felt that your treatment takes up too much of your free time? | ☐ | ☐ | ☐ | ☐ | ☐ |
| 10. | Do you feel bothered that you have to stop playing or doing things for treatment? | ☐ | ☐ | ☐ | ☐ | ☐ |

DISABKIDS © - CF Module · Young people 8-18 page 2

The last three questions are about how much trouble you have had with your cystic fibroses **in the last year**.

## About symptoms

Think about the last year

| | not at all | a little bit | mode-rately | quite a bit | extre-mely |
|---|---|---|---|---|---|
| a. How severe was your cystic fibrosis during the last year? | ☐ | ☐ | ☐ | ☐ | ☐ |

| | never | 1 time | 2 times | 3 times | more than 3 times |
|---|---|---|---|---|---|
| b. How often did you have a bad time because of your cystic fibrosis symptoms during the last year? | ☐ | ☐ | ☐ | ☐ | ☐ |

| | never | in the last year | last 6 months | last month | last week |
|---|---|---|---|---|---|
| c. When was the last time you had blood in your sputum? | ☐ | ☐ | ☐ | ☐ | ☐ |

**Thank you for your assistance!**

DISABKIDS ® • CF Module • Young people 8-18 page 3

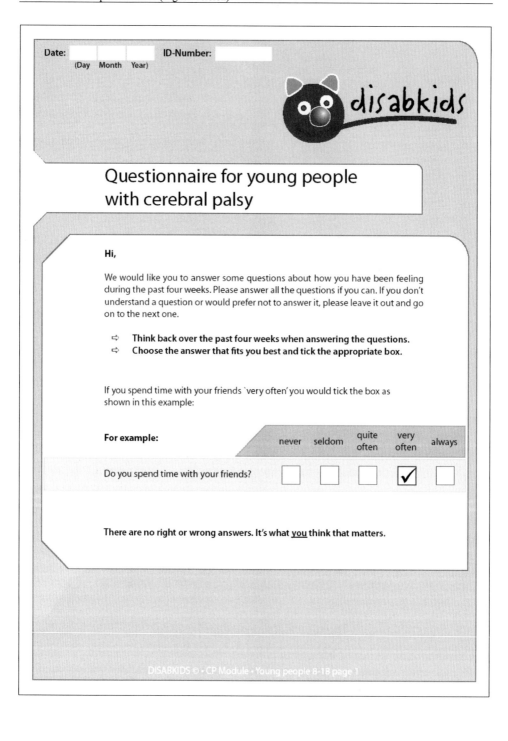

Date: ____ ____ ____     ID-Number: _____
      (Day  Month  Year)

disabkids

## Questionnaire for young people with cerebral palsy

**Hi,**

We would like you to answer some questions about how you have been feeling during the past four weeks. Please answer all the questions if you can. If you don't understand a question or would prefer not to answer it, please leave it out and go on to the next one.

⇨  **Think back over the past four weeks when answering the questions.**
⇨  **Choose the answer that fits you best and tick the appropriate box.**

If you spend time with your friends `very often' you would tick the box as shown in this example:

| **For example:** | never | seldom | quite often | very often | always |
|---|---|---|---|---|---|
| Do you spend time with your friends? | ☐ | ☐ | ☐ | ✓ | ☐ |

**There are no right or wrong answers. It's what <u>you</u> think that matters.**

DISABKIDS © · CP Module · Young people 8-18 page 1

## About your cerebral palsy

**Think about the last four weeks!**

| | | never | seldom | quite often | very often | always |
|---|---|---|---|---|---|---|
| 1. | Is it frustrating to be unable to keep up with other children? | ☐ | ☐ | ☐ | ☐ | ☐ |
| 2. | Do you wish that you could run around like everyone else? | ☐ | ☐ | ☐ | ☐ | ☐ |
| 3. | Do you wish that you could swim as well as other children? | ☐ | ☐ | ☐ | ☐ | ☐ |
| 4. | Does it bother you that getting dressed takes a long time? | ☐ | ☐ | ☐ | ☐ | ☐ |
| 5. | Do people think that you are not as clever as you are? | ☐ | ☐ | ☐ | ☐ | ☐ |
| 6. | Do you have trouble getting in and out of buildings? | ☐ | ☐ | ☐ | ☐ | ☐ |
| 7. | Are you able to do most things even though your legs don't move well? | ☐ | ☐ | ☐ | ☐ | ☐ |

| | | never | seldom | quite often | very often | always | I don't have any problems with... |
|---|---|---|---|---|---|---|---|
| 8. | Does it upset you that you are unable to walk without help? | ☐ | ☐ | ☐ | ☐ | ☐ | ☐ ...walking without help |
| 9. | Do you dislike being washed and dressed by other people? | ☐ | ☐ | ☐ | ☐ | ☐ | ☐ ...washing and dressing without help |
| 10. | Does it upset you that you need help to use the toilet? | ☐ | ☐ | ☐ | ☐ | ☐ | ☐ ...using the toilet without help |

## About your cerebral palsy

**Think about the last four weeks!**

| | | never | seldom | quite often | very often | always | I don't have any problems with... |
|---|---|---|---|---|---|---|---|
| 11. | Can you communicate as well as you'd like? | ☐ | ☐ | ☐ | ☐ | ☐ | ☐ ...talking |
| 12. | Does it upset you that you can't talk as well as other children? | ☐ | ☐ | ☐ | ☐ | ☐ | ☐ ...talking |

## Thank you for your assistance!

DISABKIDS © · CP Module · Young people 8-18 page 2

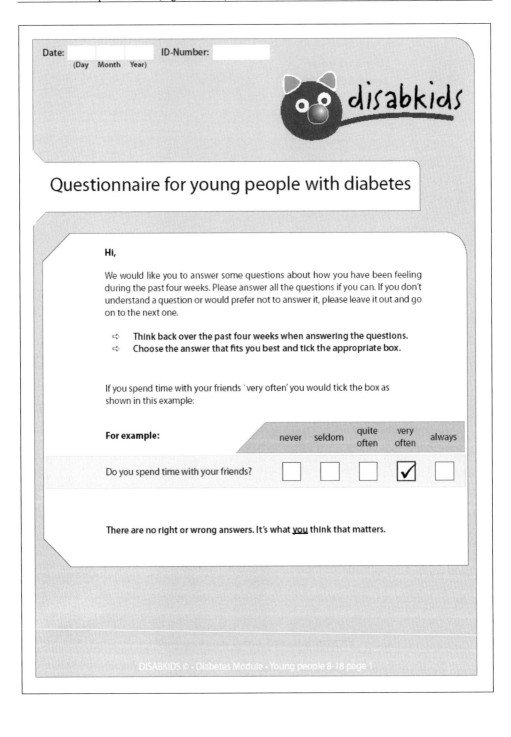

Date: _____    ID-Number: _____
(Day  Month  Year)

# disabkids

## Questionnaire for young people with diabetes

**HI,**

We would like you to answer some questions about how you have been feeling during the past four weeks. Please answer all the questions if you can. If you don't understand a question or would prefer not to answer it, please leave it out and go on to the next one.

⇨  **Think back over the past four weeks when answering the questions.**
⇨  **Choose the answer that fits you best and tick the appropriate box.**

If you spend time with your friends `very often' you would tick the box as shown in this example:

| For example: | never | seldom | quite often | very often | always |
|---|:---:|:---:|:---:|:---:|:---:|
| Do you spend time with your friends? | ☐ | ☐ | ☐ | ✓ | ☐ |

**There are no right or wrong answers. It's what <u>you</u> think that matters.**

## About your diabetes

**Think about the last four weeks!**

| | | never | seldom | quite often | very often | always |
|---|---|---|---|---|---|---|
| 1. | Does diabetes stop you from doing the things you want to do? | ☐ | ☐ | ☐ | ☐ | ☐ |
| 2. | Does diabetes rule your day? | ☐ | ☐ | ☐ | ☐ | ☐ |
| 3. | Does it bother you that you have to be careful about what you eat? | ☐ | ☐ | ☐ | ☐ | ☐ |
| 4. | Is it difficult for you to stick to your diet? | ☐ | ☐ | ☐ | ☐ | ☐ |
| 5. | Do you worry about your blood sugar level? | ☐ | ☐ | ☐ | ☐ | ☐ |
| 6. | Does it bother you that others can always eat and drink as much as they like? | ☐ | ☐ | ☐ | ☐ | ☐ |

## About your diabetes

**Think about the last four weeks!**

| | | never | seldom | quite often | very often | always |
|---|---|---|---|---|---|---|
| 7. | Do you mind taking insulin? | ☐ | ☐ | ☐ | ☐ | ☐ |
| 8. | Do you get fed up with measuring your blood sugar levels? | ☐ | ☐ | ☐ | ☐ | ☐ |
| 9. | Are you annoyed that you have to carry the testing equipment with you? | ☐ | ☐ | ☐ | ☐ | ☐ |
| 10. | Are you bothered that you have to plan everything? | ☐ | ☐ | ☐ | ☐ | ☐ |

DISABKIDS © - Diabetes Module - Young people 8-18 page 2

The last three questions are about how much trouble you have had with your diabetes **in the last year.**

## About symptoms

**Think about the last year**

| | never | once | a few times | often | all the time |
|---|---|---|---|---|---|
| a. How often did you have problems with your diabetes during the last year? | ☐ | ☐ | ☐ | ☐ | ☐ |

| | not at all | a little bit | mode- rately | quite a bit | ex- tremly |
|---|---|---|---|---|---|
| b. How severe have your problems with your diabetes been during the last year? | ☐ | ☐ | ☐ | ☐ | ☐ |

| | never | in the last year | last six months | last month | last week |
|---|---|---|---|---|---|
| c. When was the last time you have had a bad hypo attack (low blood sugar)? | ☐ | ☐ | ☐ | ☐ | ☐ |

**Thank you for your assistance!**

Date: _____  ID-Number: _____

(Day   Month   Year)

**disabkids**

# Questionnaire for young people with epilepsy

**Hi,**

We would like you to answer some questions about how you have been feeling during the past four weeks. Please answer all the questions if you can. If you don't understand a question or would prefer not to answer it, please leave it out and go on to the next one.

⇨   **Think back over the past four weeks when answering the questions.**
⇨   **Choose the answer that fits you best and tick the appropriate box.**

If you spend time with your friends `very often' you would tick the box as shown in this example:

| For example: | never | seldom | quite often | very often | always |
|---|---|---|---|---|---|
| Do you spend time with your friends? | ☐ | ☐ | ☐ | ✓ | ☐ |

**There are no right or wrong answers. It's what you think that matters.**

## About your epilepsy

**Think about the last four weeks!**

| | | never | seldom | quite often | very often | always |
|---|---|---|---|---|---|---|
| 1. | Are you afraid that you might hurt yourself during a seizure? | ☐ | ☐ | ☐ | ☐ | ☐ |
| 2. | Are you worried that you might have a seizure in public? | ☐ | ☐ | ☐ | ☐ | ☐ |
| 3. | Are you afraid of having a seizure? | ☐ | ☐ | ☐ | ☐ | ☐ |
| 4. | Do your seizures make you feel helpless? | ☐ | ☐ | ☐ | ☐ | ☐ |
| 5. | Are you scared that you could have a seizure at any time? | ☐ | ☐ | ☐ | ☐ | ☐ |

## About your epilepsy

**Think about the last four weeks!**

| | | never | seldom | quite often | very often | always |
|---|---|---|---|---|---|---|
| 6. | Does it embarrass you when people take care of you when you have a seizure? | ☐ | ☐ | ☐ | ☐ | ☐ |
| 7. | Are you worried that people make fun of you when you have a seizure? | ☐ | ☐ | ☐ | ☐ | ☐ |
| 8. | Are you afraid that you can't remember what happens during a seizure? | ☐ | ☐ | ☐ | ☐ | ☐ |
| 9. | Are you ashamed of having seizures? | ☐ | ☐ | ☐ | ☐ | ☐ |
| 10. | Are you worried that other children will see you having a seizure? | ☐ | ☐ | ☐ | ☐ | ☐ |

DISABKIDS © · Epilepsy Module · Young people 8-18 page 2

134

The last three questions are about how much trouble you have had with your epilepsy **in the last year.**

### About symptoms

**Think about the last year**

| | | not in the last year | in the last year | last 6 months | last 4 weeks | last week |
|---|---|---|---|---|---|---|
| a. | When was the last time you had an epileptic fit or seizure? | ☐ | ☐ | ☐ | ☐ | ☐ |

| | | not at all | a little bit | mode-rately | quite a bit | extre-mely |
|---|---|---|---|---|---|---|
| b. | How severe has your epilepsy been during the last year? | ☐ | ☐ | ☐ | ☐ | ☐ |

| | | none | one | a couple | quite a few | loads |
|---|---|---|---|---|---|---|
| c. | How many seizures have you had during the last year? | ☐ | ☐ | ☐ | ☐ | ☐ |

**Thank you for your assistance!**

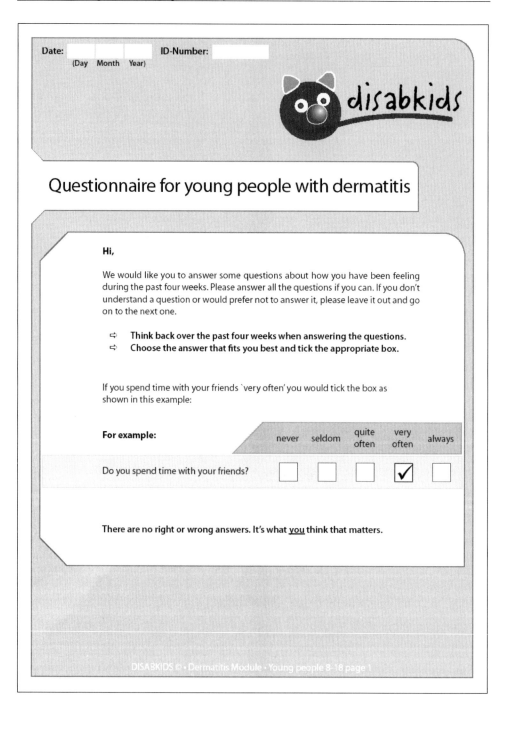

Date: _____    ID-Number: _____
(Day  Month  Year)

# disabkids

## Questionnaire for young people with dermatitis

**Hi,**

We would like you to answer some questions about how you have been feeling during the past four weeks. Please answer all the questions if you can. If you don't understand a question or would prefer not to answer it, please leave it out and go on to the next one.

⇨   **Think back over the past four weeks when answering the questions.**
⇨   **Choose the answer that fits you best and tick the appropriate box.**

If you spend time with your friends `very often' you would tick the box as shown in this example:

**For example:**

|  | never | seldom | quite often | very often | always |
|---|---|---|---|---|---|
| Do you spend time with your friends? | ☐ | ☐ | ☐ | ✓ | ☐ |

**There are no right or wrong answers. It's what <u>you</u> think that matters.**

## About your skin

**Think about the last four weeks!**

| | | never | seldom | quite often | very often | always |
|---|---|---|---|---|---|---|
| 1. | Does the itching bother you? | ☐ | ☐ | ☐ | ☐ | ☐ |
| 2. | Does the appearance of your skin bother you? | ☐ | ☐ | ☐ | ☐ | ☐ |
| 3. | Does itching bother you during the night? | ☐ | ☐ | ☐ | ☐ | ☐ |
| 4. | Does your skin condition affect your concentration at school? | ☐ | ☐ | ☐ | ☐ | ☐ |
| 5. | Does looking at your skin scare you? | ☐ | ☐ | ☐ | ☐ | ☐ |
| 6. | Does your skin get worse when you are under stress? | ☐ | ☐ | ☐ | ☐ | ☐ |
| 7. | Does your skin condition affect your free-time (sports, playing)? | ☐ | ☐ | ☐ | ☐ | ☐ |
| 8. | Do you feel comfortable with the way your skin is? | ☐ | ☐ | ☐ | ☐ | ☐ |

## About your skin

**Think about the last four weeks!**

| | | never | seldom | quite often | very often | always |
|---|---|---|---|---|---|---|
| 9. | Do you try to hide your skin condition? | ☐ | ☐ | ☐ | ☐ | ☐ |
| 10. | Are you annoyed by others giving you strange looks? | ☐ | ☐ | ☐ | ☐ | ☐ |
| 11. | Do you dislike it when your friends see your cream being applied? | ☐ | ☐ | ☐ | ☐ | ☐ |
| 12. | Do you feel uncomfortable when others look at you? | ☐ | ☐ | ☐ | ☐ | ☐ |

DISABKIDS © · Dermatitis Module · Young people 8-16 page 2

The last three questions are about how much trouble you have had with your dermatitis **in the last year.**

## About symptoms

**Think about the last year**

| | not at all | only once | a few days a month | several days a week | most days |
|---|---|---|---|---|---|
| a. How often did you have problems with your skin during the last year? | ☐ | ☐ | ☐ | ☐ | ☐ |

| | not at all | a little bit | mode-rately | quite a bit | ex-tremely |
|---|---|---|---|---|---|
| b. How severe was your skin problem during the last year? | ☐ | ☐ | ☐ | ☐ | ☐ |

| | never | in the last year | last 6 months | last month | last week |
|---|---|---|---|---|---|
| c. When was the last time your skin became sore and itchy? | ☐ | ☐ | ☐ | ☐ | ☐ |

**Thank you for your assistance!**

**Proxy version**

The DISABKIDS proxy version modules are shown on the following pages.

Date: _____ ID-Number: _____
(Day  Month  Year)

**disabkids**

# Questionnaire for parents of children with chronic conditions

**Dear Parent,**

Thank you very much for taking the time to complete this questionnaire about your child's well-being and health-related quality of life.

We would like you to complete this questionnaire on behalf of your child, but please complete the questionnaire without asking your child for any help with the answers. All the answers you give will be treated with the strictest confidentiality.

When answering the questions, unless instructed otherwise, please think about how your child has been feeling **over the past 4 weeks**.

| **For example:** | never | seldom | quite often | very often | always |
|---|---|---|---|---|---|
| Does your child spend time with his/her friends? | ☐ | ☐ | ☐ | ✓ | ☐ |

## Some questions about your child

A. Is your child male or female? ☐ female ☐ male

B. How old is your child? ☐ years

C. What is your child's condition?

☐ asthma ☐ arthritis ☐ dermatitis

☐ cerebral palsy ☐ diabetes ☐ cystic fibrosis

☐ epilepsy ☐ other ⟶ Which? ☐

D. Who is filling in the questionnaire?

☐ mother ☐ father ☐ stepmother/father's partner

☐ stepfather/mother's partner ☐ others ⟶ Who? ☐

**In some questions we use the word „condition". When you see „condition", please think about what you filled in above.**

## About your child's life

**Think about the past four weeks!**

| | | never | seldom | quite often | very often | always |
|---|---|---|---|---|---|---|
| 1. | Is your child confident about his/her future? | ☐ | ☐ | ☐ | ☐ | ☐ |
| 2. | Does your child enjoy his/her life? | ☐ | ☐ | ☐ | ☐ | ☐ |
| 3. | Is your child able to do everything they want to do even though they have their condition? | ☐ | ☐ | ☐ | ☐ | ☐ |
| 4. | Does your child feel like everyone else even though they have their condition? | ☐ | ☐ | ☐ | ☐ | ☐ |
| 5. | Does your child feel free to lead the life they want even though they have their condition? | ☐ | ☐ | ☐ | ☐ | ☐ |
| 6. | Does your child feel able to do things without you? | ☐ | ☐ | ☐ | ☐ | ☐ |

DISABKIDS © - Chronic Generic Module - Parent Version (young people aged 8-18) page 2

141

## About your child's typical day

**Think about the past four weeks!**

| | | never | seldom | quite often | very often | always |
|---|---|---|---|---|---|---|
| 7. | Does your child feel able to run and move as he/she likes? | ☐ | ☐ | ☐ | ☐ | ☐ |
| 8. | Does your child feel tired because of their condition? | ☐ | ☐ | ☐ | ☐ | ☐ |
| 9. | Does your child feel that their life is ruled by their condition? | ☐ | ☐ | ☐ | ☐ | ☐ |
| 10. | Does it bother your child that they have to explain to others what they can and can't do? | ☐ | ☐ | ☐ | ☐ | ☐ |
| 11. | Does your child find it difficult to sleep because of their condition? | ☐ | ☐ | ☐ | ☐ | ☐ |
| 12. | Does your child's condition bother them when they play or do other activities? | ☐ | ☐ | ☐ | ☐ | ☐ |

## About the way your child feels

**Think about the past four weeks!**

| | | never | seldom | quite often | very often | always |
|---|---|---|---|---|---|---|
| 13. | Does your child's condition make them feel bad about themselves? | ☐ | ☐ | ☐ | ☐ | ☐ |
| 14. | Does your child feel unhappy because of his/her condition? | ☐ | ☐ | ☐ | ☐ | ☐ |
| 15. | Does your child worry about his/her condition? | ☐ | ☐ | ☐ | ☐ | ☐ |
| 16. | Does your child's condition make him/her angry? | ☐ | ☐ | ☐ | ☐ | ☐ |
| 17. | Does your child have fears about the future because of his/her condition? | ☐ | ☐ | ☐ | ☐ | ☐ |
| 18. | Does your child's condition get him/her down? | ☐ | ☐ | ☐ | ☐ | ☐ |
| 19. | Does it bother your child that his/her life has to be planned? | ☐ | ☐ | ☐ | ☐ | ☐ |

DISABKIDS © · Chronic Generic Module · Parent Version (young people aged 8-18) page 3

## About your child and other people

**Think about the past four weeks!**

| | | never | seldom | quite often | very often | always |
|---|---|---|---|---|---|---|
| 20. | Does your child feel lonely because of his/her condition? | ☐ | ☐ | ☐ | ☐ | ☐ |
| 21. | Does your child feel that their teachers behave differently towards them than towards others? | ☐ | ☐ | ☐ | ☐ | ☐ |
| 22. | Does your child feel that they have problems concentrating at school because of their condition? | ☐ | ☐ | ☐ | ☐ | ☐ |
| 23. | Does your child feel that others have something against him/her? | ☐ | ☐ | ☐ | ☐ | ☐ |
| 24. | Does your child think that others stare at him/her? | ☐ | ☐ | ☐ | ☐ | ☐ |
| 25. | Does your child feel different from other children/adolescents? | ☐ | ☐ | ☐ | ☐ | ☐ |

## About your child's friendships

**Think about the past four weeks!**

| | | never | seldom | quite often | very often | always |
|---|---|---|---|---|---|---|
| 26. | Does your child feel that other children/adolescents understand their condition? | ☐ | ☐ | ☐ | ☐ | ☐ |
| 27. | Does your child go out with his/her friends? | ☐ | ☐ | ☐ | ☐ | ☐ |
| 28. | Does your child feel able to play or do things with other children (like sports)? | ☐ | ☐ | ☐ | ☐ | ☐ |
| 29. | Does your child think that he/she can do most things as well as other children? | ☐ | ☐ | ☐ | ☐ | ☐ |
| 30. | Does your child feel that their friends enjoy being with them? | ☐ | ☐ | ☐ | ☐ | ☐ |
| 31. | Does your child find it easy to talk about his/her condition to other people? | ☐ | ☐ | ☐ | ☐ | ☐ |

DISABKIDS © - Chronic Generic Module - Parent Version (young people aged 8-18) page 4

## About your child's medical treatment

Does your child take any medicine for their condition? (by medicine we mean tablets, cream, spray, insulin or any other medicine)   yes ☐   no ☐

**Think about the past four weeks!**

| If yes, please fill in the following questions, if no, please skip this section. | never | seldom | quite often | very often | always |
|---|---|---|---|---|---|
| 32. Does having to get help with medication from others bother your child? | ☐ | ☐ | ☐ | ☐ | ☐ |
| 33. Is it annoying for your child to have to remember his/her medication? | ☐ | ☐ | ☐ | ☐ | ☐ |
| 34. Is your child worried about his/her medication? | ☐ | ☐ | ☐ | ☐ | ☐ |
| 35. Does taking medication bother your child? | ☐ | ☐ | ☐ | ☐ | ☐ |
| 36. Does your child hate taking his/her medicine? | ☐ | ☐ | ☐ | ☐ | ☐ |
| 37. Does your child feel that taking medication disrupts his/her everyday life? | ☐ | ☐ | ☐ | ☐ | ☐ |

**Thank you for your assistance!**

DISABKIDS © · Chronic Generic Module · Parent Version (young people aged 8-18) page 5

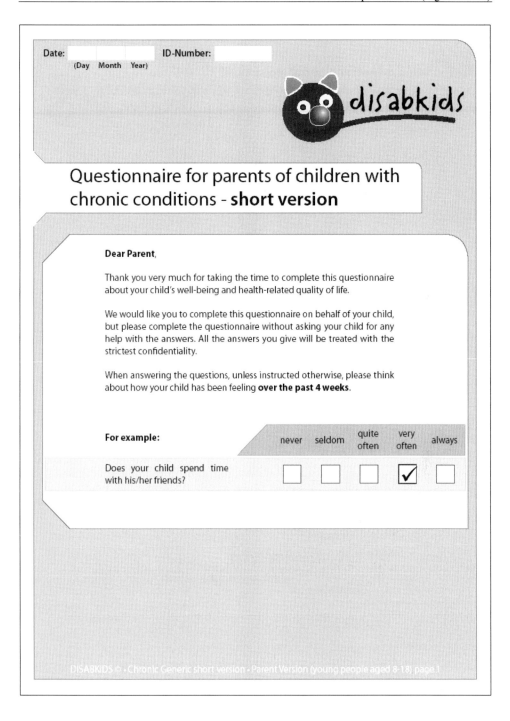

Date: _____  ID-Number: _____
(Day  Month  Year)

**disabkids**

# Questionnaire for parents of children with chronic conditions - **short version**

**Dear Parent**,

Thank you very much for taking the time to complete this questionnaire about your child's well-being and health-related quality of life.

We would like you to complete this questionnaire on behalf of your child, but please complete the questionnaire without asking your child for any help with the answers. All the answers you give will be treated with the strictest confidentiality.

When answering the questions, unless instructed otherwise, please think about how your child has been feeling **over the past 4 weeks**.

| **For example:** | never | seldom | quite often | very often | always |
|---|---|---|---|---|---|
| Does your child spend time with his/her friends? | ☐ | ☐ | ☐ | ☑ | ☐ |

DISABKIDS © - Chronic Generic short version - Parent Version (young people aged 8-18) page 1

## Some questions about your child

| | | | |
|---|---|---|---|
| A. | Is your child male or female? | ☐ female | ☐ male |
| B. | How old is your child? | ☐ years | |

C. What is your child's condition?

| ☐ asthma | ☐ arthritis | ☐ dermatitis |
|---|---|---|
| ☐ cerebral palsy | ☐ diabetes | ☐ cystic fibrosis |
| ☐ epilepsy | ☐ other ⟶ Which? | |

D. Who is filling in the questionnaire?

| ☐ mother | ☐ father | ☐ stepmother/father's partner |
|---|---|---|
| ☐ stepfather/ mother's partner | ☐ others ⟶ Who? | |

**In some questions we use the word „condition". When you see „condition", please think about what you filled in above.**

## About your child's life

**Think about the last four weeks!**

| | | never | seldom | quite often | very often | always |
|---|---|---|---|---|---|---|
| 1. | Does your child feel like everyone else even though they have their condition? | ☐ | ☐ | ☐ | ☐ | ☐ |
| 2. | Does your child feel free to lead the life they want even though they have their condition? | ☐ | ☐ | ☐ | ☐ | ☐ |
| 3. | Does your child feel that their life is ruled by their condition? | ☐ | ☐ | ☐ | ☐ | ☐ |
| 4. | Does your child's condition bother them when they play or do other activities? | ☐ | ☐ | ☐ | ☐ | ☐ |

DISABKIDS © · Chronic Generic short version · Parent Version (young people aged 8-18) page 2

## About your child's life

**Think about the past four weeks!**

| | never | seldom | quite often | very often | always |
|---|---|---|---|---|---|
| 5. Does your child feel unhappy because of his/her condition? | ☐ | ☐ | ☐ | ☐ | ☐ |
| 6. Does your child's condition get him/her down? | ☐ | ☐ | ☐ | ☐ | ☐ |
| 7. Does your child feel lonely because of his/her condition? | ☐ | ☐ | ☐ | ☐ | ☐ |
| 8. Does your child feel different from other children/adolescents? | ☐ | ☐ | ☐ | ☐ | ☐ |
| 9. Does your child think that he/she can do most things as well as other children? | ☐ | ☐ | ☐ | ☐ | ☐ |
| 10. Does your child feel that their friends enjoy being with them? | ☐ | ☐ | ☐ | ☐ | ☐ |

## About your child's medical treatment

Does your child take any medicine for their condition? (by medicine we mean tablets, cream, spray, insulin or any other medicine)     yes ☐     no ☐

**Think about the past four weeks!**

| If yes, please fill in the following questions, if no, please skip this section. | never | seldom | quite often | very often | always |
|---|---|---|---|---|---|
| 11. Does taking medication bother your child? | ☐ | ☐ | ☐ | ☐ | ☐ |
| 12. Does your child hate taking his/her medicine? | ☐ | ☐ | ☐ | ☐ | ☐ |

## Thank you for your assistance!

DISABKIDS © • Chronic Generic short version • Parent Version (young people aged 8-18) page 3

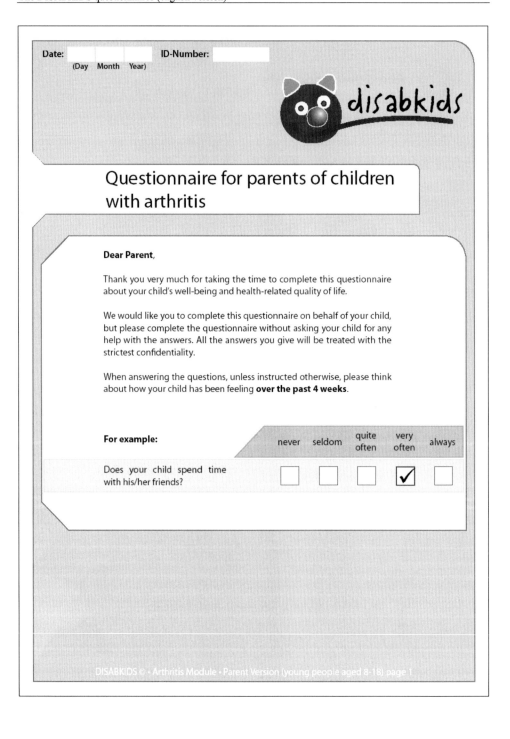

Date: _____    ID-Number: _____
(Day  Month  Year)

**disabkids**

## Questionnaire for parents of children with arthritis

**Dear Parent**,

Thank you very much for taking the time to complete this questionnaire about your child's well-being and health-related quality of life.

We would like you to complete this questionnaire on behalf of your child, but please complete the questionnaire without asking your child for any help with the answers. All the answers you give will be treated with the strictest confidentiality.

When answering the questions, unless instructed otherwise, please think about how your child has been feeling **over the past 4 weeks**.

| For example: | never | seldom | quite often | very often | always |
|---|---|---|---|---|---|
| Does your child spend time with his/her friends? | ☐ | ☐ | ☐ | ☑ | ☐ |

DISABKIDS © · Arthritis Module · Parent Version (young people aged 8-18) page 1

## About your child's arthritis

**Think about the last four weeks!**

| | | never | seldom | quite often | very often | always |
|---|---|---|---|---|---|---|
| 1. | Did your child feel stiff in the mornings (like an old grandma/granddad)? | ☐ | ☐ | ☐ | ☐ | ☐ |
| 2. | Did your child get exhausted easily? | ☐ | ☐ | ☐ | ☐ | ☐ |
| 3. | Does arthritis make your child feel too exhausted to be with his/her friends? | ☐ | ☐ | ☐ | ☐ | ☐ |
| 4. | Does your child hate being in pain? | ☐ | ☐ | ☐ | ☐ | ☐ |
| 5. | Does it annoy your child that the pain sometimes comes on so suddenly? | ☐ | ☐ | ☐ | ☐ | ☐ |
| 6. | Does pain stop your child from doing what he/she wants? | ☐ | ☐ | ☐ | ☐ | ☐ |
| 7. | Does it bother your child that they can't do all sports/hobbies because of their arthritis? | ☐ | ☐ | ☐ | ☐ | ☐ |
| 8. | Does your child hate being restricted in movement? | ☐ | ☐ | ☐ | ☐ | ☐ |
| 9. | Does it bother your child that he/she has trouble writing/ drawing? | ☐ | ☐ | ☐ | ☐ | ☐ |

## About your child's arthritis

**Think about the last four weeks!**

| | | never | seldom | quite often | very often | always |
|---|---|---|---|---|---|---|
| 10. | Does your child feel that others understand that their symptoms may change suddenly? | ☐ | ☐ | ☐ | ☐ | ☐ |
| 11. | Does your child feel that their friends understand that they may feel poorly quite suddenly? | ☐ | ☐ | ☐ | ☐ | ☐ |
| 12. | Does your child feel that their teachers understand that sometimes they can't join in? | ☐ | ☐ | ☐ | ☐ | ☐ |

DISABKIDS © · Arthritis Module · Parent Version (young people aged 8-18) page 2

The last three questions are about how much trouble your child has had with his/her arthritis **in the last year**.

### About your child's symptoms

Think about the last year

| | | never | few times | every month | every week | daily |
|---|---|---|---|---|---|---|
| a. | How often did your child have problems with his/her arthritis during the last year? | ☐ | ☐ | ☐ | ☐ | ☐ |

| | | not at all | a little bit | mode-rately | quite a bit | ex-tremely |
|---|---|---|---|---|---|---|
| b. | How severe was your child's arthritis during the last year? | ☐ | ☐ | ☐ | ☐ | ☐ |

| | | never | seldom | quite often | very often | always |
|---|---|---|---|---|---|---|
| c. | How often did your child have pain in his/her joints or muscles during the last year? | ☐ | ☐ | ☐ | ☐ | ☐ |

**Thank you for your assistance!**

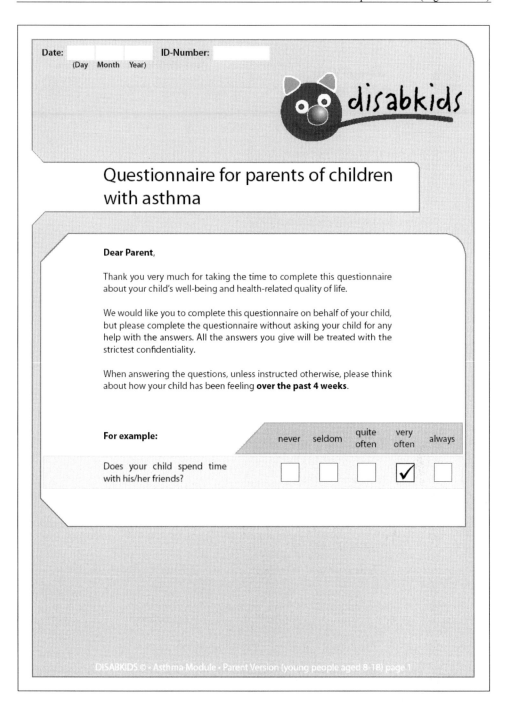

Date: _____    ID-Number: _____
(Day   Month   Year)

disabkids

# Questionnaire for parents of children with asthma

**Dear Parent,**

Thank you very much for taking the time to complete this questionnaire about your child's well-being and health-related quality of life.

We would like you to complete this questionnaire on behalf of your child, but please complete the questionnaire without asking your child for any help with the answers. All the answers you give will be treated with the strictest confidentiality.

When answering the questions, unless instructed otherwise, please think about how your child has been feeling **over the past 4 weeks**.

| **For example:** | never | seldom | quite often | very often | always |
|---|---|---|---|---|---|
| Does your child spend time with his/her friends? |  |  |  | ✓ |  |

DISABKIDS © · Asthma Module · Parent Version (young people aged 8-18) page 1

## About your child's asthma

**Think about the last four weeks!**

| | | never | seldom | quite often | very often | always |
|---|---|---|---|---|---|---|
| 1. | Does your child feel that he/she gets easily exhausted? | ☐ | ☐ | ☐ | ☐ | ☐ |
| 2. | Does asthma bother your child if he/she wants to go out? | ☐ | ☐ | ☐ | ☐ | ☐ |
| 3. | Does your child not feel able to take part in certain sports (like long-distance running)? | ☐ | ☐ | ☐ | ☐ | ☐ |
| 4. | Does your child feel short of breath when he/she does sports? | ☐ | ☐ | ☐ | ☐ | ☐ |
| 5. | Is your child bothered by the amount of time he/she spends wheezing? | ☐ | ☐ | ☐ | ☐ | ☐ |
| 6. | Does your child feel terrible when he/she is out of breath? | ☐ | ☐ | ☐ | ☐ | ☐ |

## About your child's asthma

**Think about the last four weeks!**

| | | never | seldom | quite often | very often | always |
|---|---|---|---|---|---|---|
| 7. | Is your child worried that he/she might have an asthma attack? | ☐ | ☐ | ☐ | ☐ | ☐ |
| 8. | Is your child worried that others do not know what to do if he/she have an attack? | ☐ | ☐ | ☐ | ☐ | ☐ |
| 9. | Does your child feel scared that he/she might have difficulty breathing? | ☐ | ☐ | ☐ | ☐ | ☐ |
| 10. | Is your child scared that he/she might have to go to the emergency ward? | ☐ | ☐ | ☐ | ☐ | ☐ |
| 11. | Is your child scared at night because of his/her asthma? | ☐ | ☐ | ☐ | ☐ | ☐ |

The last three questions are about how much trouble your child has had with his/her asthma **in the last year.**

### About your child's symptoms

Think about the last year

| | never | in the last year | last 6 months | last month | last week |
|---|---|---|---|---|---|
| a. When was the last time your child had an asthma attack? | ☐ | ☐ | ☐ | ☐ | ☐ |

| | never | 1 time | 2 times | 3 times | more than 3 times |
|---|---|---|---|---|---|
| b. How many asthma attacks did your child have during the last year? | ☐ | ☐ | ☐ | ☐ | ☐ |

| | not at all | a little bit | mode-rately | quite a bit | ex-tremely |
|---|---|---|---|---|---|
| c. How severe was your child's asthma during the last year? | ☐ | ☐ | ☐ | ☐ | ☐ |

**Thank you for your assistance!**

Date: _____    ID-Number: _____
(Day  Month  Year)

**disabkids**

## Questionnaire for parents of children with cystic fibrosis

**Dear Parent,**

Thank you very much for taking the time to complete this questionnaire about your child's well-being and health-related quality of life.

We would like you to complete this questionnaire on behalf of your child, but please complete the questionnaire without asking your child for any help with the answers. All the answers you give will be treated with the strictest confidentiality.

When answering the questions, unless instructed otherwise, please think about how your child has been feeling **over the past 4 weeks**.

| For example: | never | seldom | quite often | very often | always |
|---|---|---|---|---|---|
| Does your child spend time with his/her friends? | ☐ | ☐ | ☐ | ☑ | ☐ |

## About your child's cystic fibrosis

**Think about the last four weeks!**

| | | never | seldom | quite often | very often | always |
|---|---|---|---|---|---|---|
| 1. | Does your child get exhausted when he/she does sports? | ☐ | ☐ | ☐ | ☐ | ☐ |
| 2. | Does your child feel tired during the day? | ☐ | ☐ | ☐ | ☐ | ☐ |
| 3. | Does your child get out of breath? | ☐ | ☐ | ☐ | ☐ | ☐ |
| 4. | Does your child need to rest more than others? | ☐ | ☐ | ☐ | ☐ | ☐ |

## About your child's cystic fibrosis

**Think about the last four weeks!**

| | | never | seldom | quite often | very often | always |
|---|---|---|---|---|---|---|
| 5. | Does it bother your child that they must take enzymes before every meal? | ☐ | ☐ | ☐ | ☐ | ☐ |
| 6. | Does it bother your child that they have to eat a special diet to keep them healthy? | ☐ | ☐ | ☐ | ☐ | ☐ |
| 7. | Does it bother your child that he/she has to spend a lot of time having treatment? | ☐ | ☐ | ☐ | ☐ | ☐ |
| 8. | Is your child bothered because he/she has to do physiotherapy everyday? | ☐ | ☐ | ☐ | ☐ | ☐ |
| 9. | Has your child felt that their treatment takes up too much of their free time? | ☐ | ☐ | ☐ | ☐ | ☐ |
| 10. | Does your child feel bothered that he/she has to stop playing or doing things for treatment? | ☐ | ☐ | ☐ | ☐ | ☐ |

DISABKIDS © - CF Module - Parent Version (young people aged 8-18) page 2

The last three questions are about how much trouble your child has had with his/her cystic fibroses **in the last year.**

### About your child's symptoms

| | | **Think about the last year** | | | | |
|---|---|---|---|---|---|---|
| | | not at all | a little bit | moderately | quite a bit | extremely |
| a. | How severe was your child's cystic fibrosis during the last year? | ☐ | ☐ | ☐ | ☐ | ☐ |
| | | never | 1 time | 2 times | 3 times | more than 3 times |
| b. | How often did your child have a bad time because of his/her cystic fibrosis symptoms during the last year? | ☐ | ☐ | ☐ | ☐ | ☐ |
| | | never | in the last year | last 6 months | last month | last week |
| c. | When was the last time your child has had blood in their sputum? | ☐ | ☐ | ☐ | ☐ | ☐ |

**Thank you for your assistance!**

Date: _____ ID-Number: _____

(Day   Month   Year)

# disabkids

## Questionnaire for parents of children with cerebral palsy

**Dear Parent,**

Thank you very much for taking the time to complete this questionnaire about your child's well-being and health-related quality of life.

We would like you to complete this questionnaire on behalf of your child, but please complete the questionnaire without asking your child for any help with the answers. All the answers you give will be treated with the strictest confidentiality.

When answering the questions, unless instructed otherwise, please think about how your child has been feeling **over the past 4 weeks**.

| **For example:** | never | seldom | quite often | very often | always |
|---|---|---|---|---|---|
| Does your child spend time with his/her friends? | ☐ | ☐ | ☐ | ☑ | ☐ |

## About your child's cerebral palsy

**Think about the last four weeks!**

| | | never | seldom | quite often | very often | always |
|---|---|---|---|---|---|---|
| 1. | Does your child find it frustrating to be unable to keep up with other children? | ☐ | ☐ | ☐ | ☐ | ☐ |
| 2. | Does your child wish that he/she could run around like everyone else? | ☐ | ☐ | ☐ | ☐ | ☐ |
| 3. | Does your child wish that he/she could swim as well as other children? | ☐ | ☐ | ☐ | ☐ | ☐ |
| 4. | Does it bother your child that getting dressed takes a long time? | ☐ | ☐ | ☐ | ☐ | ☐ |
| 5. | Does your child feel that people think they are not as clever as he/she is? | ☐ | ☐ | ☐ | ☐ | ☐ |
| 6. | Does your child have trouble getting in and out of buildings? | ☐ | ☐ | ☐ | ☐ | ☐ |
| 7. | Is your child able to do most things even though his/her legs don't move well? | ☐ | ☐ | ☐ | ☐ | ☐ |

| | | never | seldom | quite often | very often | always | He/she doesn't have any problems with... |
|---|---|---|---|---|---|---|---|
| 8. | Does it upset your child that he/she is unable to walk without help? | ☐ | ☐ | ☐ | ☐ | ☐ | ☐ ...walking without help |
| 9. | Does your child dislike being washed and dressed by other people? | ☐ | ☐ | ☐ | ☐ | ☐ | ☐ ...washing and dressing without help |
| 10. | Does it upset your child that he/she needs help to use the toilet? | ☐ | ☐ | ☐ | ☐ | ☐ | ☐ ...using the toilet without help |

## About your child's cerebral palsy

**Think about the last four weeks!**

| | | never | seldom | quite often | very often | always | He/she doesn't have any problems with... |
|---|---|---|---|---|---|---|---|
| 11. | Does your child feel they can communicate as well as they like? | ☐ | ☐ | ☐ | ☐ | ☐ | ☐ ...talking |
| 12. | Does it upset your child that he/she can't talk as well as other children? | ☐ | ☐ | ☐ | ☐ | ☐ | ☐ ...talking |

### Thank you for your assistance!

DISABKIDS © · CP Module · Parent Version (young people aged 8-18) page 2

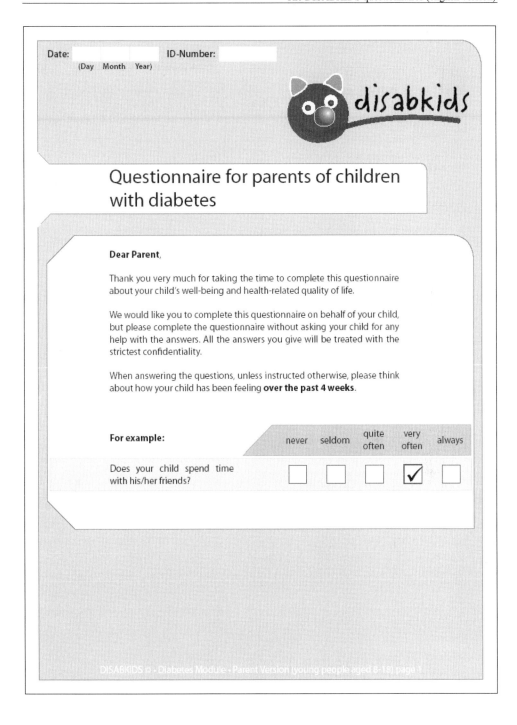

Date: _____     ID-Number: _____
(Day  Month  Year)

# disabkids

## Questionnaire for parents of children with diabetes

**Dear Parent**,

Thank you very much for taking the time to complete this questionnaire about your child's well-being and health-related quality of life.

We would like you to complete this questionnaire on behalf of your child, but please complete the questionnaire without asking your child for any help with the answers. All the answers you give will be treated with the strictest confidentiality.

When answering the questions, unless instructed otherwise, please think about how your child has been feeling **over the past 4 weeks**.

| For example: | never | seldom | quite often | very often | always |
|---|---|---|---|---|---|
| Does your child spend time with his/her friends? | ☐ | ☐ | ☐ | ☑ | ☐ |

DISABKIDS © - Diabetes Module - Parent Version (young people aged 8-18) page 1

## About your child's diabetes

**Think about the last four weeks!**

| | | never | seldom | quite often | very often | always |
|---|---|---|---|---|---|---|
| 1. | Does diabetes stop your child from doing the things he/she wants to do? | ☐ | ☐ | ☐ | ☐ | ☐ |
| 2. | Does your child feel that diabetes rules his/her day? | ☐ | ☐ | ☐ | ☐ | ☐ |
| 3. | Does it bother your child that they have to be careful about what they eat? | ☐ | ☐ | ☐ | ☐ | ☐ |
| 4. | Is it difficult for your child to stick to his/her diet? | ☐ | ☐ | ☐ | ☐ | ☐ |
| 5. | Does your child worry about his/her blood sugar level? | ☐ | ☐ | ☐ | ☐ | ☐ |
| 6. | Does it bother your child that others can always eat and drink as much as they like? | ☐ | ☐ | ☐ | ☐ | ☐ |

## About your child's diabetes

**Think about the last four weeks!**

| | | never | seldom | quite often | very often | always |
|---|---|---|---|---|---|---|
| 7. | Does your child mind taking insulin? | ☐ | ☐ | ☐ | ☐ | ☐ |
| 8. | Does your child get fed up with measuring his/her blood sugar levels? | ☐ | ☐ | ☐ | ☐ | ☐ |
| 9. | Is your child annoyed that they have to carry the testing equipment with them? | ☐ | ☐ | ☐ | ☐ | ☐ |
| 10. | Is your child bothered that he/she has to plan everything? | ☐ | ☐ | ☐ | ☐ | ☐ |

The last three questions are about how much trouble your child has had with his/her diabetes **in the last year.**

### About your child's symptoms

Think about the last year

| | never | once | a few times | often | all the time |
|---|---|---|---|---|---|
| a. How often did your child have problems with his/her diabetes during the last year? | ☐ | ☐ | ☐ | ☐ | ☐ |

| | not at all | a little bit | mode-rately | quite a bit | ex-tremely |
|---|---|---|---|---|---|
| b. How severe were your child's diabetes problems during the last year? | ☐ | ☐ | ☐ | ☐ | ☐ |

| | never | in the last year | last six months | last month | last week |
|---|---|---|---|---|---|
| c. When was the last time your child had a bad hypo attack (low blood sugar)? | ☐ | ☐ | ☐ | ☐ | ☐ |

**Thank you for your assistance!**

DISABKIDS © · CF Module · Parent Version (young people aged 8-18) page 3

161

Date: _____    ID-Number: _____
(Day   Month   Year)

**disabkids**

# Questionnaire for parents of children with epilepsy

**Dear Parent**,

Thank you very much for taking the time to complete this questionnaire about your child's well-being and health-related quality of life.

We would like you to complete this questionnaire on behalf of your child, but please complete the questionnaire without asking your child for any help with the answers. All the answers you give will be treated with the strictest confidentiality.

When answering the questions, unless instructed otherwise, please think about how your child has been feeling **over the past 4 weeks**.

| For example: | never | seldom | quite often | very often | always |
|---|---|---|---|---|---|
| Does your child spend time with his/her friends? | ☐ | ☐ | ☐ | ✓ | ☐ |

DISABKIDS © · Epilepsy Module · Parent Version (young people aged 8-18) page 1

## About your child's epilepsy

**Think about the last four weeks!**

| | | never | seldom | quite often | very often | always |
|---|---|---|---|---|---|---|
| 1. | Is your child afraid that they might hurt themselves during a seizure? | ☐ | ☐ | ☐ | ☐ | ☐ |
| 2. | Is your child worried that they might have a seizure in public? | ☐ | ☐ | ☐ | ☐ | ☐ |
| 3. | Is your child afraid of having a seizure? | ☐ | ☐ | ☐ | ☐ | ☐ |
| 4. | Do seizures make your child feel helpless? | ☐ | ☐ | ☐ | ☐ | ☐ |
| 5. | Is your child scared that he/she could have a seizure at any time? | ☐ | ☐ | ☐ | ☐ | ☐ |

## About your child's epilepsy

**Think about the last four weeks!**

| | | never | seldom | quite often | very often | always |
|---|---|---|---|---|---|---|
| 6. | Does it embarrass your child when people take care of them when they have a seizure? | ☐ | ☐ | ☐ | ☐ | ☐ |
| 7. | Is your child worried that people make fun of them when they have a seizure? | ☐ | ☐ | ☐ | ☐ | ☐ |
| 8. | Is your child afraid that they can't remember what happens during a seizure? | ☐ | ☐ | ☐ | ☐ | ☐ |
| 9. | Is your child ashamed of having seizures? | ☐ | ☐ | ☐ | ☐ | ☐ |
| 10. | Is your child worried that other children will see him/her having a seizure? | ☐ | ☐ | ☐ | ☐ | ☐ |

DISABKIDS © - Epilepsy Module - Parent Version (young people aged 8-16) page 2

## About your child's epilepsy

**Think about the last four weeks!**

| | | never | seldom | quite often | very often | always |
|---|---|---|---|---|---|---|
| 1. | Is your child afraid that they might hurt themselves during a seizure? | ☐ | ☐ | ☐ | ☐ | ☐ |
| 2. | Is your child worried that they might have a seizure in public? | ☐ | ☐ | ☐ | ☐ | ☐ |
| 3. | Is your child afraid of having a seizure? | ☐ | ☐ | ☐ | ☐ | ☐ |
| 4. | Do seizures make your child feel helpless? | ☐ | ☐ | ☐ | ☐ | ☐ |
| 5. | Is your child scared that he/she could have a seizure at any time? | ☐ | ☐ | ☐ | ☐ | ☐ |

## About your child's epilepsy

**Think about the last four weeks!**

| | | never | seldom | quite often | very often | always |
|---|---|---|---|---|---|---|
| 6. | Does it embarrass your child when people take care of them when they have a seizure? | ☐ | ☐ | ☐ | ☐ | ☐ |
| 7. | Is your child worried that people make fun of them when they have a seizure? | ☐ | ☐ | ☐ | ☐ | ☐ |
| 8. | Is your child afraid that they can't remember what happens during a seizure? | ☐ | ☐ | ☐ | ☐ | ☐ |
| 9. | Is your child ashamed of having seizures? | ☐ | ☐ | ☐ | ☐ | ☐ |
| 10. | Is your child worried that other children will see him/her having a seizure? | ☐ | ☐ | ☐ | ☐ | ☐ |

DISABKIDS © - Epilepsy Module - Parent Version (young people aged 8-18) page 2

Date: _____    ID-Number: _____

(Day   Month   Year)

**disabkids**

# Questionnaire for parents of children with dermatitis

**Dear Parent,**

Thank you very much for taking the time to complete this questionnaire about your child's well-being and health-related quality of life.

We would like you to complete this questionnaire on behalf of your child, but please complete the questionnaire without asking your child for any help with the answers. All the answers you give will be treated with the strictest confidentiality.

When answering the questions, unless instructed otherwise, please think about how your child has been feeling **over the past 4 weeks**.

| **For example:** | never | seldom | quite often | very often | always |
|---|---|---|---|---|---|
| Does your child spend time with his/her friends? | ☐ | ☐ | ☐ | ☑ | ☐ |

DISABKIDS © · Dermatitis Module · Parent Version (young people aged 8-18) page 1

## About your child's skin

**Think about the last four weeks!**

| | never | seldom | quite often | very often | always |
|---|---|---|---|---|---|
| 1. Does the itching bother your child? | ☐ | ☐ | ☐ | ☐ | ☐ |
| 2. Does the appearance of your child's skin bother him/her? | ☐ | ☐ | ☐ | ☐ | ☐ |
| 3. Does itching bother your child during the night? | ☐ | ☐ | ☐ | ☐ | ☐ |
| 4. Does your child's skin condition affect his/her concentration at school? | ☐ | ☐ | ☐ | ☐ | ☐ |
| 5. Does looking at his/her skin scare your child? | ☐ | ☐ | ☐ | ☐ | ☐ |
| 6. Does your child's skin get worse when he/she is under stress? | ☐ | ☐ | ☐ | ☐ | ☐ |
| 7. Does your child's skin condition affect his/her free-time (sports, playing)? | ☐ | ☐ | ☐ | ☐ | ☐ |
| 8. Does your child feel comfortable with the way his/her skin is? | ☐ | ☐ | ☐ | ☐ | ☐ |

## About your child's skin

**Think about the last four weeks!**

| | never | seldom | quite often | very often | always |
|---|---|---|---|---|---|
| 9. Does your child try to hide his/her skin condition? | ☐ | ☐ | ☐ | ☐ | ☐ |
| 10. Is your child annoyed by others giving him/her strange looks? | ☐ | ☐ | ☐ | ☐ | ☐ |
| 11. Does your child dislike it when his/her friends see their cream being applied? | ☐ | ☐ | ☐ | ☐ | ☐ |
| 12. Does your child feel uncomfortable when others look at him/her? | ☐ | ☐ | ☐ | ☐ | ☐ |

DISABKIDS © - Dermatitis Module - Parent Version (young people aged 8-18) page 2

The last three questions are about how much trouble your child has had with his/her dermatitis **in the last year**.

### About your child's symptoms

| | | Think about the last year | | | | |
|---|---|---|---|---|---|---|
| | | not at all | only once | a few days a month | several days a week | most days |
| a. | How often did your child have problems with his/her skin during the last year? | ☐ | ☐ | ☐ | ☐ | ☐ |
| | | not at all | a little bit | mode-rately | quite a bit | ex-tremely |
| b. | How severe was your child's skin problem during the last year? | ☐ | ☐ | ☐ | ☐ | ☐ |
| | | never | in the last year | last 6 months | last month | last week |
| c. | When was the last time your child's skin became sore and itchy? | ☐ | ☐ | ☐ | ☐ | ☐ |

**Thank you for your assistance!**

## A-II      Reference Data (DISBKIDS field study sample)

**Table 1  DISABKIDS chronic generic module, sub-scale "independence" (self-report) – DCGM-37-S**

| DCGM-37-S INDEPENDENCE SELF-REPORT | | Total sample 8-12 (n = 513) | | Total sample 13-16 (n = 437) | | Total sample Overall (n = 950) | | Females 8-12 (n = 233) | | Females 13-16 (n =215) | | Females Overall (n = 448) | | Males 8-12 (n = 280) | | Males 13-16 (n = 222) | | Males Overall (n = 502) | |
|---|---|---|---|---|---|---|---|---|---|---|---|---|---|---|---|---|---|---|---|
| **RS** | **TRS** | PR | TS | PR | TS | PR | TS | PR | TS | PR | TS | PR | TS | PR | TS | PR | TS | PR | TS |
| 6 | **0.00** | .2 | 6,83 | - | - | .1 | 5,41 | - | - | - | - | - | - | .4 | 7,98 | - | - | .2 | 5,90 |
| 7 | **4.17** | .4 | 9,15 | - | - | .2 | 7,81 | - | - | - | - | - | - | .7 | 10,25 | - | - | .4 | 8,27 |
| 8 | **8.33** | .4 | 9,15 | - | - | .2 | 7,81 | - | - | - | - | - | - | .7 | 10,25 | - | - | .4 | 8,27 |
| 9 | **12.50** | .6 | 13,80 | - | - | .3 | 12,61 | .4 | 12,59 | - | - | .2 | 12,18 | .7 | 10,25 | - | - | .4 | 8,27 |
| 10 | **16.67** | .8 | 16,13 | .2 | 13,59 | .5 | 15,01 | .9 | 14,97 | .5 | 14,22 | .7 | 14,62 | .7 | 10,25 | - | - | .4 | 8,27 |
| 11 | **20.83** | 1.0 | 18,45 | .2 | 13,59 | .6 | 17,41 | .9 | 14,97 | .5 | 14,22 | .7 | 14,62 | 1.1 | 19,34 | - | - | .6 | 17,74 |
| 12 | **25.00** | 1.4 | 20,77 | .7 | 18,59 | 1.1 | 19,81 | 1.3 | 19,75 | 1.4 | 19,22 | 1.3 | 19,50 | 1.4 | 21,61 | - | - | .8 | 20,11 |
| 13 | **29.17** | 1.9 | 23,10 | 1.6 | 21,09 | 1.8 | 22,22 | 2.1 | 22,14 | 1.9 | 21,71 | 2.0 | 21,94 | 1.8 | 23,88 | 1.4 | 20,47 | 1.6 | 22,47 |
| 14 | **33.33** | 2.5 | 25,42 | 1.8 | 23,59 | 2.2 | 24,62 | 3.0 | 24,52 | 2.3 | 24,21 | 2.7 | 24,38 | 2.1 | 26,15 | 1.4 | 20,47 | 1.8 | 24,84 |
| 15 | **37.50** | 3.3 | 27,74 | 2.1 | 26,09 | 2.7 | 27,02 | 4.3 | 26,91 | 2.3 | 24,21 | 3.3 | 26,81 | 2.5 | 28,42 | 1.8 | 25,48 | 2.2 | 27,21 |
| 16 | **41.67** | 4.9 | 30,07 | 4.1 | 28,59 | 4.5 | 29,42 | 6.0 | 29,30 | 4.2 | 29,20 | 5.1 | 29,25 | 3.9 | 30,69 | 4.1 | 27,99 | 4.0 | 29,58 |
| 17 | **45.83** | 7.6 | 32,39 | 6.6 | 31,10 | 7.2 | 31,82 | 8.6 | 31,69 | 7.4 | 31,69 | 8.0 | 31,69 | 6.8 | 32,96 | 5.9 | 30,50 | 6.4 | 31,95 |
| 18 | **50.00** | 10.9 | 34,72 | 9.4 | 33,60 | 10.2 | 34,22 | 10.7 | 34,08 | 9.8 | 34,19 | 10.3 | 34,13 | 11.1 | 35,24 | 9.0 | 33,00 | 10.2 | 34,31 |
| 19 | **54.17** | 13.5 | 37,04 | 11.9 | 36,10 | 12.7 | 36,62 | 11.6 | 36,46 | 13.0 | 36,69 | 12.3 | 36,57 | 15.0 | 37,51 | 10.8 | 35,51 | 13.1 | 36,68 |
| 20 | **58.33** | 16.8 | 39,36 | 16.9 | 38,60 | 16.8 | 39,03 | 13.7 | 38,85 | 18.6 | 39,18 | 16.1 | 39,01 | 19.3 | 39,78 | 15.3 | 38,02 | 17.5 | 39,05 |
| 21 | **62.50** | 21.1 | 41,69 | 22.2 | 41,10 | 21.6 | 41,43 | 17.2 | 41,24 | 22.8 | 41,68 | 19.9 | 41,44 | 24.3 | 42,05 | 21.6 | 40,53 | 23.1 | 41,42 |
| 22 | **66.67** | 26.7 | 44,01 | 26.8 | 43,60 | 26.7 | 43,83 | 22.7 | 43,63 | 27.0 | 44,17 | 24.8 | 43,88 | 30.0 | 44,32 | 26.6 | 43,03 | 28.5 | 43,79 |
| 23 | **70.83** | 33.5 | 46,34 | 33.2 | 46,10 | 33.4 | 46,23 | 30.9 | 46,01 | 33.0 | 46,67 | 31.9 | 46,32 | 35.7 | 46,59 | 33.3 | 45,54 | 34.7 | 46,16 |
| 24 | **75.00** | 40.2 | 48,66 | 40.5 | 48,60 | 40.3 | 48,63 | 39.1 | 48,40 | 40.5 | 49,16 | 39.7 | 48,76 | 41.1 | 48,86 | 40.5 | 48,05 | 40.8 | 48,52 |
| 25 | **79.17** | 48.9 | 50,98 | 51.0 | 51,10 | 49.9 | 51,03 | 49.8 | 50,79 | 52.6 | 51,66 | 51.1 | 51,20 | 48.2 | 51,14 | 49.5 | 50,55 | 48.8 | 50,89 |
| 26 | **83.33** | 60.4 | 53,31 | 63.6 | 53,60 | 61.9 | 53,44 | 60.5 | 53,18 | 68.4 | 54,16 | 64.3 | 53,64 | 60.4 | 53,41 | 59.0 | 53,06 | 59.8 | 53,26 |
| 27 | **87.50** | 71.7 | 55,63 | 74.8 | 56,10 | 73.2 | 55,84 | 73.0 | 55,56 | 80.5 | 56,65 | 76.6 | 56,07 | 70.7 | 55,68 | 69.4 | 55,57 | 70.1 | 55,63 |
| 28 | **91.67** | 81.5 | 57,95 | 84.2 | 58,60 | 82.7 | 58,24 | 83.3 | 57,95 | 85.6 | 59,15 | 84.4 | 58,51 | 80.0 | 57,95 | 82.9 | 58,07 | 81.3 | 58,00 |
| 29 | **95.83** | 92.2 | 60,28 | 92.0 | 61,10 | 92.1 | 60,64 | 93.1 | 60,34 | 94.4 | 61,64 | 93.8 | 60,95 | 91.4 | 60,22 | 89.6 | 60,58 | 90.6 | 60,36 |
| 30 | **100.00** | 100.0 | 62,60 | 100.0 | 63,60 | 100.0 | 63,04 | 100.0 | 62,73 | 100.0 | 64,14 | 100.0 | 63,39 | 100.0 | 62,49 | 100.0 | 63,09 | 100.0 | 62,73 |

*Note: Calculation of scores was restricted to complete cases. RS = raw score; TRS = transformed raw score (range 0-100); PR = percentile; TS = T-score (M = 50, SD = 10).*

**Table 2   DISABKIDS chronic generic module, sub-scale "emotion" (self-report) – DCGM-37-S**

| DCGM-37-S EMOTION SELF-REPORT | | Total sample 8-12 (n = 529) | | Total sample 13-16 (n = 428) | | Total sample Overall (n = 957) | | Females 8-12 (n = 245) | | Females 13-16 (n = 219) | | Females Overall (n = 464) | | Males 8-12 (n = 284) | | Males 13-16 (n = 209) | | Males Overall (n = 493) | |
|---|---|---|---|---|---|---|---|---|---|---|---|---|---|---|---|---|---|---|---|
| RS | TRS | PR | TS | PR | TS | PR | TS | PR | TS | PR | TS | PR | TS | PR | TS | PR | TS | PR | TS |
| 7 | 0.00 | – | – | .2 | 14,55 | .1 | 12,45 | – | – | – | – | – | – | – | – | – | – | .2 | 10,38 |
| 8 | 3.57 | – | – | .2 | 14,55 | .1 | 12,45 | – | – | – | – | – | – | – | – | – | – | .2 | 10,38 |
| 9 | 7.14 | .2 | 13,96 | .2 | 14,55 | .2 | 15,94 | – | – | – | – | – | – | .4 | 14,26 | .5 | 9,95 | .4 | 13,93 |
| 10 | 10.71 | .6 | 15,76 | .2 | 14,55 | .4 | 17,68 | .4 | 15,76 | – | – | .2 | 19,12 | .7 | 16,02 | .5 | 9,95 | .6 | 15,71 |
| 11 | 14.29 | .8 | 17,57 | .7 | 21,32 | .7 | 19,43 | .4 | 15,76 | .9 | 23,76 | .6 | 20,86 | 1.1 | 17,78 | .5 | 9,95 | .8 | 17,49 |
| 12 | 17.86 | .9 | 19,37 | 1.4 | 23,01 | 1.1 | 21,17 | .4 | 15,76 | 1.4 | 25,43 | .9 | 22,61 | 1.4 | 19,54 | .5 | 9,95 | 1.4 | 19,27 |
| 13 | 21.43 | 1.7 | 21,17 | 1.6 | 24,71 | 1.7 | 22,92 | 1.6 | 21,17 | 1.8 | 27,10 | 1.7 | 24,35 | 1.8 | 21,29 | 1.4 | 18,96 | 1.6 | 21,05 |
| 14 | 25.00 | 1.9 | 22,98 | 2.8 | 26,40 | 2.3 | 24,67 | 2.0 | 22,98 | 3.7 | 28,77 | 2.8 | 26,10 | 1.8 | 21,29 | 1.4 | 18,96 | 1.8 | 22,82 |
| 15 | 28.57 | 2.3 | 24,78 | 3.5 | 28,09 | 2.8 | 26,41 | 2.4 | 24,78 | 5.0 | 30,44 | 3.7 | 27,84 | 2.1 | 24,81 | 1.9 | 22,56 | 2.0 | 24,60 |
| 16 | 32.14 | 2.6 | 26,58 | 4.4 | 29,79 | 3.4 | 28,16 | 2.4 | 24,78 | 5.9 | 32,11 | 4.1 | 29,59 | 2.8 | 26,57 | 2.9 | 26,17 | 2.8 | 26,38 |
| 17 | 35.71 | 3.4 | 28,39 | 5.8 | 31,48 | 4.5 | 29,90 | 3.3 | 28,39 | 7.8 | 33,78 | 5.4 | 31,33 | 3.5 | 28,32 | 3.8 | 27,97 | 3.7 | 28,16 |
| 18 | 39.29 | 5.3 | 30,19 | 8.9 | 33,17 | 6.9 | 31,65 | 4.5 | 30,19 | 11.9 | 35,45 | 8.0 | 33,08 | 6.0 | 30,08 | 5.7 | 29,77 | 5.9 | 29,93 |
| 19 | 42.86 | 7.2 | 32,00 | 10.3 | 34,87 | 8.6 | 33,39 | 6.9 | 32,00 | 13.7 | 37,12 | 10.1 | 34,83 | 7.4 | 31,84 | 6.7 | 31,57 | 7.1 | 31,71 |
| 20 | 46.43 | 9.6 | 33,80 | 12.9 | 36,56 | 11.1 | 35,14 | 9.0 | 33,80 | 16.9 | 38,79 | 12.7 | 36,57 | 10.2 | 33,60 | 8.6 | 33,38 | 9.5 | 33,49 |
| 21 | 50.00 | 11.5 | 35,60 | 15.7 | 38,25 | 13.4 | 36,88 | 11.0 | 35,60 | 20.5 | 40,46 | 15.5 | 38,32 | 12.0 | 35,35 | 10.5 | 35,18 | 11.4 | 35,27 |
| 22 | 53.57 | 13.6 | 37,41 | 18.7 | 39,94 | 15.9 | 38,63 | 13.1 | 37,41 | 24.2 | 42,13 | 18.3 | 40,06 | 14.1 | 37,11 | 12.9 | 36,98 | 13.6 | 37,04 |
| 23 | 57.14 | 17.0 | 39,21 | 22.9 | 41,64 | 19.6 | 40,37 | 17.1 | 39,21 | 28.8 | 43,80 | 22.6 | 41,81 | 16.9 | 38,87 | 16.7 | 38,78 | 16.8 | 38,82 |
| 24 | 60.71 | 20.4 | 41,02 | 26.9 | 43,33 | 23.3 | 42,12 | 21.6 | 41,02 | 34.7 | 45,47 | 27.8 | 43,55 | 19.4 | 40,63 | 18.7 | 40,58 | 19.1 | 40,60 |
| 25 | 64.29 | 24.4 | 42,82 | 32.7 | 45,02 | 28.1 | 43,86 | 26.9 | 42,82 | 40.2 | 47,14 | 33.2 | 45,30 | 22.2 | 42,38 | 24.9 | 42,39 | 23.3 | 42,38 |
| 26 | 67.86 | 29.1 | 44,62 | 36.9 | 46,72 | 32.6 | 45,61 | 32.2 | 44,62 | 45.7 | 48,81 | 38.6 | 47,04 | 26.4 | 44,14 | 27.8 | 44,19 | 27.0 | 44,15 |
| 27 | 71.43 | 34.4 | 46,43 | 40.4 | 48,41 | 37.1 | 47,36 | 38.8 | 46,43 | 49.8 | 50,48 | 44.0 | 48,79 | 30.6 | 45,90 | 30.6 | 45,99 | 30.6 | 45,93 |
| 28 | 75.00 | 38.6 | 48,23 | 46.5 | 50,10 | 42.1 | 49,10 | 44.1 | 48,23 | 55.7 | 52,15 | 49.6 | 50,53 | 33.8 | 47,65 | 36.8 | 47,79 | 35.1 | 47,71 |
| 29 | 78.57 | 44.0 | 50,03 | 50.7 | 51,80 | 47.0 | 50,85 | 48.2 | 50,03 | 60.7 | 53,82 | 54.1 | 52,28 | 40.5 | 49,41 | 40.2 | 49,59 | 40.4 | 49,49 |
| 30 | 82.14 | 51.2 | 51,84 | 57.0 | 53,49 | 53.8 | 52,59 | 55.9 | 51,84 | 68.5 | 55,49 | 61.9 | 54,02 | 47.2 | 51,17 | 45.0 | 51,40 | 46.2 | 51,27 |
| 31 | 85.71 | 59.0 | 53,64 | 64.0 | 55,18 | 61.2 | 54,34 | 63.7 | 53,64 | 74.0 | 57,16 | 68.5 | 55,77 | 54.9 | 52,93 | 53.6 | 53,20 | 54.4 | 53,04 |
| 32 | 89.29 | 66.4 | 55,45 | 71.5 | 56,88 | 68.7 | 56,08 | 71.8 | 55,45 | 79.9 | 58,83 | 75.6 | 57,52 | 61.6 | 54,68 | 62.7 | 55,00 | 62.1 | 54,82 |
| 33 | 92.86 | 74.3 | 57,25 | 80.1 | 58,57 | 76.9 | 57,83 | 79.6 | 57,25 | 85.8 | 60,50 | 82.5 | 59,26 | 69.7 | 56,44 | 74.2 | 56,80 | 71.6 | 56,60 |
| 34 | 96.43 | 81.5 | 59,05 | 88.8 | 60,26 | 84.7 | 59,57 | 85.3 | 59,05 | 91.3 | 62,17 | 88.1 | 61,01 | 78.2 | 58,20 | 86.1 | 58,61 | 81.5 | 58,38 |
| 35 | 100.00 | 100.0 | 60,86 | 100.0 | 61,95 | 100.0 | 61,32 | 100.0 | 60,86 | 100.0 | 63,84 | 100.0 | 62,75 | 100.0 | 59,96 | 100.0 | 60,41 | 100.0 | 60,15 |

*Note: Calculation of scores was restricted to complete cases. RS = raw score; TRS = transformed raw score (range 0-100); PR = percentile; TS = T-score (M = 50, SD = 10).*

**Table 3  DISABKIDS chronic generic module, sub-scale "social inclusion" (self-report) – DCGM-37-S**

| DCGM-37-S INCLUSION SELF-REPORT | | Total sample 8-12 (n = 523) | | Total sample 13-16 (n = 427) | | Total sample Overall (n = 950) | | Females 8-12 (n = 242) | | Females 13-16 (n = 209) | | Females Overall (n = 451) | | Males 8-12 (n = 281) | | Males 13-16 (n = 218) | | Males Overall (n = 499) | |
|---|---|---|---|---|---|---|---|---|---|---|---|---|---|---|---|---|---|---|---|
| RS | TRS | PR | TS | PR | TS | PR | TS | PR | TS | PR | TS | PR | TS | PR | TS | PR | TS | PR | TS |
| 6 | 0.00 | | | .2 | 4,05 | .1 | 7,81 | | | | | | | | | .5 | 5,45 | .2 | 8,18 |
| 7 | 4.17 | | | .2 | 4,05 | .1 | 7,81 | | | | | | | | | .5 | 5,45 | .2 | 8,18 |
| 8 | 8.33 | | | .2 | 4,05 | .1 | 7,81 | | | | | | | | | .5 | 5,45 | .2 | 8,18 |
| 9 | 12.50 | .2 | 16,86 | .2 | 4,05 | .2 | 14,85 | .4 | 17,32 | | | .2 | 14,85 | | | .5 | 5,45 | .2 | 8,18 |
| 10 | 16.67 | .8 | 19,15 | .5 | 13,93 | .6 | 17,19 | 1.7 | 19,61 | | | .9 | 17,19 | | | .9 | 14,91 | .4 | 17,38 |
| 11 | 20.83 | 1.1 | 21,44 | .5 | 13,93 | .8 | 19,54 | 1.7 | 19,61 | | | .9 | 17,19 | .7 | 21,04 | .9 | 14,91 | .8 | 19,68 |
| 12 | 25.00 | 1.9 | 23,73 | .7 | 13,93 | 1.3 | 21,88 | 1.7 | 19,61 | | | .9 | 17,19 | 2.1 | 23,33 | .9 | 14,91 | 1.6 | 21,98 |
| 13 | 29.17 | 2.5 | 26,01 | 1.9 | 21,34 | 1.7 | 24,23 | 1.7 | 19,61 | | | .9 | 17,19 | 3.2 | 25,62 | 1.4 | 22,00 | 2.4 | 24,28 |
| 14 | 33.33 | 3.4 | 28,30 | 4.0 | 23,81 | 2.7 | 26,57 | 3.3 | 28,76 | 1.0 | 23,07 | 2.2 | 26,57 | 3.6 | 27,91 | 2.8 | 24,36 | 3.2 | 26,59 |
| 15 | 37.50 | 4.2 | 30,59 | 4.7 | 26,28 | 4.1 | 28,92 | 4.5 | 31,05 | 2.9 | 25,67 | 3.8 | 28,92 | 3.9 | 30,19 | 5.0 | 26,73 | 4.4 | 28,89 |
| 16 | 41.67 | 6.9 | 32,88 | 6.3 | 28,75 | 5.9 | 31,26 | 7.9 | 33,33 | 3.8 | 28,28 | 6.0 | 31,26 | 6.0 | 32,48 | 5.5 | 29,09 | 5.8 | 31,19 |
| 17 | 45.83 | 10.9 | 35,16 | 8.0 | 31,22 | 8.8 | 33,61 | 12.8 | 35,62 | 6.2 | 30,88 | 9.8 | 33,61 | 9.3 | 34,77 | 6.4 | 31,46 | 8.0 | 33,49 |
| 18 | 50.00 | 14.5 | 37,45 | 10.8 | 33,69 | 11.6 | 35,96 | 16.1 | 37,91 | 8.6 | 33,48 | 12.6 | 35,96 | 13.2 | 37,06 | 7.3 | 33,82 | 10.6 | 35,79 |
| 19 | 54.17 | 19.1 | 39,74 | 15.0 | 36,16 | 15.4 | 38,30 | 20.2 | 40,20 | 12.0 | 36,08 | 16.4 | 38,30 | 18.1 | 39,34 | 9.6 | 36,18 | 14.4 | 38,09 |
| 20 | 58.33 | 23.9 | 42,03 | 22.2 | 38,63 | 19.9 | 40,65 | 24.4 | 42,48 | 16.3 | 38,68 | 20.6 | 40,65 | 23.5 | 41,63 | 13.8 | 38,55 | 19.2 | 40,39 |
| 21 | 62.50 | 29.1 | 44,31 | 27.4 | 41,10 | 26.0 | 42,99 | 29.3 | 44,77 | 25.4 | 41,28 | 27.5 | 42,99 | 28.8 | 43,92 | 19.3 | 40,91 | 24.6 | 42,69 |
| 22 | 66.67 | 37.7 | 46,60 | 33.3 | 43,57 | 33.1 | 45,34 | 37.6 | 47,06 | 30.1 | 43,88 | 34.1 | 45,34 | 37.7 | 46,21 | 24.8 | 43,28 | 32.1 | 44,99 |
| 23 | 70.83 | 44.6 | 48,89 | 42.4 | 46,04 | 39.5 | 47,68 | 45.0 | 49,35 | 34.9 | 46,48 | 40.4 | 47,68 | 44.1 | 48,49 | 31.7 | 45,64 | 38.7 | 47,29 |
| 24 | 75.00 | 52.6 | 51,18 | 49.6 | 48,51 | 48.0 | 50,03 | 56.2 | 51,64 | 46.4 | 49,08 | 51.7 | 50,03 | 49.5 | 50,78 | 38.5 | 48,00 | 44.7 | 49,59 |
| 25 | 79.17 | 61.6 | 53,46 | 61.1 | 50,98 | 56.2 | 52,37 | 63.6 | 53,92 | 54.1 | 51,68 | 59.2 | 52,37 | 59.8 | 53,07 | 45.4 | 50,37 | 53.5 | 51,90 |
| 26 | 83.33 | 73.0 | 55,75 | 74.7 | 53,45 | 67.7 | 54,72 | 72.7 | 56,21 | 63.6 | 54,28 | 68.5 | 54,72 | 73.3 | 55,36 | 58.7 | 52,73 | 66.9 | 54,20 |
| 27 | 87.50 | 80.7 | 58,04 | 83.6 | 55,92 | 78.0 | 57,06 | 82.6 | 58,50 | 79.4 | 56,88 | 81.2 | 57,06 | 79.0 | 57,64 | 70.2 | 55,10 | 75.2 | 56,50 |
| 28 | 91.67 | 88.3 | 60,33 | 91.6 | 58,39 | 86.2 | 59,41 | 90.9 | 60,79 | 86.1 | 59,48 | 88.7 | 59,41 | 86.1 | 59,93 | 81.2 | 57,46 | 84.0 | 58,80 |
| 29 | 95.83 | 94.5 | 62,61 | | 60,86 | 93.2 | 61,75 | 97.1 | 63,07 | 93.8 | 62,08 | 95.6 | 61,75 | 92.2 | 62,22 | 89.4 | 59,83 | 91.0 | 61,10 |
| 30 | 100.00 | 100.0 | 64,90 | 100.0 | 63,33 | 100.0 | 64,10 | 100.0 | 65,36 | 100.0 | 64,68 | 100.0 | 64,10 | 100.0 | 64,51 | 100.0 | 62,19 | 100.0 | 63,40 |

*Note: Calculation of scores was restricted to complete cases. RS = raw score; TRS = transformed raw score (range 0-100); PR = percentile; TS = T-score (M = 50, SD = 10).*

172

Table 4    DISABKIDS chronic generic module, sub-scale "social exclusion" (self-report) – DCGM-37-S

| DCGM-37-S EXCLUSION SELF-REPORT | | Total sample 8-12 (n = 530) | | Total sample 13-16 (n = 435) | | Total sample Overall (n = 965) | | Females 8-12 (n = 242) | | Females 13-16 (n =219) | | Females Overall (n = 461) | | Males 8-12 (n = 288) | | Males 13-16 (n = 216) | | Males Overall (n = 504) | |
|---|---|---|---|---|---|---|---|---|---|---|---|---|---|---|---|---|---|---|---|
| RS | TRS | PR | TS | PR | TS | PR | TS | PR | TS | PR | TS | PR | TS | PR | TS | PR | TS | PR | TS |
| 6 | 0.00 | - | - | - | - | - | - | - | - | - | - | - | - | - | - | - | - | - | - |
| 7 | 4.17 | - | - | - | - | - | - | - | - | - | - | - | - | - | - | - | - | - | - |
| 8 | 8.33 | .4 | - | - | - | .2 | ,69 | .4 | 2,85 | - | - | .2 | 2,41 | - | - | - | - | .2 | -1,20 |
| 9 | 12.50 | .4 | - | - | - | .2 | ,69 | .4 | 2,85 | - | - | .2 | 2,41 | - | ,70 | - | - | .2 | -1,20 |
| 10 | 16.67 | .6 | 1,68 | .2 | - | .3 | 6,06 | .4 | 2,85 | - | - | .2 | 2,41 | .3 | ,70 | - | - | .4 | 4,29 |
| 11 | 20.83 | .6 | 1,68 | .5 | 7,69 | .4 | 8,74 | .4 | 2,85 | - | - | .2 | 2,41 | .3 | 6,01 | - | 4,66 | .6 | 7,04 |
| 12 | 25.00 | .8 | 6,91 | .5 | 10,47 | .6 | 11,42 | .8 | 13,12 | .5 | 12,54 | .7 | 12,94 | .7 | 6,01 | .5 | 4,66 | .6 | 7,04 |
| 13 | 29.17 | 1.1 | 12,14 | .7 | 10,47 | .8 | 14,10 | 1.2 | 15,69 | .5 | 12,54 | .9 | 15,57 | .7 | 13,98 | .5 | 4,66 | .8 | 12,53 |
| 14 | 33.33 | 1.1 | 14,76 | 1.1 | 16,01 | .9 | 16,79 | 1.2 | 15,69 | .9 | 17,98 | 1.1 | 18,20 | 1.0 | 13,98 | .5 | 4,66 | .8 | 12,53 |
| 15 | 37.50 | 1.3 | 19,99 | 1.1 | 18,78 | 1.2 | 19,47 | 1.7 | 20,83 | 1.4 | 20,70 | 1.5 | 20,83 | 1.0 | 13,98 | .9 | 16,17 | 1.0 | 18,02 |
| 16 | 41.67 | 1.9 | 22,60 | 2.1 | 21,55 | 2.0 | 22,15 | 2.5 | 23,39 | 2.7 | 23,41 | 2.6 | 23,46 | 1.4 | 21,94 | 1.4 | 19,05 | 1.4 | 20,76 |
| 17 | 45.83 | 3.4 | 25,22 | 2.8 | 24,32 | 3.1 | 24,83 | 3.7 | 25,96 | 3.7 | 26,13 | 3.7 | 26,09 | 3.1 | 24,60 | 1.9 | 21,92 | 2.6 | 23,51 |
| 18 | 50.00 | 4.5 | 27,84 | 3.9 | 27,09 | 4.2 | 27,52 | 5.4 | 28,53 | 5.0 | 28,85 | 5.2 | 28,72 | 3.8 | 27,25 | 2.8 | 24,80 | 3.4 | 26,25 |
| 19 | 54.17 | 6.4 | 30,45 | 5.5 | 29,86 | 6.0 | 30,20 | 7.4 | 31,10 | 6.8 | 31,56 | 7.2 | 31,35 | 5.6 | 29,91 | 4.2 | 27,68 | 5.0 | 29,00 |
| 20 | 58.33 | 8.3 | 33,07 | 7.8 | 32,63 | 8.1 | 32,88 | 9.5 | 33,67 | 9.1 | 34,28 | 9.3 | 33,98 | 7.3 | 32,56 | 6.5 | 30,55 | 6.9 | 31,74 |
| 21 | 62.50 | 10.2 | 35,68 | 11.5 | 35,40 | 10.8 | 35,56 | 10.7 | 36,24 | 12.8 | 37,00 | 11.7 | 36,62 | 9.7 | 35,22 | 10.2 | 33,43 | 9.9 | 34,49 |
| 22 | 66.67 | 15.3 | 38,30 | 15.4 | 38,17 | 15.3 | 38,25 | 15.3 | 38,80 | 17.8 | 39,71 | 16.5 | 39,25 | 15.3 | 37,87 | 13.0 | 36,31 | 14.3 | 37,23 |
| 23 | 70.83 | 19.4 | 40,91 | 20.2 | 40,94 | 19.8 | 40,93 | 19.4 | 41,37 | 23.3 | 42,43 | 21.3 | 41,88 | 19.4 | 40,52 | 17.1 | 39,18 | 18.5 | 39,98 |
| 24 | 75.00 | 24.9 | 43,53 | 26.4 | 43,71 | 25.6 | 43,61 | 24.4 | 43,94 | 32.0 | 45,15 | 28.0 | 44,51 | 25.3 | 43,18 | 20.8 | 42,06 | 23.4 | 42,72 |
| 25 | 79.17 | 29.6 | 46,15 | 32.0 | 46,48 | 30.7 | 46,29 | 29.8 | 46,51 | 36.5 | 47,87 | 33.0 | 47,14 | 29.5 | 45,83 | 27.3 | 44,94 | 28.6 | 45,47 |
| 26 | 83.33 | 37.5 | 48,76 | 43.0 | 49,25 | 40.0 | 48,98 | 38.8 | 49,08 | 50.2 | 50,58 | 44.3 | 49,77 | 36.5 | 48,49 | 35.6 | 47,82 | 36.1 | 48,21 |
| 27 | 87.50 | 48.1 | 51,38 | 54.0 | 52,03 | 50.8 | 51,66 | 50.4 | 51,64 | 60.7 | 53,30 | 55.3 | 52,40 | 46.2 | 51,14 | 47.2 | 50,69 | 46.6 | 50,96 |
| 28 | 91.67 | 61.1 | 53,99 | 66.9 | 54,80 | 63.7 | 54,34 | 64.0 | 54,21 | 73.5 | 56,02 | 68.5 | 55,03 | 58.7 | 53,80 | 60.2 | 53,57 | 59.3 | 53,70 |
| 29 | 95.83 | 75.7 | 56,61 | 78.6 | 57,57 | 77.0 | 57,02 | 76.0 | 56,78 | 84.0 | 58,73 | 79.8 | 57,67 | 75.3 | 56,45 | 73.1 | 56,45 | 74.4 | 56,45 |
| 30 | 100.00 | 100.0 | 59,22 | 100.0 | 60,34 | 100.0 | 59,71 | 100.0 | 59,35 | 100.0 | 61,45 | 100.0 | 60,30 | 100.0 | 59,11 | 100.0 | 59,32 | 100.0 | 59,19 |

Note: Calculation of z-cores was restricted to complete cases. RS = raw score; TRS = transformed raw score (range 0-100); PR = percentile; TS = T-score (M = 50, SD = 10).

**Table 5   DISABKIDS chronic generic module, sub-scale "physical limitation" (self-report) – DCGM-37-S**

| DCGM-37-S LIMITATION SELF-REPORT | | Total sample 8-12 (n = 536) | | Total sample 13-16 (n = 438) | | Total sample Overall (n = 974) | | Females 8-12 (n = 246) | | Females 13-16 (n = 216) | | Females Overall (n = 462) | | Males 8-12 (n = 290) | | Males 13-16 (n = 222) | | Males Overall (n = 512) | |
|---|---|---|---|---|---|---|---|---|---|---|---|---|---|---|---|---|---|---|---|
| RS | TRS | PR | TS | PR | TS | PR | TS | PR | TS | PR | TS | PR | TS | PR | TS | PR | TS | PR | TS |
| 6 | 0.00 | - | - | - | - | - | - | - | - | - | - | - | - | - | - | - | - | - | - |
| 7 | 4.17 | - | - | - | - | - | - | - | - | - | - | - | - | - | - | - | - | - | - |
| 8 | 8.33 | .2 | 14,43 | .2 | 15,42 | .2 | 14,86 | - | - | .5 | - | .2 | - | .3 | 15,97 | - | - | .2 | 14,39 |
| 9 | 12.50 | .4 | 16,67 | .2 | 15,42 | .3 | 17,09 | - | - | .5 | - | .2 | - | .7 | 18,09 | - | - | .4 | 16,58 |
| 10 | 16.67 | .6 | 18,92 | .2 | 15,42 | .4 | 19,31 | - | - | .5 | 17,65 | .2 | 15,01 | 1.0 | 20,21 | - | - | .6 | 18,78 |
| 11 | 20.83 | .9 | 21,16 | .9 | 22,02 | .9 | 21,54 | .4 | 19,43 | 1.9 | 24,16 | 1.1 | 21,88 | 1.4 | 22,34 | - | - | .8 | 20,97 |
| 12 | 25.00 | 2.1 | 23,41 | 1.6 | 24,22 | 1.8 | 23,77 | 1.2 | 21,86 | 2.8 | 26,33 | 1.9 | 24,17 | 2.8 | 24,46 | .5 | 21,26 | 1.8 | 23,16 |
| 13 | 29.17 | 2.4 | 25,65 | 2.3 | 26,42 | 2.4 | 25,99 | 1.2 | 24,28 | 3.7 | 28,50 | 2.4 | 26,45 | 3.4 | 26,58 | .9 | 23,56 | 2.3 | 25,36 |
| 14 | 33.33 | 3.7 | 27,90 | 3.9 | 28,62 | 3.8 | 28,22 | 2.8 | 26,70 | 5.1 | 30,67 | 3.9 | 28,74 | 4.5 | 28,71 | 2.7 | 25,86 | 3.7 | 27,55 |
| 15 | 37.50 | 5.0 | 30,15 | 6.8 | 30,82 | 5.9 | 30,44 | 4.1 | 29,12 | 8.3 | 32,84 | 6.1 | 31,03 | 5.9 | 30,83 | 5.4 | 28,15 | 5.7 | 29,75 |
| 16 | 41.67 | 7.1 | 32,39 | 9.4 | 33,02 | 8.1 | 32,67 | 5.7 | 31,54 | 11.1 | 35,01 | 8.2 | 33,32 | 8.3 | 32,95 | 7.7 | 30,45 | 8.0 | 31,94 |
| 17 | 45.83 | 9.9 | 34,64 | 11.0 | 35,22 | 10.4 | 34,90 | 9.3 | 33,96 | 13.9 | 37,18 | 11.5 | 35,61 | 10.3 | 35,08 | 8.1 | 32,75 | 9.4 | 34,13 |
| 18 | 50.00 | 11.8 | 36,88 | 14.4 | 37,42 | 12.9 | 37,12 | 11.4 | 36,39 | 17.6 | 39,34 | 14.3 | 37,90 | 12.1 | 37,20 | 11.3 | 35,05 | 11.7 | 36,33 |
| 19 | 54.17 | 17.0 | 39,13 | 18.0 | 39,62 | 17.5 | 39,35 | 17.9 | 38,81 | 20.8 | 41,51 | 19.3 | 40,18 | 16.2 | 39,32 | 15.3 | 37,35 | 15.8 | 38,52 |
| 20 | 58.33 | 21.3 | 41,37 | 22.4 | 41,82 | 21.8 | 41,57 | 22.8 | 41,23 | 25.9 | 43,68 | 24.2 | 42,47 | 20.0 | 41,45 | 18.9 | 39,65 | 19.5 | 40,71 |
| 21 | 62.50 | 27.2 | 43,62 | 28.8 | 44,02 | 27.9 | 43,80 | 27.2 | 43,65 | 35.2 | 45,85 | 31.0 | 44,76 | 27.2 | 43,57 | 22.5 | 41,95 | 25.2 | 42,91 |
| 22 | 66.67 | 34.5 | 45,86 | 33.6 | 46,22 | 34.1 | 46,03 | 35.4 | 46,07 | 41.2 | 48,02 | 38.1 | 47,05 | 33.8 | 45,69 | 26.1 | 44,25 | 30.5 | 45,10 |
| 23 | 70.83 | 42.5 | 48,11 | 41.1 | 48,42 | 41.9 | 48,25 | 44.3 | 48,49 | 49.5 | 50,19 | 46.8 | 49,34 | 41.0 | 47,82 | 32.9 | 46,55 | 37.5 | 47,30 |
| 24 | 75.00 | 50.4 | 50,36 | 49.3 | 50,62 | 49.9 | 50,48 | 54.9 | 50,92 | 56.9 | 52,36 | 55.8 | 51,62 | 46.6 | 49,94 | 41.9 | 48,85 | 44.5 | 49,49 |
| 25 | 79.17 | 58.6 | 52,60 | 60.3 | 52,82 | 59.3 | 52,70 | 63.4 | 53,34 | 67.6 | 54,53 | 65.4 | 53,91 | 54.5 | 52,06 | 53.2 | 51,15 | 53.9 | 51,68 |
| 26 | 83.33 | 66.2 | 54,85 | 69.9 | 55,02 | 67.9 | 54,93 | 70.7 | 55,76 | 75.9 | 56,70 | 73.2 | 56,20 | 62.4 | 54,19 | 64.0 | 53,45 | 63.1 | 53,88 |
| 27 | 87.50 | 76.3 | 57,09 | 77.2 | 57,22 | 76.7 | 57,16 | 80.1 | 58,18 | 83.8 | 58,87 | 81.8 | 58,49 | 73.1 | 56,31 | 70.7 | 55,75 | 72.1 | 56,07 |
| 28 | 91.67 | 85.6 | 59,34 | 85.6 | 59,42 | 85.6 | 59,38 | 90.2 | 60,60 | 90.7 | 61,04 | 90.5 | 60,78 | 81.7 | 58,43 | 80.6 | 58,05 | 81.3 | 58,27 |
| 29 | 95.83 | 92.2 | 61,58 | 91.3 | 61,63 | 91.8 | 61,61 | 94.7 | 63,02 | 95.4 | 63,21 | 95.0 | 63,07 | 90.0 | 60,56 | 87.4 | 60,35 | 88.9 | 60,46 |
| 30 | 100.00 | 100.0 | 63,83 | 100.0 | 63,83 | 100.0 | 63,83 | 100.0 | 65,45 | 100.0 | 65,37 | 100.0 | 65,35 | 100.0 | 62,68 | 100.0 | 62,65 | 100.0 | 62,65 |

Note: Calculation of scores was restricted to complete cases. RS = raw score; TRS = transformed raw score (range 0-100); PR = percentile; TS = T-score (M = 50, SD = 10).

174

**Table 6   DISABKIDS chronic generic module, sub-scale "treatment/ medication" (self-report) – DCGM-37-S**

| DCGM-37-S TREATMENT SELF-REPORT | | Total sample 8-12 (n = 472) | | Total sample 13-16 (n = 373) | | Total sample Overall (n = 845) | | Females 8-12 (n = 215) | | Females 13-16 (n = 190) | | Females Overall (n = 405) | | Males 8-12 (n = 257) | | Males 13-16 (n = 183) | | Males Overall (n = 440) | |
|---|---|---|---|---|---|---|---|---|---|---|---|---|---|---|---|---|---|---|---|
| RS | TRS | PR | TS | PR | TS | PR | TS | PR | TS | PR | TS | PR | TS | PR | TS | PR | TS | PR | TS |
| 6 | 0.00 | .2 | 15,07 | - | - | .1 | 17,65 | - | - | - | - | - | - | .3 | 14,06 | - | - | .2 | 16,80 |
| 7 | 4.17 | .2 | 17,01 | .3 | 21,98 | .2 | 19,50 | - | - | .5 | 22,23 | .2 | 20,07 | .3 | 16,00 | - | - | .2 | 18,64 |
| 8 | 8.33 | .6 | 18,96 | .5 | 23,75 | .6 | 21,35 | .5 | 19,73 | 1.1 | 24,04 | .7 | 21,96 | .4 | 17,93 | .5 | 25,01 | .5 | 20,47 |
| 9 | 12.50 | .6 | 20,90 | 1.3 | 25,51 | .9 | 23,20 | .5 | 21,71 | 2.1 | 25,86 | 1.2 | 23,85 | .4 | 19,87 | 2.2 | 26,75 | .7 | 22,31 |
| 10 | 16.67 | 1.7 | 22,84 | 2.7 | 27,28 | 2.1 | 25,06 | 1.4 | 23,69 | 3.2 | 27,67 | 2.2 | 25,74 | 1.9 | 21,80 | 2.2 | 28,49 | 2.0 | 24,15 |
| 11 | 20.83 | 1.9 | 24,78 | 3.8 | 29,05 | 2.7 | 26,91 | 1.9 | 25,68 | 5.3 | 29,48 | 3.5 | 27,63 | 1.9 | 23,74 | 2.2 | 30,22 | 2.0 | 25,98 |
| 12 | 25.00 | 3.2 | 26,72 | 4.8 | 30,82 | 3.9 | 28,76 | 3.7 | 27,66 | 7.4 | 31,29 | 5.4 | 29,52 | 2.7 | 25,67 | 4.4 | 31,96 | 2.5 | 27,82 |
| 13 | 29.17 | 4.4 | 28,67 | 6.7 | 32,59 | 5.4 | 30,61 | 5.6 | 29,64 | 8.9 | 33,11 | 7.2 | 31,41 | 3.5 | 27,60 | 9.3 | 33,69 | 3.9 | 29,65 |
| 14 | 33.33 | 5.3 | 30,61 | 9.9 | 34,36 | 7.3 | 32,46 | 6.5 | 31,62 | 10.5 | 34,92 | 8.4 | 33,30 | 4.3 | 29,54 | 14.8 | 35,43 | 6.4 | 31,49 |
| 15 | 37.50 | 6.4 | 32,55 | 13.4 | 36,13 | 9.5 | 34,31 | 7.9 | 33,60 | 12.1 | 36,73 | 9.9 | 35,20 | 5.1 | 31,47 | 16.9 | 37,17 | 9.1 | 33,33 |
| 16 | 41.67 | 8.9 | 34,49 | 15.8 | 37,89 | 12.0 | 36,16 | 10.2 | 35,58 | 14.7 | 38,54 | 12.3 | 37,09 | 7.8 | 33,41 | 20.2 | 38,91 | 11.6 | 35,16 |
| 17 | 45.83 | 11.7 | 36,43 | 19.3 | 39,66 | 15.0 | 38,01 | 13.0 | 37,56 | 18.4 | 40,36 | 15.6 | 38,98 | 10.5 | 35,34 | 23.5 | 40,64 | 14.5 | 37,00 |
| 18 | 50.00 | 17.4 | 38,38 | 23.1 | 41,43 | 19.9 | 39,86 | 20.5 | 39,54 | 22.6 | 42,17 | 21.5 | 40,87 | 14.8 | 37,28 | 26.8 | 42,38 | 18.4 | 38,83 |
| 19 | 54.17 | 21.0 | 40,32 | 26.8 | 43,20 | 23.6 | 41,71 | 22.8 | 41,52 | 26.8 | 43,98 | 24.7 | 42,76 | 19.5 | 39,21 | 29.5 | 44,12 | 22.5 | 40,67 |
| 20 | 58.33 | 24.6 | 42,26 | 31.9 | 44,97 | 27.8 | 43,56 | 26.5 | 43,50 | 34.2 | 45,79 | 30.1 | 44,65 | 23.0 | 41,15 | 36.1 | 45,85 | 25.7 | 42,51 |
| 21 | 62.50 | 29.2 | 44,20 | 37.3 | 46,74 | 32.8 | 45,41 | 32.6 | 45,49 | 38.4 | 47,61 | 35.3 | 46,54 | 26.5 | 43,08 | 41.0 | 47,59 | 30.5 | 44,34 |
| 22 | 66.67 | 35.8 | 46,14 | 44.0 | 48,51 | 39.4 | 47,26 | 40.0 | 47,47 | 46.8 | 49,42 | 43.2 | 48,43 | 32.3 | 45,02 | 45.9 | 49,33 | 35.9 | 46,18 |
| 23 | 70.83 | 39.8 | 48,09 | 50.4 | 50,28 | 44.5 | 49,11 | 45.1 | 49,45 | 54.7 | 51,23 | 49.6 | 50,32 | 35.4 | 46,95 | 50.8 | 51,06 | 39.8 | 48,01 |
| 24 | 75.00 | 46.2 | 50,03 | 56.8 | 52,04 | 50.9 | 50,96 | 54.4 | 51,43 | 62.6 | 53,04 | 58.3 | 52,21 | 39.3 | 48,89 | 54.1 | 52,80 | 44.1 | 49,85 |
| 25 | 79.17 | 52.1 | 51,97 | 61.7 | 53,81 | 56.3 | 52,81 | 60.9 | 53,41 | 68.9 | 54,86 | 64.7 | 54,10 | 44.7 | 50,82 | 60.1 | 54,54 | 48.6 | 51,69 |
| 26 | 83.33 | 60.8 | 53,91 | 66.2 | 55,58 | 63.2 | 54,66 | 69.3 | 55,39 | 72.1 | 56,67 | 70.6 | 55,99 | 53.7 | 52,76 | 64.5 | 56,27 | 56.4 | 53,52 |
| 27 | 87.50 | 68.0 | 55,85 | 72.1 | 57,35 | 69.8 | 56,51 | 75.8 | 57,37 | 79.5 | 58,48 | 77.5 | 57,89 | 61.5 | 54,69 | 73.8 | 58,01 | 62.7 | 55,36 |
| 28 | 91.67 | 76.5 | 57,80 | 80.2 | 59,12 | 78.1 | 58,36 | 83.3 | 59,35 | 86.3 | 60,29 | 84.7 | 59,78 | 70.8 | 56,62 | 82.5 | 59,75 | 72.0 | 57,19 |
| 29 | 95.83 | 85.0 | 59,74 | 86.6 | 60,89 | 85.7 | 60,21 | 89.8 | 61,33 | 90.5 | 62,11 | 90.1 | 61,67 | 80.9 | 58,56 | 82.5 | 59,75 | 81.6 | 59,03 |
| 30 | 100.00 | 100.0 | 61,68 | 100.0 | 62,66 | 100.0 | 62,06 | 100.0 | 63,31 | 100.0 | 63,92 | 100.0 | 63,56 | 100.0 | 60,49 | 100.0 | 61,48 | 100.0 | 60,87 |

*Note: Calculation of scores was restricted to complete cases. RS = raw score; TRS = transformed raw score (range 0-100); PR = percentile; TS = T-score (M = 50, SD = 10).*

**Table 7  Total score of the DISABKIDS chronic generic module (if the "treatment" scale is included*; self-report) – DCGM-37-S**

| DCGM-37-S TOTAL SCORE SELF-REPORT | | Total sample 8-12 (n = 405) | | Total sample 13-16 (n = 332) | | Total sample Overall (n = 737) | | Females 8-12 (n = 178) | | Females 13-16 (n = 169) | | Females Overall (n = 347) | | Males 8-12 (n = 227) | | Males 13-16 (n = 163) | | Males Overall (n = 390) | |
| RS | TRS | PR | TS | PR | TS | PR | TS | PR | TS | PR | TS | PR | TS | PR | TS | PR | TS | PR | TS |
|---|---|---|---|---|---|---|---|---|---|---|---|---|---|---|---|---|---|---|---|
| <= 90 | 35.81 | 1.0 | 19,53 | .9 | 21,01 | .9 | 21,21 | .6 | 12,35 | 1.8 | 23,30 | 1.2 | 22,72 | 1.3 | 18,98 | - | - | .8 | 17,54 |
| 91 | 36.49 | 1.0 | 19,53 | .9 | 21,01 | .9 | 21,21 | .6 | 12,35 | 1.8 | 23,30 | 1.2 | 22,72 | 1.3 | 18,98 | - | - | .8 | 17,54 |
| 92 | 37.16 | 1.0 | 19,53 | .9 | 21,01 | 1.1 | 23,08 | .6 | 12,35 | 1.8 | 23,30 | 1.2 | 22,72 | 1.3 | 18,98 | - | - | .8 | 17,54 |
| 93 | 37.84 | 1.2 | 23,19 | 1.5 | 23,40 | 1.4 | 23,55 | 1.1 | 23,84 | 1.8 | 23,30 | 1.4 | 24,57 | 1.3 | 18,98 | .6 | 19,83 | .8 | 17,54 |
| 94 | 38.51 | 1.2 | 23,19 | 1.5 | 23,40 | 1.4 | 23,55 | 1.1 | 23,84 | 1.8 | 23,30 | 1.7 | 25,03 | 1.3 | 18,98 | .6 | 19,83 | 1.0 | 21,82 |
| 95 | 39.19 | 1.2 | 23,19 | 1.5 | 23,40 | 1.4 | 23,55 | 1.1 | 23,84 | 2.4 | 25,65 | 1.7 | 25,03 | 1.3 | 18,98 | .6 | 19,83 | 1.0 | 21,82 |
| 96 | 39.86 | 1.2 | 23,19 | 1.5 | 23,40 | 1.4 | 23,55 | 1.1 | 23,84 | 2.4 | 25,65 | 1.7 | 25,03 | 1.3 | 18,98 | .6 | 19,83 | 1.0 | 21,82 |
| 97 | 40.54 | 1.2 | 23,19 | 1.5 | 23,40 | 1.4 | 23,55 | 1.1 | 23,84 | 2.4 | 25,65 | 1.7 | 25,03 | 1.3 | 18,98 | .6 | 19,83 | 1.0 | 21,82 |
| 98 | 41.22 | 1.5 | 25,49 | 1.5 | 23,40 | 1.5 | 25,41 | 1.1 | 23,84 | 2.4 | 25,65 | 2.6 | 27,35 | 1.8 | 24,94 | .6 | 19,83 | 1.3 | 23,72 |
| 99 | 41.90 | 1.7 | 25,94 | 2.1 | 25,78 | 1.9 | 25,88 | 1.7 | 26,60 | 3.6 | 28,01 | 2.9 | 27,82 | 1.8 | 24,94 | .6 | 19,83 | 1.3 | 23,72 |
| 100 | 42.57 | 2.0 | 26,40 | 2.1 | 25,78 | 2.0 | 26,35 | 2.2 | 27,06 | 3.6 | 28,01 | 3.5 | 28,28 | 1.8 | 24,94 | .6 | 19,83 | 1.3 | 23,72 |
| 101 | 43.24 | 2.2 | 26,86 | 2.4 | 26,74 | 2.3 | 26,81 | 2.8 | 27,52 | 4.1 | 28,95 | 3.7 | 28,74 | 1.8 | 24,94 | .6 | 19,83 | 1.3 | 23,72 |
| 102 | 43.92 | 2.2 | 26,86 | 2.7 | 27,21 | 2.4 | 27,28 | 2.8 | 27,52 | 4.7 | 29,42 | 4.6 | 29,21 | 1.8 | 24,94 | .6 | 19,83 | 1.3 | 23,72 |
| 103 | 44.60 | 2.5 | 27,78 | 3.3 | 27,69 | 2.8 | 27,75 | 3.4 | 28,44 | 5.9 | 29,89 | 5.2 | 29,67 | 1.8 | 24,94 | .6 | 19,83 | 1.3 | 23,72 |
| 104 | 45.27 | 3.0 | 28,24 | 3.3 | 27,69 | 3.1 | 28,21 | 4.5 | 28,90 | 5.9 | 29,89 | 6.1 | 30,13 | 1.8 | 24,94 | .6 | 19,83 | 1.3 | 23,72 |
| 105 | 45.94 | 3.5 | 28,70 | 3.6 | 28,64 | 3.5 | 28,21 | 5.6 | 29,36 | 6.5 | 30,83 | 6.1 | 30,13 | 1.8 | 24,94 | .6 | 19,83 | 1.3 | 23,72 |
| 106 | 46.62 | 3.5 | 28,70 | 3.6 | 28,64 | 3.5 | 28,68 | 5.6 | 29,36 | 6.5 | 30,83 | 6.3 | 31,06 | 1.8 | 24,94 | .6 | 19,83 | 1.3 | 23,72 |
| 107 | 47.30 | 3.5 | 28,70 | 3.9 | 29,60 | 3.7 | 29,61 | 5.6 | 29,36 | 7.1 | 31,77 | 6.3 | 31,06 | 2.2 | 29,52 | 1.8 | 27,37 | 1.5 | 28,48 |
| 108 | 47.97 | 3.7 | 30,07 | 3.9 | 29,60 | 3.8 | 30,08 | 5.6 | 29,36 | 7.1 | 31,77 | 6.9 | 31,99 | 2.6 | 29,98 | 2.5 | 27,88 | 2.3 | 28,96 |
| 109 | 48.65 | 4.4 | 30,53 | 4.5 | 30,55 | 4.5 | 30,55 | 6.7 | 31,20 | 7.1 | 31,77 | 6.9 | 31,99 | 3.1 | 30,44 | 3.1 | 28,38 | 2.8 | 29,43 |
| 110 | 49.32 | 4.7 | 30,99 | 4.8 | 31,03 | 4.7 | 31,01 | 6.7 | 31,20 | 7.1 | 31,77 | 6.9 | 31,99 | 3.5 | 30,90 | 3.1 | 28,89 | 3.3 | 29,91 |
| 111 | 50.00 | 5.2 | 31,45 | 5.4 | 31,51 | 5.3 | 31,48 | 7.3 | 32,12 | 7.7 | 33,66 | 7.5 | 32,92 | 3.5 | 30,90 | 4.3 | 29,39 | 3.3 | 29,91 |
| 112 | 50.67 | 5.2 | 31,45 | 5.4 | 31,51 | 6.1 | 32,41 | 7.3 | 32,12 | 7.7 | 33,66 | 7.5 | 32,92 | 4.0 | 31,81 | 4.3 | 29,90 | 4.1 | 30,86 |
| 113 | 51.35 | 5.4 | 32,36 | 6.9 | 32,46 | 6.1 | 32,41 | 7.3 | 32,12 | 9.5 | 34,60 | 8.4 | 33,84 | 4.8 | 32,27 | 4.3 | 30,40 | 4.6 | 31,33 |
| 114 | 52.02 | 6.2 | 32,82 | 6.9 | 32,46 | 6.5 | 32,88 | 7.9 | 33,50 | 9.5 | 34,60 | 8.6 | 34,31 | 4.8 | 32,27 | 4.3 | 30,91 | 4.6 | 31,33 |
| 115 | 52.70 | 6.4 | 33,28 | 7.5 | 33,42 | 6.9 | 33,35 | 8.4 | 33,96 | 10.7 | 35,54 | 9.5 | 34,77 | 5.3 | 33,19 | 4.6 | 31,41 | 4.9 | 32,29 |
| 116 | 53.38 | 6.9 | 33,74 | 8.1 | 33,89 | 7.5 | 33,81 | 9.0 | 34,42 | 11.8 | 36,01 | 10.4 | 35,23 | 5.7 | 33,65 | 4.9 | 31,90 | 5.1 | 32,76 |
| 117 | 54.05 | 7.4 | 34,20 | 8.1 | 33,89 | 7.7 | 34,28 | 9.6 | 34,88 | 11.8 | 36,01 | 10.7 | 35,70 | 6.6 | 34,10 | 5.1 | 32,40 | 6.9 | 33,24 |
| 118 | 54.73 | 7.9 | 34,66 | 9.6 | 34,85 | 8.7 | 34,74 | 9.6 | 34,88 | 11.8 | 36,01 | 10.7 | 35,70 | 6.9 | 34,56 | 6.9 | 32,91 | 7.9 | 33,71 |
| 119 | 55.40 | 8.9 | 35,12 | 10.2 | 35,32 | 9.5 | 35,21 | 10.1 | 35,80 | 12.4 | 37,42 | 11.2 | 36,62 | 7.9 | 35,02 | 7.4 | 33,41 | 9.0 | 34,19 |
| 120 | 56.08 | 9.9 | 35,57 | 10.8 | 35,80 | 10.3 | 35,68 | 11.2 | 36,26 | 12.4 | 37,42 | 11.8 | 37,09 | 8.8 | 35,48 | 8.0 | 33,91 | 10.0 | 34,67 |
| 121 | 56.76 | 10.9 | 36,03 | 11.1 | 36,28 | 11.0 | 36,14 | 11.8 | 36,72 | 14.2 | 38,84 | 12.1 | 37,55 | 10.1 | 35,94 | 9.2 | 34,42 | 10.8 | 35,14 |
| 122 | 57.43 | 11.6 | 36,49 | 12.3 | 36,75 | 11.9 | 36,61 | 12.4 | 37,17 | 14.8 | 39,31 | 13.3 | 38,02 | 11.0 | 36,40 | 9.8 | 34,92 | 11.3 | 35,62 |
| 123 | 58.10 | 11.9 | 36,95 | 13.0 | 37,23 | 12.3 | 37,08 | 12.4 | 37,17 | 16.0 | 39,78 | 13.5 | 38,48 | 11.5 | 36,85 | 10.4 | 35,43 | 12.8 | 36,09 |
| 124 | 58.78 | 13.3 | 37,41 | 14.2 | 37,71 | 13.7 | 37,54 | 13.5 | 38,09 | 17.8 | 40,25 | 14.7 | 38,94 | 13.2 | 37,31 | 11.0 | 35,93 | 13.6 | 36,57 |
| 125 | 59.46 | 14.1 | 37,87 | 15.1 | 38,19 | 14.5 | 38,01 | 13.5 | 38,09 | 18.3 | 40,72 | 15.6 | 39,41 | 14.5 | 37,77 | 12.3 | 36,43 | 14.4 | 37,04 |
| 126 | 60.13 | 15.6 | 38,33 | 16.0 | 38,66 | 15.7 | 38,48 | 16.3 | 39,01 | 18.9 | 41,19 | 17.3 | 39,87 | 15.0 | 37,77 | 13.5 | 36,94 | 14.6 | 37,52 |
| 127 | 60.81 | 15.8 | 38,78 | 16.6 | 39,14 | 16.1 | 38,94 | 16.9 | 39,47 | 20.1 | 41,66 | 17.9 | 40,33 | 15.0 | 38,69 | 14.1 | 37,44 | 15.4 | 38,00 |
| 128 | 61.49 | 17.3 | 39,24 | 17.5 | 39,62 | 17.4 | 39,41 | 19.1 | 39,93 | 20.1 | 41,66 | 19.6 | 40,80 | 15.9 | 39,14 | 14.7 | 37,94 | 15.4 | 38,00 |
| 129 | 62.16 | 17.8 | 39,70 | 17.8 | 40,09 | 17.8 | 39,88 | 19.7 | 40,39 | 20.1 | 41,66 | 19.9 | 41,26 | 16.3 | 39,14 | 15.3 | 38,45 | 15.9 | 38,47 |

**Table 7    continued**

| DCGM-37-S TOTAL SCORE SELF-REPORT | | Total sample 8-12 (n = 405) | | Total sample 13-16 (n = 332) | | Total sample Overall (n = 737) | | Females 8-12 (n = 178) | | Females 13-16 (n = 169) | | Females Overall (n = 347) | | Males 8-12 (n = 227) | | Males 13-16 (n = 163) | | Males Overall (n = 390) | |
|---|---|---|---|---|---|---|---|---|---|---|---|---|---|---|---|---|---|---|---|
| RS | TRS | PR | TS | PR | TS | PR | TS | PR | TS | RS | TRS | PR | TS | PR | TS | PR | TS | PR | TS |
| 130 | 62,83 | 18,8 | 40,16 | 18,1 | 40,57 | 18,5 | 40,34 | 20,8 | 40,85 | 20,7 | 42,60 | 20,7 | 41,72 | 17,2 | 39,60 | 15,3 | 36,43 | 16,4 | 38,95 |
| 131 | 63,51 | 20,2 | 40,62 | 19,3 | 41,05 | 19,8 | 40,81 | 21,3 | 41,31 | 21,3 | 43,08 | 21,3 | 42,19 | 19,4 | 40,06 | 17,2 | 36,93 | 18,5 | 39,42 |
| 132 | 64,19 | 21,0 | 41,08 | 20,2 | 41,53 | 20,6 | 41,28 | 22,5 | 41,77 | 22,5 | 43,55 | 22,5 | 42,65 | 19,8 | 40,52 | 17,8 | 37,44 | 19,0 | 39,90 |
| 133 | 64,86 | 21,5 | 41,53 | 21,1 | 42,00 | 21,3 | 41,74 | 23,0 | 42,23 | 24,3 | 44,02 | 23,6 | 43,11 | 20,3 | 40,98 | 17,8 | 37,44 | 19,2 | 40,38 |
| 134 | 65,54 | 21,7 | 41,99 | 21,7 | 42,48 | 21,7 | 42,21 | 23,6 | 42,69 | 25,4 | 44,49 | 24,5 | 43,58 | 20,3 | 40,98 | 17,8 | 37,44 | 19,2 | 40,38 |
| 135 | 66,22 | 22,7 | 42,45 | 22,3 | 42,96 | 22,5 | 42,68 | 24,2 | 43,15 | 26,0 | 44,96 | 25,1 | 44,04 | 21,6 | 41,89 | 18,4 | 38,44 | 20,3 | 41,33 |
| 136 | 66,89 | 23,7 | 42,91 | 23,2 | 43,43 | 23,5 | 43,14 | 24,7 | 43,61 | 26,6 | 45,43 | 25,6 | 44,51 | 22,9 | 42,35 | 19,6 | 38,94 | 21,5 | 41,80 |
| 137 | 67,57 | 24,4 | 43,37 | 23,5 | 43,91 | 24,0 | 43,61 | 24,7 | 43,61 | 27,2 | 45,90 | 25,9 | 44,97 | 24,2 | 42,81 | 19,6 | 38,94 | 22,3 | 42,28 |
| 138 | 68,24 | 25,4 | 43,83 | 25,6 | 44,39 | 25,5 | 44,08 | 25,8 | 44,53 | 29,0 | 46,37 | 27,4 | 45,43 | 25,1 | 43,27 | 22,1 | 40,45 | 23,8 | 42,75 |
| 139 | 68,92 | 26,4 | 44,29 | 26,8 | 44,86 | 26,6 | 44,54 | 27,5 | 44,99 | 30,2 | 46,84 | 28,8 | 45,90 | 25,6 | 43,73 | 23,3 | 40,96 | 24,6 | 43,23 |
| 140 | 69,59 | 28,1 | 44,74 | 28,6 | 45,34 | 28,4 | 45,01 | 28,7 | 45,45 | 33,1 | 47,31 | 30,8 | 46,36 | 27,8 | 44,18 | 23,9 | 41,96 | 26,2 | 43,71 |
| 141 | 70,27 | 28,9 | 45,20 | 30,7 | 45,82 | 29,7 | 45,48 | 29,2 | 45,91 | 35,5 | 47,78 | 32,3 | 46,82 | 28,6 | 44,64 | 25,8 | 42,47 | 27,4 | 44,18 |
| 142 | 70,94 | 30,4 | 45,66 | 32,2 | 46,30 | 31,4 | 45,94 | 31,5 | 46,37 | 37,3 | 48,26 | 34,3 | 47,29 | 29,5 | 45,10 | 27,0 | 42,97 | 28,5 | 44,66 |
| 143 | 71,62 | 32,6 | 46,12 | 34,3 | 46,77 | 33,4 | 46,41 | 34,3 | 46,83 | 40,2 | 48,73 | 37,2 | 47,75 | 31,3 | 45,56 | 28,2 | 43,47 | 30,0 | 45,13 |
| 144 | 72,23 | 32,8 | 46,58 | 35,8 | 47,25 | 34,2 | 46,88 | 34,3 | 46,83 | 42,6 | 49,20 | 38,3 | 48,21 | 31,7 | 46,02 | 28,8 | 43,98 | 30,5 | 45,61 |
| 145 | 72,98 | 34,6 | 47,04 | 36,7 | 47,73 | 35,5 | 47,34 | 35,4 | 47,75 | 43,2 | 49,67 | 39,2 | 48,68 | 33,9 | 46,48 | 30,1 | 44,48 | 32,3 | 46,08 |
| 146 | 73,65 | 37,0 | 47,50 | 38,3 | 48,20 | 37,6 | 47,81 | 38,8 | 48,21 | 46,2 | 50,14 | 42,4 | 49,14 | 35,7 | 46,93 | 30,1 | 44,98 | 33,3 | 46,56 |
| 147 | 74,32 | 37,8 | 47,95 | 41,3 | 48,68 | 39,3 | 48,27 | 39,9 | 48,67 | 50,3 | 50,61 | 45,0 | 49,60 | 36,1 | 47,39 | 31,9 | 45,48 | 34,4 | 47,04 |
| 148 | 75,00 | 39,0 | 48,41 | 42,8 | 49,16 | 40,7 | 48,74 | 40,4 | 49,13 | 52,7 | 51,08 | 46,4 | 50,07 | 37,9 | 47,85 | 32,5 | 46,49 | 35,6 | 47,51 |
| 149 | 75,67 | 40,5 | 48,87 | 44,0 | 49,64 | 42,1 | 49,21 | 42,1 | 49,59 | 53,3 | 51,55 | 47,6 | 50,53 | 39,2 | 48,31 | 34,4 | 46,99 | 37,2 | 47,99 |
| 150 | 76,35 | 41,2 | 49,33 | 46,4 | 50,11 | 43,6 | 49,67 | 42,1 | 49,59 | 55,0 | 52,02 | 48,4 | 51,00 | 40,5 | 48,77 | 37,4 | 47,50 | 39,2 | 48,46 |
| 151 | 77,03 | 43,0 | 49,79 | 48,2 | 50,59 | 45,3 | 50,14 | 44,9 | 50,51 | 57,4 | 52,49 | 51,0 | 51,46 | 41,4 | 49,22 | 38,7 | 48,00 | 40,3 | 48,94 |
| 152 | 77,70 | 43,5 | 50,25 | 49,4 | 51,07 | 46,1 | 50,61 | 45,5 | 50,97 | 59,2 | 52,96 | 52,2 | 51,92 | 41,9 | 49,68 | 39,3 | 48,50 | 40,8 | 49,42 |
| 153 | 52,50 | 43,7 | 50,71 | 50,3 | 51,54 | 46,7 | 51,07 | 45,5 | 50,97 | 60,4 | 53,44 | 52,7 | 52,39 | 42,3 | 50,14 | 39,9 | 49,01 | 41,3 | 49,89 |
| 154 | 79,05 | 46,4 | 51,16 | 51,2 | 52,02 | 48,6 | 51,54 | 47,8 | 51,89 | 60,9 | 53,91 | 54,2 | 52,85 | 45,4 | 50,60 | 41,1 | 49,51 | 43,6 | 50,37 |
| 155 | 79,73 | 47,2 | 51,62 | 53,3 | 52,50 | 49,9 | 52,01 | 49,4 | 52,35 | 63,3 | 54,38 | 56,2 | 53,31 | 45,4 | 50,60 | 42,9 | 50,02 | 44,4 | 50,84 |
| 156 | 80,40 | 48,6 | 52,08 | 55,7 | 52,97 | 51,8 | 52,47 | 50,6 | 52,81 | 67,5 | 54,85 | 58,8 | 53,78 | 47,1 | 51,52 | 43,6 | 50,52 | 45,6 | 51,32 |
| 157 | 81,08 | 50,6 | 52,54 | 58,4 | 53,45 | 54,1 | 52,94 | 53,4 | 53,27 | 71,0 | 55,32 | 62,0 | 54,24 | 48,5 | 51,97 | 45,4 | 51,02 | 47,2 | 51,79 |
| 158 | 81,76 | 52,8 | 53,00 | 62,0 | 53,93 | 57,0 | 53,41 | 53,9 | 53,73 | 72,8 | 55,79 | 63,1 | 54,70 | 52,0 | 52,43 | 50,9 | 51,52 | 51,5 | 52,27 |
| 159 | 82,43 | 54,8 | 53,46 | 64,2 | 54,41 | 59,0 | 53,87 | 56,7 | 54,19 | 74,0 | 56,26 | 65,1 | 55,17 | 53,3 | 52,89 | 54,0 | 52,02 | 53,6 | 52,75 |
| 160 | 83,10 | 57,5 | 53,92 | 65,4 | 54,88 | 61,1 | 54,34 | 60,1 | 54,65 | 75,1 | 56,73 | 67,4 | 55,63 | 55,5 | 53,35 | 55,2 | 52,53 | 55,4 | 53,22 |
| 161 | 83,78 | 60,5 | 54,37 | 68,1 | 55,36 | 63,3 | 54,81 | 62,4 | 55,11 | 77,5 | 57,20 | 69,7 | 56,09 | 59,0 | 53,81 | 58,3 | 53,03 | 58,7 | 53,70 |
| 162 | 84,46 | 62,5 | 54,83 | 69,3 | 55,84 | 65,5 | 55,27 | 64,0 | 55,57 | 78,1 | 57,67 | 70,9 | 56,56 | 61,2 | 54,27 | 60,1 | 53,53 | 60,8 | 54,17 |
| 163 | 85,13 | 66,2 | 55,29 | 70,8 | 56,31 | 68,2 | 55,74 | 69,7 | 56,03 | 79,3 | 58,14 | 74,4 | 57,02 | 63,4 | 54,72 | 62,0 | 54,04 | 62,8 | 54,65 |
| 164 | 85,81 | 67,4 | 55,75 | 72,6 | 56,79 | 69,7 | 56,21 | 71,3 | 56,49 | 81,1 | 58,62 | 76,1 | 57,49 | 64,3 | 55,18 | 63,8 | 54,54 | 64,1 | 55,13 |
| 165 | 86,49 | 68,6 | 56,21 | 74,4 | 57,27 | 71,2 | 56,67 | 71,9 | 56,95 | 82,8 | 59,09 | 77,2 | 57,95 | 66,1 | 55,64 | 65,6 | 55,04 | 65,9 | 55,60 |
| 166 | 87,16 | 71,1 | 56,67 | 75,9 | 57,74 | 73,3 | 57,14 | 75,8 | 57,41 | 83,4 | 59,56 | 79,5 | 58,41 | 67,4 | 56,10 | 68,1 | 55,55 | 67,7 | 56,08 |
| 167 | 87,84 | 73,3 | 57,12 | 76,5 | 58,22 | 74,8 | 57,61 | 78,1 | 57,87 | 83,4 | 59,56 | 80,7 | 58,88 | 69,6 | 56,56 | 69,3 | 56,05 | 69,5 | 56,55 |
| 168 | 88,51 | 75,6 | 57,58 | 78,6 | 58,70 | 76,9 | 58,00 | 79,8 | 58,33 | 84,6 | 60,50 | 82,1 | 59,34 | 72,2 | 57,01 | 72,4 | 56,55 | 72,3 | 57,03 |
| 169 | 89,19 | 78,8 | 58,04 | 80,7 | 59,18 | 79,6 | 58,54 | 83,1 | 58,79 | 85,8 | 60,97 | 84,4 | 59,80 | 75,3 | 57,47 | 75,5 | 57,06 | 75,4 | 57,50 |

**Table 7** continued

| DCGM-37-S TOTAL SCORE SELF-REPORT | | Total sample 8-12 (n = 405) | | Total sample 13-16 (n = 332) | | Total sample Overall (n = 737) | | Females 8-12 (n = 178) | | Females 13-16 (n = 169) | | Females Overall (n = 347) | | Males 8-12 (n = 227) | | Males 13-16 (n = 163) | | Males Overall (n = 390) | |
|------|--------|------|------|------|------|------|------|------|------|------|------|------|------|------|------|------|------|------|------|
| RS | TRS | PR | TS | PR | TS | PR | TS | PR | TS | RS | TRS | PR | TS | PR | TS | PR | TS | PR | TS |
| 170 | 89.87 | 80.5 | 58,50 | 82.8 | 59,65 | 81.5 | 59,01 | 83.7 | 59,24 | 88.2 | 61,44 | 85.9 | 60,27 | 78.0 | 57,93 | 77.3 | 57,56 | 77.7 | 57,98 |
| 171 | 90.54 | 82.0 | 58,96 | 84.6 | 60,13 | 83.2 | 59,47 | 86.5 | 59,70 | 89.3 | 61,91 | 87.9 | 60,73 | 78.4 | 58,39 | 79.8 | 58,06 | 79.0 | 58,46 |
| 172 | 91.22 | 83.7 | 59,42 | 88.6 | 60,61 | 85.9 | 59,94 | 87.6 | 60,16 | 94.1 | 62,38 | 90.8 | 61,19 | 80.6 | 58,85 | 82.8 | 58,56 | 81.5 | 58,93 |
| 173 | 91.89 | 85.7 | 59,88 | 89.8 | 61,08 | 87.5 | 60,41 | 88.8 | 60,62 | 94.7 | 62,85 | 91.6 | 61,66 | 83.3 | 59,31 | 84.7 | 59,07 | 83.8 | 59,41 |
| 174 | 92.57 | 87.4 | 60,33 | 91.0 | 61,56 | 89.0 | 60,87 | 91.0 | 61,08 | 95.9 | 63,32 | 93.4 | 62,12 | 84.6 | 59,76 | 85.9 | 59,57 | 85.1 | 59,88 |
| 175 | 93.24 | 88.9 | 60,79 | 91.6 | 62,04 | 90.1 | 61,34 | 92.1 | 61,54 | 96.4 | 63,80 | 94.2 | 62,58 | 86.3 | 60,22 | 86.5 | 60,07 | 86.4 | 60,36 |
| 176 | 93.92 | 90.6 | 61,25 | 92.8 | 62,52 | 91.6 | 61,80 | 93.8 | 62,00 | 96.4 | 63,80 | 95.1 | 63,05 | 88.1 | 60,68 | 89.0 | 60,58 | 88.5 | 60,84 |
| 177 | 94.59 | 93.1 | 61,71 | 93.7 | 62,99 | 93.4 | 62,27 | 96.6 | 62,46 | 96.4 | 63,80 | 96.5 | 63,51 | 90.3 | 61,14 | 90.8 | 61,08 | 90.5 | 61,31 |
| 178 | 95.27 | 95.1 | 62,17 | 94.6 | 63,47 | 94.8 | 62,74 | 98.3 | 62,92 | 96.4 | 63,80 | 97.4 | 63,98 | 92.5 | 61,60 | 92.6 | 61,58 | 92.6 | 61,79 |
| 179 | 95.94 | 96.0 | 62,63 | 96.4 | 63,95 | 96.2 | 63,20 | 98.9 | 63,38 | 97.0 | 65,68 | 98.0 | 64,44 | 93.8 | 62,05 | 95.7 | 62,09 | 94.6 | 62,26 |
| 180 | 96.62 | 96.8 | 63,09 | 97.3 | 64,42 | 97.0 | 63,67 | 98.9 | 63,38 | 97.0 | 65,68 | 98.0 | 64,44 | 95.2 | 62,51 | 97.5 | 62,59 | 96.2 | 62,74 |
| 181 | 97.23 | 97.3 | 63,54 | 97.6 | 64,90 | 97.4 | 64,14 | 99.4 | 64,30 | 97.6 | 66,62 | 98.6 | 65,37 | 95.6 | 62,97 | 97.5 | 63,09 | 96.4 | 63,21 |
| 182 | 97.97 | 98.0 | 64,00 | 98.5 | 65,38 | 98.2 | 64,60 | 99.4 | 64,30 | 98.8 | 67,09 | 99.1 | 65,83 | 96.9 | 63,43 | 98.2 | 64,10 | 97.4 | 63,69 |
| 183 | 98.65 | 98.3 | 64,46 | 99.4 | 65,85 | 98.8 | 65,07 | 99.4 | 64,30 | 98.8 | 67,09 | 99.1 | 65,83 | 97.4 | 63,89 | 100.0 | 60,58 | 98.5 | 64,17 |
| 184 | 99.32 | 99.0 | 64,92 | 99.7 | 66,33 | 99.3 | 65,54 | 100.0 | 65,68 | 99.4 | 68,03 | 99.7 | 66,76 | 98.2 | 64,35 | 100.0 | 64,60 | 99.0 | 64,64 |
| 185 | 100.00 | 100.0 | 65,38 | 100.0 | 66,81 | 100.0 | 66,00 | 100.0 | 65,68 | 100.0 | 68,51 | 100.0 | 67,22 | 100.0 | 64,80 | 100.0 | 64,60 | 100.0 | 65,12 |

*Note: Calculation of scores was restricted to complete cases.* **RS** *= raw score;* **TRS** *= transformed raw score (range 0-100);* **PR** *= percentile;* **TS** *= T-score (M = 50, SD = 10).*
\* *This reference table should be used when treatment/medication applies to children.*

**Table 8** The total score of the DISABKIDS chronic generic module (if the "treatment" scale is not applicable; self-report) – DCGM-37-S (V-31)

| DCGM-37-S (V-31) TOTAL SCORE (V-31) SELF-REPORT | | Total sample 8-12 (n=462) | | Total sample 13-16 (n=387) | | Total sample Overall (n=849) | | Females 8-12 (n=206) | | Females 13-16 (n=194) | | Females Overall (n=400) | | Males 8-12 (n=256) | | Males 13-16 (n=193) | | Males Overall (n=449) | |
|---|---|---|---|---|---|---|---|---|---|---|---|---|---|---|---|---|---|---|---|
| RS | TRS | PR | TS | PR | TS | PR | TS | PR | TS | PR | TS | PR | TS | PR | TS | PR | TS | PR | TS |
| <= 75 | 35,48 | 1,1 | 21,26 | ,5 | 18,68 | 1,2 | 21,87 | 1,0 | 20,77 | 1,0 | 21,22 | 1,0 | 21,90 | 1,2 | 20,60 | - | - | ,7 | 18,56 |
| 76 | 36,29 | 1,3 | 21,80 | ,8 | 20,95 | 1,4 | 22,41 | 1,0 | 20,77 | 1,5 | 23,45 | 1,3 | 22,46 | 1,6 | 22,19 | - | - | ,9 | 20,24 |
| 77 | 37,10 | 1,5 | 22,35 | 1,0 | 21,52 | 1,6 | 22,95 | 1,5 | 21,88 | 2,1 | 24,00 | 1,8 | 23,01 | 1,6 | 22,19 | - | - | ,9 | 20,24 |
| 78 | 37,90 | 1,9 | 22,89 | 1,0 | 21,52 | 1,8 | 23,49 | 1,9 | 22,44 | 2,1 | 24,00 | 2,0 | 23,57 | 2,0 | 23,25 | ,5 | 18,90 | 1,1 | 21,36 |
| 79 | 38,71 | 2,2 | 23,43 | 1,3 | 22,65 | 2,0 | 24,03 | 1,9 | 22,44 | 2,1 | 24,00 | 2,0 | 23,57 | 2,3 | 23,79 | ,5 | 18,90 | 1,6 | 21,91 |
| 80 | 39,52 | 2,2 | 23,43 | 1,6 | 23,22 | 2,1 | 24,57 | 1,9 | 22,44 | 2,6 | 25,67 | 2,3 | 24,68 | 2,3 | 23,79 | ,5 | 18,90 | 1,6 | 21,91 |
| 81 | 40,32 | 2,2 | 23,43 | 1,6 | 23,22 | 2,1 | 24,57 | 1,9 | 22,44 | 2,6 | 25,67 | 2,3 | 24,68 | 2,3 | 23,79 | ,5 | 18,90 | 1,6 | 21,91 |
| 82 | 41,13 | 2,2 | 23,43 | 1,6 | 23,22 | 2,2 | 25,64 | 1,9 | 22,44 | 2,6 | 25,67 | 2,3 | 24,68 | 2,3 | 23,79 | ,5 | 18,90 | 1,6 | 21,91 |
| 83 | 41,94 | 2,2 | 23,43 | 2,3 | 24,92 | 2,7 | 26,18 | 1,9 | 22,44 | 4,1 | 27,33 | 3,0 | 26,34 | 2,3 | 23,79 | ,5 | 18,90 | 1,6 | 21,91 |
| 84 | 42,74 | 2,2 | 23,43 | 2,3 | 24,92 | 2,7 | 26,18 | 1,9 | 22,44 | 4,1 | 27,33 | 3,0 | 26,34 | 2,3 | 23,79 | ,5 | 18,90 | 1,6 | 21,91 |
| 85 | 43,55 | 2,2 | 23,43 | 2,8 | 26,06 | 3,0 | 27,26 | 1,9 | 22,44 | 4,6 | 28,44 | 3,3 | 27,45 | 2,3 | 23,79 | 1,0 | 22,51 | 1,8 | 25,26 |
| 86 | 44,35 | 2,6 | 27,24 | 3,1 | 26,63 | 3,4 | 27,80 | 2,9 | 26,91 | 5,2 | 29,00 | 4,0 | 28,01 | 2,3 | 23,79 | 1,0 | 22,51 | 1,8 | 25,26 |
| 87 | 45,16 | 2,6 | 27,24 | 3,1 | 26,63 | 3,4 | 27,80 | 2,9 | 26,91 | 5,2 | 29,00 | 4,0 | 28,01 | 2,3 | 23,79 | 1,0 | 22,51 | 1,8 | 25,26 |
| 88 | 45,97 | 3,0 | 28,32 | 3,4 | 27,76 | 3,8 | 28,88 | 3,9 | 28,03 | 5,7 | 30,11 | 4,8 | 29,12 | 2,3 | 23,79 | 1,0 | 22,51 | 1,8 | 25,26 |
| 89 | 46,77 | 3,2 | 28,87 | 3,4 | 27,76 | 3,9 | 29,42 | 3,9 | 28,03 | 5,7 | 30,11 | 4,8 | 29,12 | 2,7 | 29,10 | 1,0 | 22,51 | 2,0 | 27,50 |
| 90 | 47,58 | 3,9 | 29,41 | 3,4 | 27,76 | 4,3 | 29,96 | 4,9 | 29,14 | 5,7 | 30,11 | 5,3 | 30,23 | 3,1 | 29,63 | 1,0 | 22,51 | 2,2 | 28,05 |
| 91 | 48,39 | 4,8 | 29,95 | 3,6 | 29,46 | 4,8 | 30,50 | 6,3 | 29,70 | 6,2 | 31,78 | 6,3 | 30,78 | 3,5 | 30,16 | 1,0 | 22,51 | 2,4 | 28,61 |
| 92 | 49,19 | 5,0 | 30,50 | 3,9 | 30,03 | 5,2 | 31,04 | 6,8 | 30,26 | 6,7 | 32,33 | 6,8 | 31,34 | 3,5 | 30,16 | 1,0 | 22,51 | 2,4 | 28,61 |
| 93 | 50,00 | 5,4 | 31,04 | 3,9 | 30,03 | 5,5 | 31,58 | 7,3 | 30,82 | 6,7 | 32,33 | 7,0 | 31,89 | 3,9 | 31,23 | 1,0 | 22,51 | 2,7 | 29,73 |
| 94 | 50,81 | 5,6 | 31,58 | 4,4 | 31,16 | 5,9 | 32,12 | 7,8 | 31,38 | 6,7 | 32,33 | 7,3 | 32,45 | 3,9 | 31,23 | 2,1 | 27,93 | 3,1 | 30,29 |
| 95 | 51,61 | 6,1 | 32,13 | 4,7 | 31,73 | 6,2 | 32,66 | 8,3 | 31,93 | 6,7 | 32,33 | 7,5 | 33,00 | 4,3 | 31,23 | 2,6 | 28,54 | 3,6 | 30,84 |
| 96 | 52,42 | 6,5 | 32,67 | 5,4 | 32,30 | 6,8 | 33,20 | 8,7 | 32,49 | 7,7 | 34,56 | 8,3 | 33,56 | 4,7 | 32,29 | 3,1 | 29,14 | 4,0 | 31,40 |
| 97 | 53,23 | 6,9 | 33,21 | 5,9 | 32,86 | 7,4 | 33,74 | 9,2 | 33,05 | 8,2 | 35,11 | 8,8 | 34,11 | 5,1 | 32,82 | 3,6 | 29,74 | 4,5 | 31,96 |
| 98 | 54,03 | 7,1 | 33,76 | 6,7 | 33,43 | 8,0 | 34,28 | 9,2 | 33,05 | 8,2 | 35,11 | 8,8 | 34,11 | 5,2 | 33,35 | 5,2 | 30,34 | 5,3 | 32,52 |
| 99 | 54,84 | 7,6 | 34,30 | 8,5 | 34,00 | 8,9 | 34,82 | 9,2 | 33,05 | 11,3 | 36,22 | 10,3 | 35,22 | 6,3 | 33,88 | 5,7 | 30,95 | 6,0 | 33,08 |
| 100 | 55,65 | 8,9 | 34,84 | 9,0 | 34,57 | 9,9 | 35,35 | 9,2 | 33,05 | 11,9 | 36,78 | 10,5 | 35,78 | 8,6 | 34,42 | 6,2 | 31,55 | 7,6 | 33,64 |
| 101 | 56,45 | 10,0 | 35,39 | 9,8 | 35,13 | 10,9 | 35,89 | 9,2 | 33,05 | 12,9 | 37,33 | 11,0 | 36,33 | 10,5 | 34,95 | 6,7 | 32,15 | 8,9 | 34,19 |
| 102 | 57,26 | 10,6 | 35,93 | 11,4 | 35,70 | 12,0 | 36,43 | 9,7 | 35,84 | 13,9 | 37,89 | 11,8 | 36,89 | 11,3 | 35,48 | 8,8 | 32,75 | 10,2 | 34,75 |
| 103 | 58,06 | 11,0 | 36,47 | 12,4 | 36,27 | 12,8 | 36,97 | 10,2 | 36,40 | 14,9 | 38,44 | 12,5 | 37,44 | 11,7 | 36,01 | 9,8 | 33,36 | 10,9 | 35,31 |
| 104 | 58,87 | 11,3 | 37,02 | 12,7 | 36,84 | 13,2 | 37,51 | 10,7 | 36,96 | 15,5 | 39,00 | 13,0 | 37,99 | 11,7 | 36,54 | 9,8 | 33,36 | 10,9 | 35,31 |
| 105 | 59,68 | 12,6 | 37,56 | 13,7 | 37,40 | 14,3 | 38,05 | 11,7 | 37,52 | 16,5 | 39,55 | 14,0 | 38,55 | 13,3 | 37,60 | 10,9 | 34,56 | 12,2 | 36,43 |
| 106 | 60,48 | 13,2 | 38,10 | 15,0 | 37,97 | 15,1 | 38,59 | 12,1 | 38,08 | 17,5 | 40,11 | 14,8 | 39,10 | 14,1 | 38,14 | 12,4 | 35,16 | 13,4 | 36,99 |
| 107 | 61,29 | 14,3 | 38,65 | 15,8 | 38,54 | 16,0 | 39,13 | 13,1 | 38,63 | 19,1 | 40,67 | 16,0 | 39,66 | 15,2 | 38,67 | 12,4 | 35,16 | 14,0 | 37,54 |
| 108 | 62,10 | 15,4 | 39,19 | 17,6 | 39,10 | 17,4 | 39,67 | 13,6 | 39,19 | 20,1 | 41,22 | 16,8 | 40,21 | 16,8 | 39,20 | 15,0 | 36,37 | 16,0 | 38,10 |
| 109 | 62,90 | 17,5 | 39,73 | 18,6 | 39,67 | 18,8 | 40,21 | 16,0 | 39,75 | 21,1 | 41,78 | 18,5 | 40,77 | 18,8 | 39,73 | 16,1 | 36,97 | 17,6 | 38,66 |
| 110 | 63,71 | 19,0 | 40,28 | 19,1 | 40,24 | 19,8 | 40,75 | 18,0 | 40,31 | 21,1 | 41,78 | 19,5 | 41,32 | 19,9 | 40,26 | 17,1 | 37,57 | 18,7 | 39,22 |
| 111 | 64,52 | 20,8 | 40,82 | 19,9 | 40,81 | 21,0 | 41,29 | 18,4 | 40,87 | 22,2 | 42,89 | 20,3 | 41,88 | 22,7 | 40,79 | 17,6 | 38,17 | 20,5 | 39,78 |
| 112 | 65,32 | 21,6 | 41,36 | 20,7 | 41,37 | 22,0 | 41,83 | 18,9 | 41,43 | 23,7 | 43,44 | 21,3 | 42,43 | 23,8 | 41,32 | 17,6 | 38,17 | 21,2 | 40,33 |
| 113 | 66,13 | 22,3 | 41,91 | 21,2 | 41,94 | 22,5 | 42,37 | 20,4 | 41,98 | 24,2 | 44,00 | 22,3 | 42,99 | 23,8 | 41,32 | 18,1 | 39,38 | 21,4 | 40,89 |
| 114 | 66,94 | 22,7 | 42,45 | 22,0 | 42,51 | 23,1 | 42,91 | 21,4 | 42,54 | 24,2 | 44,00 | 22,8 | 43,54 | 23,8 | 41,32 | 19,7 | 39,98 | 22,0 | 41,45 |
| 115 | 67,74 | 23,2 | 43,00 | 23,5 | 43,07 | 24,0 | 43,45 | 21,4 | 42,54 | 27,3 | 45,11 | 24,3 | 44,10 | 24,6 | 42,92 | 19,7 | 39,98 | 22,5 | 42,01 |

# Reference tables

## Table 8  continued

| DCGM-37-S (V-31) TOTAL SCORE (V-31) SELF-REPORT | | Total sample 8-12 (n =462) | | Total sample 13-16 (n =387) | | Total sample Overall (n =849) | | Females 8-12 (n =206) | | Females 13-16 (n =194) | | Females Overall (n =400) | | Males 8-12 (n =256) | | Males 13-16 (n =193) | | Males Overall (n =449) | |
|---|---|---|---|---|---|---|---|---|---|---|---|---|---|---|---|---|---|---|---|
| RS | TRS | PR | TS | PR | TS | PR | TS | PR | TS | RS | TRS | PR | TS | PR | TS | PR | TS | PR | TS |
| 116 | 68,55 | 24,5 | 43,54 | 25,3 | 43,64 | 25,6 | 43,99 | 22,8 | 43,66 | 30,9 | 45,66 | 26,8 | 44,65 | 25,8 | 43,45 | 19,7 | 39,98 | 23,2 | 42,57 |
| 117 | 69,35 | 26,2 | 44,08 | 26,4 | 44,21 | 26,9 | 44,53 | 24,8 | 44,22 | 31,4 | 46,22 | 28,0 | 45,21 | 27,3 | 43,98 | 21,2 | 41,79 | 24,7 | 43,13 |
| 118 | 70,16 | 28,4 | 44,63 | 27,9 | 44,78 | 28,8 | 45,07 | 27,2 | 44,78 | 33,5 | 46,78 | 30,3 | 45,76 | 29,3 | 44,51 | 22,3 | 42,39 | 26,3 | 43,68 |
| 119 | 70,97 | 29,2 | 45,17 | 30,0 | 45,34 | 30,2 | 45,60 | 27,2 | 44,78 | 36,1 | 47,33 | 31,5 | 46,32 | 30,9 | 45,04 | 23,8 | 42,99 | 27,8 | 44,24 |
| 120 | 71,77 | 30,7 | 45,71 | 31,3 | 45,91 | 31,5 | 46,14 | 29,6 | 45,89 | 38,7 | 47,89 | 34,0 | 46,87 | 31,6 | 45,58 | 23,8 | 42,99 | 28,3 | 44,80 |
| 121 | 72,58 | 31,6 | 46,26 | 32,8 | 46,48 | 32,8 | 46,68 | 31,1 | 46,45 | 40,2 | 48,44 | 35,5 | 47,43 | 32,0 | 46,11 | 25,4 | 44,20 | 29,2 | 45,36 |
| 122 | 73,39 | 32,7 | 46,80 | 33,9 | 47,05 | 33,8 | 47,22 | 33,0 | 47,01 | 40,7 | 49,00 | 36,8 | 47,98 | 32,4 | 46,64 | 26,9 | 44,80 | 30,1 | 45,92 |
| 123 | 74,19 | 33,5 | 47,34 | 34,6 | 47,61 | 34,6 | 47,76 | 33,5 | 47,57 | 41,8 | 49,55 | 37,5 | 48,54 | 33,6 | 47,17 | 27,5 | 45,40 | 31,0 | 46,47 |
| 124 | 75,00 | 34,6 | 47,89 | 36,4 | 48,18 | 36,4 | 48,30 | 34,5 | 48,13 | 44,8 | 50,11 | 39,5 | 49,09 | 34,8 | 47,70 | 28,0 | 46,01 | 31,8 | 47,03 |
| 125 | 75,81 | 36,6 | 48,43 | 39,8 | 48,75 | 38,7 | 48,84 | 37,4 | 48,69 | 47,4 | 50,66 | 42,3 | 49,65 | 35,9 | 48,23 | 32,1 | 46,61 | 34,3 | 47,59 |
| 126 | 76,61 | 38,1 | 48,97 | 40,8 | 49,31 | 39,9 | 49,38 | 39,8 | 49,24 | 48,5 | 51,22 | 44,0 | 50,20 | 36,7 | 48,76 | 33,2 | 47,21 | 35,2 | 48,15 |
| 127 | 77,42 | 40,0 | 49,52 | 43,7 | 49,88 | 42,1 | 49,92 | 40,8 | 49,80 | 51,0 | 51,78 | 45,8 | 50,76 | 39,5 | 49,30 | 36,3 | 47,81 | 38,1 | 48,71 |
| 128 | 78,23 | 41,8 | 50,06 | 44,4 | 50,45 | 43,3 | 50,46 | 42,7 | 50,36 | 52,1 | 52,33 | 47,3 | 51,31 | 41,0 | 49,83 | 36,8 | 48,41 | 39,2 | 49,27 |
| 129 | 79,03 | 43,7 | 50,60 | 47,5 | 51,02 | 45,8 | 51,00 | 45,6 | 50,92 | 54,6 | 52,89 | 50,0 | 51,87 | 42,2 | 50,36 | 40,4 | 49,02 | 41,4 | 49,82 |
| 130 | 79,84 | 45,7 | 51,15 | 49,1 | 51,58 | 47,5 | 51,54 | 49,0 | 51,48 | 56,2 | 53,44 | 52,5 | 52,42 | 43,0 | 50,89 | 42,0 | 49,62 | 42,5 | 50,38 |
| 131 | 80,65 | 47,8 | 51,69 | 51,4 | 52,15 | 49,8 | 52,08 | 51,0 | 52,04 | 58,8 | 54,00 | 54,8 | 52,98 | 45,3 | 51,42 | 44,0 | 50,22 | 44,8 | 50,94 |
| 132 | 81,45 | 50,0 | 52,23 | 55,3 | 52,72 | 52,7 | 52,62 | 52,4 | 52,59 | 62,9 | 54,55 | 57,5 | 53,53 | 48,0 | 51,95 | 47,7 | 50,82 | 47,9 | 51,50 |
| 133 | 82,26 | 52,6 | 52,78 | 58,1 | 53,28 | 55,4 | 53,16 | 54,9 | 53,15 | 67,0 | 55,11 | 60,8 | 54,09 | 50,8 | 52,48 | 49,2 | 51,43 | 50,1 | 52,06 |
| 134 | 83,06 | 55,4 | 53,32 | 60,2 | 53,85 | 58,0 | 53,70 | 57,3 | 53,71 | 69,6 | 55,66 | 63,3 | 54,64 | 53,9 | 53,02 | 50,8 | 52,03 | 52,6 | 52,61 |
| 135 | 83,87 | 58,0 | 53,86 | 62,3 | 54,42 | 60,6 | 54,24 | 60,2 | 54,27 | 72,2 | 56,22 | 66,0 | 55,20 | 56,3 | 53,55 | 52,3 | 52,63 | 54,6 | 53,17 |
| 136 | 84,68 | 60,6 | 54,41 | 64,6 | 54,99 | 63,0 | 54,78 | 62,6 | 54,83 | 74,2 | 56,77 | 68,3 | 55,75 | 59,0 | 54,08 | 54,9 | 53,23 | 57,2 | 53,73 |
| 137 | 85,48 | 63,2 | 54,95 | 66,1 | 55,55 | 65,0 | 55,31 | 66,0 | 55,39 | 76,3 | 57,33 | 71,0 | 56,31 | 60,9 | 54,61 | 56,0 | 53,84 | 58,8 | 54,29 |
| 138 | 86,29 | 66,2 | 55,49 | 68,2 | 56,12 | 67,4 | 55,85 | 68,9 | 55,94 | 78,9 | 57,89 | 73,8 | 56,86 | 64,1 | 55,14 | 57,5 | 54,44 | 61,2 | 54,85 |
| 139 | 87,10 | 68,2 | 56,04 | 71,3 | 56,69 | 70,0 | 56,39 | 71,8 | 56,50 | 80,4 | 58,44 | 76,0 | 57,42 | 65,2 | 55,67 | 62,2 | 55,04 | 63,9 | 55,41 |
| 140 | 87,90 | 72,5 | 56,58 | 73,1 | 57,26 | 73,2 | 56,93 | 74,8 | 57,06 | 81,4 | 59,00 | 78,0 | 57,97 | 70,7 | 56,21 | 64,8 | 55,64 | 68,2 | 55,96 |
| 141 | 88,71 | 75,1 | 57,12 | 76,7 | 57,82 | 76,0 | 57,47 | 78,2 | 57,62 | 85,1 | 59,55 | 81,5 | 58,53 | 72,7 | 56,74 | 68,4 | 56,25 | 70,8 | 56,52 |
| 142 | 89,52 | 78,4 | 57,67 | 78,8 | 58,39 | 78,8 | 58,01 | 81,1 | 58,18 | 86,1 | 60,11 | 83,5 | 59,08 | 76,2 | 57,27 | 71,5 | 56,85 | 74,2 | 57,08 |
| 143 | 90,32 | 80,1 | 58,21 | 81,1 | 58,96 | 80,7 | 58,55 | 82,0 | 58,74 | 88,1 | 60,66 | 85,0 | 59,64 | 78,5 | 57,80 | 74,1 | 57,45 | 76,6 | 57,64 |
| 144 | 91,13 | 81,2 | 58,75 | 83,7 | 59,52 | 82,3 | 59,09 | 83,0 | 59,29 | 90,7 | 61,22 | 86,8 | 60,19 | 79,7 | 58,33 | 76,7 | 58,05 | 78,4 | 58,20 |
| 145 | 91,94 | 83,5 | 59,30 | 87,1 | 60,09 | 85,4 | 59,63 | 85,0 | 59,85 | 93,3 | 61,77 | 89,0 | 60,75 | 82,4 | 58,86 | 80,8 | 58,65 | 81,7 | 58,75 |
| 146 | 92,74 | 85,3 | 59,84 | 88,4 | 60,66 | 86,9 | 60,17 | 87,9 | 60,41 | 93,8 | 62,33 | 90,8 | 61,30 | 83,2 | 59,39 | 82,9 | 59,26 | 83,1 | 59,31 |
| 147 | 93,55 | 88,5 | 60,38 | 90,4 | 61,23 | 89,5 | 60,71 | 92,7 | 60,97 | 94,8 | 62,89 | 93,8 | 61,86 | 85,2 | 59,93 | 86,0 | 59,86 | 85,5 | 59,87 |
| 148 | 94,35 | 92,2 | 60,93 | 92,2 | 61,79 | 92,2 | 61,25 | 95,6 | 61,53 | 95,9 | 63,44 | 95,8 | 62,41 | 89,5 | 60,46 | 88,6 | 60,46 | 89,1 | 60,43 |
| 149 | 95,16 | 93,3 | 61,47 | 94,1 | 62,36 | 93,5 | 61,79 | 96,6 | 62,09 | 96,4 | 64,00 | 96,5 | 62,97 | 90,6 | 60,99 | 91,7 | 61,06 | 91,1 | 60,99 |
| 150 | 95,97 | 95,0 | 62,01 | 95,3 | 62,93 | 95,1 | 62,33 | 97,1 | 62,64 | 96,9 | 64,55 | 97,0 | 63,52 | 93,4 | 61,52 | 93,8 | 61,67 | 93,5 | 61,55 |
| 151 | 96,77 | 96,1 | 62,56 | 96,9 | 63,49 | 96,2 | 62,87 | 98,1 | 63,20 | 97,4 | 65,11 | 97,8 | 64,08 | 94,5 | 62,05 | 96,4 | 62,27 | 95,3 | 62,10 |
| 152 | 97,58 | 97,0 | 63,10 | 97,9 | 64,06 | 97,1 | 63,41 | 98,5 | 63,76 | 97,9 | 65,66 | 98,3 | 64,63 | 95,7 | 62,58 | 96,9 | 62,87 | 96,2 | 62,66 |
| 153 | 98,39 | 98,1 | 63,64 | 98,4 | 64,63 | 98,2 | 63,95 | 99,0 | 64,32 | 98,5 | 66,22 | 98,8 | 65,19 | 97,3 | 63,11 | 98,4 | 63,47 | 97,8 | 63,22 |
| 154 | 99,19 | 98,5 | 64,19 | 99,2 | 65,20 | 98,9 | 64,49 | 99,5 | 64,88 | 99,5 | 66,77 | 99,5 | 65,74 | 97,7 | 63,65 | 99,0 | 64,08 | 98,2 | 63,78 |
| 155 | 100,00 | 100,0 | 64,73 | 100,0 | 65,76 | 100,0 | 65,02 | 100,0 | 65,44 | 100,0 | 67,33 | 100,0 | 66,30 | 100,0 | 64,18 | 100,0 | 64,68 | 100,0 | 64,34 |

Note: Calculation of scores was restricted to complete cases. RS = raw score; TRS = transformed raw score (range 0-100); PR = percentile; TS = T-score (M = 50, SD = 10).

* This reference table should be used when treatment/medication does not apply to children.

**Table 9  The DISABKIDS chronic generic short-form score (if the "treatment" scale is applicable; self-report) – DCGM-12-S**

| DCGM-12-S SCORE SELF-REPORT | | Total sample 8-12 (n = 461) | | Total sample 13-16 (n =375) | | Total sample Overall (n = 836) | | Females 8-12 (n = 206) | | Females 13-16 (n = 194) | | Females Overall (n = 400) | | Males 8-12 (n = 255) | | Males 13-16 (n = 181) | | Males Overall (n = 436) | |
|---|---|---|---|---|---|---|---|---|---|---|---|---|---|---|---|---|---|---|---|
| RS | TRS | PR | TS | PR | TS | PR | TS | PR | TS | PR | TS | PR | TS | PR | TS | PR | TS | PR | TS |
| <=25 | 27.08 | 1.1 | 19,33 | .5 | 20,79 | .8 | 20,05 | 1.5 | 20,91 | 1.0 | 21,09 | 1.3 | 21,70 | .8 | 16,50 | - | - | .5 | 16,69 |
| 26 | 29.17 | 1.1 | 19,33 | 1.3 | 22,04 | 1.2 | 21,30 | 1.5 | 20,91 | 2.6 | 22,35 | 2.0 | 22,94 | .8 | 16,50 | - | - | .5 | 16,69 |
| 27 | 31.25 | 1.3 | 21,83 | 1.6 | 23,29 | 1.4 | 22,54 | 1.9 | 23,37 | 2.6 | 23,60 | 2.3 | 24,17 | .8 | 16,50 | .6 | 20,85 | .7 | 20,53 |
| 28 | 33.33 | 1.3 | 21,83 | 1.9 | 24,54 | 1.6 | 23,79 | 1.9 | 23,37 | 3.1 | 26,10 | 2.5 | 25,41 | .8 | 16,50 | .6 | 20,85 | .7 | 20,53 |
| 29 | 35.42 | 1.5 | 24,33 | 2.1 | 25,79 | 1.8 | 25,04 | 1.9 | 23,37 | 3.1 | 28,61 | 2.5 | 25,41 | 1.2 | 22,87 | 1.1 | 23,42 | 1.1 | 23,08 |
| 30 | 37.50 | 2.6 | 25,58 | 2.4 | 27,04 | 2.5 | 26,28 | 3.9 | 27,06 | 3.6 | 29,86 | 3.8 | 27,88 | 1.6 | 24,15 | 1.1 | 23,42 | 1.4 | 24,36 |
| 31 | 39.58 | 2.8 | 26,83 | 4.0 | 28,29 | 3.3 | 27,53 | 3.9 | 27,06 | 5.2 | 31,11 | 4.5 | 29,12 | 2.0 | 25,42 | 2.8 | 25,98 | 2.3 | 25,64 |
| 32 | 41.67 | 3.0 | 28,07 | 4.8 | 29,54 | 3.8 | 28,78 | 3.9 | 27,06 | 6.7 | 32,37 | 5.3 | 30,35 | 2.4 | 26,69 | 2.8 | 25,98 | 2.5 | 26,92 |
| 33 | 43.75 | 3.9 | 29,32 | 5.9 | 30,79 | 4.8 | 30,02 | 5.3 | 30,75 | 7.2 | 33,62 | 6.3 | 31,59 | 2.7 | 27,97 | 4.4 | 28,55 | 3.4 | 28,20 |
| 34 | 45.83 | 4.6 | 30,57 | 6.7 | 32,04 | 5.5 | 31,27 | 6.8 | 31,98 | 7.7 | 33,62 | 7.3 | 32,83 | 2.7 | 27,97 | 5.5 | 29,83 | 3.9 | 29,48 |
| 35 | 47.92 | 6.1 | 31,82 | 7.2 | 33,29 | 6.6 | 32,52 | 8.3 | 33,21 | 8.8 | 34,87 | 8.5 | 34,06 | 4.3 | 30,52 | 5.5 | 29,83 | 4.8 | 30,75 |
| 36 | 50.00 | 6.9 | 33,07 | 9.1 | 34,54 | 7.9 | 33,77 | 8.7 | 34,44 | 10.8 | 36,13 | 9.8 | 35,30 | 5.5 | 31,79 | 7.2 | 32,39 | 6.2 | 32,03 |
| 37 | 52.08 | 8.5 | 34,32 | 11.2 | 35,79 | 9.7 | 35,01 | 9.7 | 35,67 | 12.9 | 37,38 | 11.3 | 36,54 | 7.5 | 33,07 | 9.4 | 33,68 | 8.3 | 33,31 |
| 38 | 54.17 | 10.8 | 35,57 | 13.1 | 37,05 | 11.8 | 36,26 | 13.6 | 36,90 | 14.9 | 38,63 | 14.3 | 37,77 | 8.6 | 34,34 | 11.0 | 34,96 | 9.6 | 34,59 |
| 39 | 56.25 | 12.4 | 36,82 | 15.5 | 38,30 | 13.8 | 37,51 | 14.6 | 38,13 | 18.0 | 39,88 | 16.3 | 39,01 | 10.6 | 35,62 | 12.7 | 36,24 | 11.5 | 35,87 |
| 40 | 58.33 | 14.5 | 38,07 | 17.3 | 39,55 | 15.8 | 38,75 | 16.5 | 39,36 | 19.6 | 41,14 | 18.0 | 40,25 | 12.9 | 36,89 | 14.9 | 37,52 | 13.8 | 37,15 |
| 41 | 60.42 | 17.1 | 39,31 | 20.5 | 40,80 | 18.7 | 40,00 | 19.4 | 40,59 | 23.2 | 42,39 | 21.3 | 41,48 | 15.3 | 38,17 | 17.7 | 38,81 | 16.3 | 38,42 |
| 42 | 62.50 | 20.0 | 40,56 | 22.9 | 42,05 | 21.3 | 41,25 | 22.3 | 41,82 | 26.3 | 43,64 | 24.3 | 42,72 | 18.0 | 39,44 | 19.3 | 40,09 | 18.6 | 39,70 |
| 43 | 64.58 | 22.3 | 41,81 | 24.0 | 43,30 | 23.1 | 42,50 | 23.8 | 43,05 | 26.8 | 44,89 | 25.3 | 43,96 | 21.2 | 40,71 | 21.0 | 41,37 | 21.1 | 40,98 |
| 44 | 66.67 | 26.0 | 43,06 | 27.7 | 44,55 | 26.8 | 43,74 | 29.1 | 44,28 | 30.4 | 46,15 | 29.8 | 45,19 | 23.5 | 41,99 | 24.9 | 42,65 | 24.1 | 42,26 |
| 45 | 68.75 | 28.0 | 44,31 | 31.2 | 45,80 | 29.4 | 44,99 | 30.6 | 45,51 | 34.5 | 47,40 | 32.5 | 46,43 | 25.9 | 43,26 | 27.6 | 43,94 | 26.6 | 43,54 |
| 46 | 70.83 | 31.0 | 45,56 | 36.3 | 47,05 | 33.4 | 46,24 | 34.5 | 46,74 | 40.7 | 48,65 | 37.5 | 47,67 | 28.2 | 44,54 | 31.5 | 45,22 | 29.6 | 44,82 |
| 47 | 72.92 | 35.6 | 46,81 | 40.0 | 48,30 | 37.6 | 47,48 | 39.3 | 47,97 | 46.4 | 49,90 | 42.8 | 48,90 | 32.5 | 45,81 | 33.1 | 46,50 | 32.8 | 46,09 |
| 48 | 75.00 | 37.7 | 48,06 | 44.5 | 49,55 | 40.8 | 48,73 | 39.8 | 49,20 | 52.1 | 51,16 | 45.8 | 50,14 | 36.1 | 47,09 | 36.5 | 47,78 | 36.2 | 47,37 |
| 49 | 77.08 | 41.4 | 49,31 | 48.5 | 50,80 | 44.6 | 49,98 | 43.2 | 50,43 | 57.2 | 52,41 | 50.0 | 51,38 | 40.0 | 48,36 | 39.2 | 49,06 | 39.7 | 48,65 |
| 50 | 79.17 | 44.9 | 50,56 | 52.8 | 52,05 | 48.4 | 51,22 | 47.1 | 51,66 | 62.4 | 53,66 | 54.5 | 52,61 | 43.1 | 49,64 | 42.5 | 50,35 | 42.9 | 49,93 |
| 51 | 81.25 | 50.1 | 51,80 | 60.0 | 53,31 | 54.5 | 52,47 | 52.9 | 52,89 | 68.0 | 54,91 | 60.3 | 53,85 | 47.8 | 50,91 | 51.4 | 51,63 | 49.3 | 51,21 |
| 52 | 83.33 | 56.8 | 53,05 | 64.5 | 54,56 | 60.3 | 53,72 | 60.7 | 54,12 | 73.2 | 56,17 | 66.8 | 55,09 | 53.7 | 52,18 | 55.2 | 52,91 | 54.4 | 52,49 |
| 53 | 85.42 | 61.6 | 54,30 | 70.4 | 55,81 | 65.6 | 54,97 | 67.0 | 55,35 | 78.9 | 57,42 | 72.8 | 56,32 | 57.3 | 53,46 | 61.3 | 54,19 | 58.9 | 53,76 |
| 54 | 87.50 | 68.5 | 55,55 | 74.1 | 57,06 | 71.1 | 56,21 | 73.8 | 56,58 | 82.0 | 58,67 | 77.8 | 57,56 | 64.3 | 54,73 | 65.7 | 55,48 | 64.9 | 55,04 |
| 55 | 89.58 | 74.2 | 56,80 | 80.3 | 58,31 | 76.9 | 57,46 | 80.1 | 57,81 | 86.6 | 59,92 | 83.3 | 58,79 | 69.4 | 56,01 | 73.5 | 56,76 | 71.1 | 56,32 |
| 56 | 91.67 | 78.3 | 58,05 | 84.3 | 59,56 | 81.0 | 58,71 | 85.4 | 59,04 | 90.7 | 61,18 | 88.0 | 60,03 | 72.5 | 57,28 | 77.3 | 58,04 | 74.5 | 57,60 |
| 57 | 93.75 | 82.2 | 59,30 | 89.1 | 60,81 | 85.3 | 59,95 | 88.8 | 60,27 | 93.3 | 62,43 | 91.0 | 61,27 | 76.9 | 58,56 | 84.5 | 59,32 | 80.0 | 58,88 |
| 58 | 95.83 | 89.8 | 60,55 | 92.3 | 62,06 | 90.9 | 61,20 | 93.7 | 61,50 | 94.3 | 63,68 | 94.0 | 62,50 | 86.7 | 59,83 | 90.1 | 60,61 | 88.1 | 60,16 |
| 59 | 97.92 | 93.9 | 61,80 | 96.0 | 63,31 | 94.9 | 62,45 | 97.1 | 62,73 | 96.9 | 64,93 | 97.0 | 63,74 | 91.4 | 61,11 | 95.0 | 61,89 | 92.9 | 61,44 |
| 60 | 100.00 | 100.0 | 63,04 | 100.0 | 64,56 | 100.0 | 63,70 | 100.0 | 63,96 | 100.0 | 66,19 | 100.0 | 64,98 | 100.0 | 62,38 | 100.0 | 63,17 | 100.0 | 62,71 |

*Note: Calculation of scores was restricted to complete cases. RS = raw score; TRS = transformed raw score (range 0-100); PR = percentile; TS = T-score (M = 50, SD = 10).*

**Table 10  The DISABKIDS chronic generic short-form score (if the "treatment" scale is not applicable; self-report) – DCGM-12-S (V-10)**

| DCGM-12-S (V-10) SCORE (V-10) SELF-REPORT | | Total sample 8-12 (n = 514) | | Total sample 13-16 (n =425) | | Total sample Overall (n = 939) | | Females 8-12 (n = 231) | | Females 13-16 (n = 213) | | Females Overall (n = 444) | | Males 8-12 (n = 283) | | Males 13-16 (n = 212) | | Males Overall (n = 495) | |
|---|---|---|---|---|---|---|---|---|---|---|---|---|---|---|---|---|---|---|---|
| RS | TRS | PR | TS | PR | TS | PR | TS | PR | TS | PR | TS | PR | TS | PR | TS | PR | TS | PR | TS |
| <= 20 | <= 25.00 | ,6 | 13,58 | ,5 | 15,39 | ,5 | 14,45 | ,4 | 14,35 | ,5 | 16,86 | ,5 | 15,72 | ,7 | 12,94 | ,5 | 13,20 | ,6 | 13,01 |
| 21 | 27.50 | ,6 | 13,58 | ,5 | 15,39 | ,5 | 14,45 | ,4 | 14,35 | ,5 | 16,86 | ,5 | 15,72 | ,7 | 12,94 | ,5 | 13,20 | ,6 | 13,01 |
| 22 | 30.00 | ,8 | 19,58 | 1,2 | 21,29 | 1,0 | 20,40 | ,4 | 14,35 | 1,4 | 22,75 | ,9 | 21,62 | 1,1 | 18,97 | ,9 | 19,21 | 1,0 | 19,04 |
| 23 | 32.50 | 1,2 | 21,08 | 1,4 | 22,76 | 1,3 | 21,88 | 1,3 | 21,79 | 1,9 | 24,22 | 1,6 | 23,09 | 1,1 | 18,97 | ,9 | 19,21 | 1,0 | 19,04 |
| 24 | 35.00 | 1,9 | 22,58 | 2,1 | 24,23 | 2,0 | 23,37 | 2,6 | 23,28 | 3,3 | 25,70 | 2,9 | 24,56 | 1,4 | 21,99 | ,9 | 19,21 | 1,2 | 22,06 |
| 25 | 37.50 | 2,5 | 24,07 | 2,6 | 25,71 | 2,6 | 24,85 | 3,0 | 24,77 | 3,3 | 25,70 | 3,2 | 26,04 | 2,1 | 23,49 | 1,9 | 23,72 | 2,0 | 23,57 |
| 26 | 40.00 | 2,7 | 25,57 | 3,5 | 27,18 | 3,1 | 26,34 | 3,5 | 26,26 | 5,2 | 28,64 | 4,3 | 27,51 | 2,1 | 23,49 | 1,9 | 23,72 | 2,0 | 23,57 |
| 27 | 42.50 | 3,7 | 27,07 | 4,2 | 28,65 | 3,9 | 27,82 | 4,3 | 27,75 | 5,6 | 30,12 | 5,0 | 28,99 | 3,2 | 26,51 | 2,8 | 26,73 | 3,0 | 26,58 |
| 28 | 45.00 | 4,3 | 28,57 | 4,9 | 30,13 | 4,6 | 29,31 | 5,2 | 29,23 | 6,6 | 31,59 | 5,9 | 30,46 | 3,5 | 28,02 | 3,3 | 28,23 | 3,4 | 28,09 |
| 29 | 47.50 | 5,6 | 30,07 | 6,8 | 31,60 | 6,2 | 30,79 | 7,4 | 30,72 | 8,5 | 33,06 | 7,9 | 31,94 | 4,2 | 29,53 | 5,2 | 29,73 | 4,6 | 29,59 |
| 30 | 50.00 | 6,0 | 31,57 | 8,7 | 33,07 | 7,2 | 32,28 | 8,2 | 32,21 | 9,9 | 34,54 | 9,0 | 33,41 | 4,2 | 29,53 | 7,5 | 31,24 | 5,7 | 31,10 |
| 31 | 52.50 | 7,8 | 33,07 | 9,4 | 34,55 | 8,5 | 33,76 | 9,1 | 33,70 | 10,3 | 36,01 | 9,7 | 34,88 | 6,7 | 32,54 | 8,5 | 32,74 | 7,5 | 32,61 |
| 32 | 55.00 | 9,7 | 34,57 | 10,6 | 36,02 | 10,1 | 35,25 | 10,4 | 35,19 | 11,3 | 37,48 | 10,8 | 36,36 | 9,2 | 34,05 | 9,9 | 34,24 | 9,5 | 34,12 |
| 33 | 57.50 | 12,6 | 36,07 | 13,4 | 37,49 | 13,0 | 36,73 | 13,0 | 36,68 | 15,0 | 38,96 | 14,0 | 37,83 | 12,4 | 35,56 | 11,8 | 35,74 | 12,1 | 35,62 |
| 34 | 60.00 | 14,4 | 37,56 | 16,5 | 38,97 | 15,3 | 38,22 | 15,6 | 38,16 | 18,3 | 40,43 | 16,9 | 39,31 | 13,4 | 37,07 | 14,6 | 37,25 | 13,9 | 37,13 |
| 35 | 62.50 | 16,1 | 39,06 | 19,8 | 40,44 | 17,8 | 39,71 | 16,5 | 39,65 | 22,5 | 41,90 | 19,4 | 40,78 | 15,9 | 38,57 | 17,0 | 38,75 | 16,4 | 38,64 |
| 36 | 65.00 | 18,9 | 40,56 | 22,1 | 41,91 | 20,3 | 41,19 | 19,0 | 41,14 | 25,4 | 43,37 | 22,1 | 42,25 | 18,7 | 40,08 | 18,9 | 40,25 | 18,8 | 40,15 |
| 37 | 67.50 | 22,4 | 42,06 | 25,9 | 43,39 | 24,0 | 42,68 | 22,1 | 42,63 | 30,5 | 44,85 | 26,1 | 43,73 | 22,6 | 41,59 | 21,2 | 41,76 | 22,0 | 41,65 |
| 38 | 70.00 | 26,1 | 43,56 | 29,2 | 44,86 | 27,5 | 44,16 | 25,5 | 44,12 | 34,3 | 46,32 | 29,7 | 45,20 | 26,5 | 43,10 | 24,1 | 43,26 | 25,5 | 43,16 |
| 39 | 72.50 | 28,8 | 45,06 | 32,7 | 46,33 | 30,6 | 45,65 | 29,4 | 45,61 | 39,0 | 47,79 | 34,0 | 46,68 | 28,3 | 44,61 | 26,4 | 44,76 | 27,5 | 44,67 |
| 40 | 75.00 | 32,7 | 46,56 | 37,2 | 47,81 | 34,7 | 47,13 | 34,2 | 47,09 | 43,2 | 49,27 | 38,5 | 48,15 | 31,4 | 46,12 | 31,1 | 46,26 | 31,3 | 46,18 |
| 41 | 77.50 | 35,8 | 48,06 | 42,1 | 49,28 | 38,7 | 48,62 | 37,2 | 48,58 | 47,9 | 50,74 | 42,3 | 49,62 | 34,6 | 47,62 | 36,3 | 47,77 | 35,4 | 47,68 |
| 42 | 80.00 | 40,7 | 49,56 | 48,5 | 50,75 | 44,2 | 50,10 | 43,3 | 50,07 | 53,5 | 52,21 | 48,2 | 51,10 | 38,5 | 49,13 | 43,4 | 49,27 | 40,6 | 49,19 |
| 43 | 82.50 | 45,1 | 51,06 | 52,0 | 52,23 | 48,2 | 51,59 | 47,2 | 51,56 | 56,8 | 53,69 | 51,8 | 52,57 | 43,5 | 50,64 | 47,2 | 50,77 | 45,1 | 50,70 |
| 44 | 85.00 | 53,5 | 52,55 | 58,4 | 53,70 | 55,7 | 53,07 | 54,5 | 53,05 | 65,3 | 55,16 | 59,7 | 54,05 | 52,7 | 52,15 | 51,4 | 52,28 | 52,1 | 52,20 |
| 45 | 87.50 | 59,5 | 54,05 | 65,4 | 55,17 | 62,2 | 54,56 | 60,6 | 54,54 | 73,7 | 56,63 | 66,9 | 55,52 | 58,7 | 53,66 | 57,1 | 53,78 | 58,0 | 53,71 |
| 46 | 90.00 | 67,7 | 55,55 | 72,9 | 56,65 | 70,1 | 56,04 | 71,4 | 56,02 | 82,2 | 58,11 | 76,6 | 57,00 | 64,7 | 55,16 | 63,7 | 55,28 | 64,2 | 55,22 |
| 47 | 92.50 | 73,5 | 57,05 | 80,2 | 58,12 | 76,6 | 57,53 | 77,1 | 57,51 | 87,8 | 59,58 | 82,2 | 58,47 | 70,7 | 56,67 | 72,6 | 56,78 | 71,5 | 56,73 |
| 48 | 95.00 | 82,5 | 58,55 | 85,4 | 59,59 | 83,8 | 59,02 | 86,1 | 59,00 | 91,5 | 61,05 | 88,7 | 59,94 | 79,5 | 58,18 | 79,2 | 58,29 | 79,4 | 58,23 |
| 49 | 97.50 | 91,4 | 60,05 | 92,0 | 61,07 | 91,7 | 60,50 | 94,8 | 60,49 | 94,4 | 62,52 | 94,6 | 61,42 | 88,7 | 59,69 | 89,6 | 59,79 | 89,1 | 59,74 |
| 50 | 100.00 | 100,0 | 61,55 | 100,0 | 62,54 | 100,0 | 61,99 | 100,0 | 61,98 | 100,0 | 64,00 | 100,0 | 62,89 | 100,0 | 61,20 | 100,0 | 61,29 | 100,0 | 61,25 |

Note: Calculation of scores was restricted to complete cases. RS = raw score; TRS = transformed raw score (range 0-100); PR = percentile; TS = T-score (M = 50, SD = 10).

Table 11   DISABKIDS smiley module (self-report I) – DSM-S

| DSM-S SMILEYS SCORE SELF-REPORT | | Total sample 4-7 (n = 338) | | Total sample 8-12 (n = 535) | | Total sample 13-16 (n = 422) | | Total sample Overall (n = 1.345) | | Females 4-7 (n = 185) | | Females 8-12 (n = 242) | | Females 13-16 (n = 210) | | Females Overall (n = 637) | |
|---|---|---|---|---|---|---|---|---|---|---|---|---|---|---|---|---|---|
| RS | TRS | PR | TS | PR | TS | PR | TS | PR | TS | PR | TS | PR | TS | PR | TS | PR | TS |
| 6 | 0.00 | - | - | - | - | .2 | 9,21 | .1 | 8,35 | - | - | - | - | - | - | - | - |
| 7 | 4.17 | - | - | - | - | .2 | 9,21 | .1 | 8,35 | - | - | - | - | - | - | - | - |
| 8 | 8.33 | - | - | - | - | .2 | 9,21 | .1 | 8,35 | - | - | - | - | - | - | - | - |
| 9 | 12.50 | - | - | - | - | .2 | 9,21 | .1 | 8,35 | - | - | - | - | - | - | - | - |
| 10 | 16.67 | - | - | .2 | 15,83 | .5 | 17,34 | .2 | 16,36 | - | - | .4 | - | .5 | 17,22 | .3 | 16,17 |
| 11 | 20.83 | .3 | 18,06 | .2 | 15,83 | .9 | 20,05 | .4 | 19,03 | - | - | .4 | - | .5 | 17,22 | .3 | 16,17 |
| 12 | 25.00 | .3 | 18,06 | .4 | 21,24 | 1.4 | 22,76 | .7 | 21,71 | - | - | .4 | 16,36 | 1.0 | 22,86 | .5 | 21,61 |
| 13 | 29.17 | .3 | 18,06 | .6 | 23,94 | 1.7 | 25,47 | .8 | 24,38 | - | - | .8 | 24,59 | 1.0 | 22,86 | .6 | 24,33 |
| 14 | 33.33 | 1.3 | 25,97 | 2.1 | 26,64 | 3.3 | 28,19 | 2.2 | 27,05 | - | - | 1.2 | 27,33 | 3.3 | 28,49 | 1.6 | 27,05 |
| 15 | 37.50 | 3.1 | 28,61 | 3.4 | 29,35 | 4.5 | 30,90 | 3.6 | 29,72 | .5 | 26,15 | 3.7 | 30,08 | 4.8 | 31,31 | 3.1 | 29,77 |
| 16 | 41.67 | 5.4 | 31,25 | 4.5 | 32,05 | 6.4 | 33,61 | 5.4 | 32,40 | 3.2 | 28,94 | 5.4 | 32,82 | 7.1 | 34,13 | 5.3 | 32,49 |
| 17 | 45.83 | 9.8 | 33,89 | 7.7 | 34,75 | 11.8 | 36,32 | 9.6 | 35,07 | 7.0 | 31,72 | 8.7 | 35,57 | 13.3 | 36,95 | 9.7 | 35,21 |
| 18 | 50.00 | 12.9 | 36,53 | 15.3 | 37,46 | 15.2 | 39,03 | 14.6 | 37,74 | 9.2 | 34,50 | 15.7 | 38,31 | 18.1 | 39,76 | 14.6 | 37,94 |
| 19 | 54.17 | 16.8 | 39,17 | 19.8 | 40,16 | 21.1 | 41,74 | 19.3 | 40,41 | 12.4 | 37,29 | 22.3 | 41,05 | 23.3 | 42,58 | 19.8 | 40,66 |
| 20 | 58.33 | 22.4 | 41,81 | 28.8 | 42,86 | 31.3 | 44,45 | 27.7 | 43,08 | 17.8 | 40,07 | 33.1 | 43,80 | 36.2 | 45,40 | 29.7 | 43,38 |
| 21 | 62.50 | 31.7 | 44,45 | 38.1 | 45,56 | 41.7 | 47,16 | 37.4 | 45,76 | 27.6 | 42,85 | 43.0 | 46,54 | 48.1 | 48,22 | 40.2 | 46,10 |
| 22 | 66.67 | 41.8 | 47,09 | 47.1 | 48,27 | 53.8 | 49,87 | 47.7 | 48,43 | 39.5 | 45,64 | 51.7 | 49,29 | 60.0 | 51,03 | 50.9 | 48,82 |
| 23 | 70.83 | 51.0 | 49,73 | 56.3 | 50,97 | 67.1 | 52,58 | 58.1 | 51,10 | 47.6 | 48,42 | 60.3 | 52,03 | 71.0 | 53,85 | 60.1 | 51,54 |
| 24 | 75.00 | 64.2 | 52,37 | 68.2 | 53,67 | 73.5 | 55,29 | 68.7 | 53,77 | 61.6 | 51,20 | 72.3 | 54,77 | 80.0 | 56,67 | 71.7 | 54,26 |
| 25 | 79.17 | 73.5 | 55,01 | 76.6 | 56,38 | 81.8 | 58,00 | 77.3 | 56,45 | 70.8 | 53,99 | 81.0 | 57,52 | 86.2 | 59,49 | 79.7 | 56,98 |
| 26 | 83.33 | 80.7 | 57,65 | 83.9 | 59,08 | 86.5 | 60,71 | 83.8 | 59,12 | 78.9 | 56,77 | 87.6 | 60,26 | 89.5 | 62,30 | 85.7 | 59,71 |
| 27 | 87.50 | 86.6 | 60,28 | 89.9 | 61,78 | 94.8 | 63,43 | 90.5 | 61,79 | 83.8 | 59,55 | 92.1 | 63,01 | 94.8 | 65,12 | 90.6 | 62,43 |
| 28 | 91.67 | 92.8 | 62,92 | 95.0 | 64,48 | 98.3 | 66,14 | 95.4 | 64,46 | 91.4 | 62,34 | 95.9 | 65,75 | 98.6 | 67,94 | 95.4 | 65,15 |
| 29 | 95.83 | 95.1 | 65,56 | 97.9 | 67,19 | 99.1 | 68,85 | 97.5 | 67,13 | 91.9 | 65,12 | 97.9 | 68,49 | 99.5 | 70,76 | 96.7 | 67,87 |
| 30 | 100.00 | 100.0 | 68,20 | 100.0 | 69,89 | 100.0 | 71,56 | 100.0 | 69,81 | 100.0 | 67,90 | 100.0 | 71,24 | 100.0 | 73,57 | 100.0 | 70,59 |

Note: Calculation of z-scores was restricted to complete cases. RS = raw score; TRS = transformed raw score (range 0-100); PR = percentile; TS = T-score (M = 50, SD = 10).

**Table 12   DISABKIDS smiley module (self-report II) – DSM-S**

| DSM-S SMILEYS SCORE SELF-REPORT | | Males 4-7 (n =203) | | Males 8-12 (n =293) | | Males 13-16 (n =212) | | Males Overall (n =708) | |
|---|---|---|---|---|---|---|---|---|---|
| RS | TRS | PR | TS | PR | TS | PR | TS | PR | TS |
| 6 | 0.00 | - | - | - | - | - | - | - | - |
| 7 | 4.17 | - | - | - | - | .5 | 9,17 | .1 | 8,60 |
| 8 | 8.33 | - | - | - | - | .5 | 9,17 | .1 | 8,60 |
| 9 | 12.50 | - | - | - | - | .5 | 9,17 | .1 | 8,60 |
| 10 | 16.67 | - | - | - | - | .5 | 9,17 | .1 | 8,60 |
| 11 | 20.83 | .5 | - | - | - | 1.4 | 19,74 | .6 | 19,13 |
| 12 | 25.00 | .5 | 20,21 | .3 | 20,56 | 1.9 | 22,38 | .8 | 21,76 |
| 13 | 29.17 | .5 | 27,86 | .3 | 20,56 | 2.4 | 25,02 | 1.0 | 24,40 |
| 14 | 33.33 | 2.5 | 30,41 | 2.7 | 25,94 | 3.3 | 27,66 | 2.8 | 27,03 |
| 15 | 37.50 | 5.4 | 32,96 | 3.1 | 28,62 | 4.2 | 30,30 | 4.1 | 29,66 |
| 16 | 41.67 | 7.4 | 35,51 | 3.8 | 31,31 | 5.7 | 32,94 | 5.4 | 32,29 |
| 17 | 45.83 | 12.3 | 38,06 | 6.8 | 34,00 | 10.4 | 35,59 | 9.5 | 34,92 |
| 18 | 50.00 | 16.3 | 40,61 | 15.0 | 36,68 | 12.3 | 38,23 | 14.5 | 37,56 |
| 19 | 54.17 | 20.7 | 43,16 | 17.7 | 39,37 | 18.9 | 40,87 | 18.9 | 40,19 |
| 20 | 58.33 | 26.6 | 45,71 | 25.3 | 42,06 | 26.4 | 43,51 | 26.0 | 42,82 |
| 21 | 62.50 | 35.5 | 48,27 | 34.1 | 44,75 | 35.4 | 46,15 | 34.9 | 45,45 |
| 22 | 66.67 | 43.8 | 48,27 | 43.3 | 47,43 | 47.6 | 48,79 | 44.8 | 48,09 |
| 23 | 70.83 | 54.2 | 50,82 | 52.9 | 50,12 | 63.2 | 51,43 | 56.4 | 50,72 |
| 24 | 75.00 | 66.5 | 53,37 | 64.8 | 52,81 | 67.0 | 54,07 | 66.0 | 53,35 |
| 25 | 79.17 | 75.9 | 55,92 | 73.0 | 55,49 | 77.4 | 56,72 | 75.1 | 55,98 |
| 26 | 83.33 | 82.3 | 58,47 | 80.9 | 58,18 | 83.5 | 59,36 | 82.1 | 58,61 |
| 27 | 87.50 | 89.2 | 61,02 | 88.1 | 60,87 | 94.8 | 62,00 | 90.4 | 61,25 |
| 28 | 91.67 | 94.1 | 63,57 | 94.2 | 63,55 | 98.1 | 64,64 | 95.3 | 63,88 |
| 29 | 95.83 | 98.0 | 66,12 | 98.0 | 66,24 | 98.6 | 67,28 | 98.2 | 66,51 |
| 30 | 100.00 | 100.0 | 68,67 | 100.0 | 68,93 | 100.0 | 69,92 | 100.0 | 69,14 |

*Note: Calculation of scores was restricted to complete cases. RS = raw score; TRS = transformed raw score (range 0-100); PR = percentile; TS = T-score (M = 50, SD = 10).*

184

**Table 13  DISABKIDS condition specific module asthma, sub-scales "impact" and "worry" (self-report) – DCSM-AsM-S**

| DCSM-AsM-S IMPACT SELF-REPORT | | Total sample 8-12 (n = 218) | | Total sample 13-16 (n = 117) | | Total sample Overall (n = 335) | |
|---|---|---|---|---|---|---|---|
| RS | TRS | PR | TS | PR | TS | PR | TS |
| 6 | 0.00 | - | - | .9 | 26.75 | .3 | 21.53 |
| 7 | 4.17 | - | - | 1.7 | 28.44 | .6 | 23.36 |
| 8 | 8.33 | - | - | 2.6 | 30.13 | .9 | 25.19 |
| 9 | 12.50 | .9 | 22.68 | 3.4 | 31.83 | 1.8 | 27.02 |
| 10 | 16.67 | 1.8 | 24.70 | 5.1 | 33.52 | 3.0 | 28.84 |
| 11 | 20.83 | 2.3 | 26.72 | 9.4 | 35.21 | 4.8 | 30.67 |
| 12 | 25.00 | 2.3 | 26.72 | 13.7 | 36.90 | 6.3 | 32.50 |
| 13 | 29.17 | 5.0 | 30.75 | 17.9 | 38.59 | 9.6 | 34.33 |
| 14 | 33.33 | 6.9 | 32.77 | 25.6 | 40.28 | 13.4 | 36.16 |
| 15 | 37.50 | 10.1 | 34.78 | 28.2 | 41.97 | 16.4 | 37.99 |
| 16 | 41.67 | 13.3 | 36.80 | 33.3 | 43.66 | 20.3 | 39.82 |
| 17 | 45.83 | 17.4 | 38.82 | 35.9 | 45.35 | 23.9 | 41.64 |
| 18 | 50.00 | 22.0 | 40.83 | 40.2 | 47.04 | 28.4 | 43.47 |
| 19 | 54.17 | 28.0 | 42.85 | 43.6 | 48.73 | 33.4 | 45.30 |
| 20 | 58.33 | 31.7 | 44.87 | 49.6 | 50.42 | 37.9 | 47.13 |
| 21 | 62.50 | 36.2 | 46.88 | 55.6 | 52.11 | 43.0 | 48.96 |
| 22 | 66.67 | 45.0 | 48.90 | 61.5 | 53.80 | 50.7 | 50.79 |
| 23 | 70.83 | 53.2 | 50.92 | 69.2 | 55.49 | 58.8 | 52.61 |
| 24 | 75.00 | 58.7 | 52.93 | 76.1 | 57.18 | 64.8 | 54.44 |
| 25 | 79.17 | 70.2 | 54.95 | 82.9 | 58.87 | 74.6 | 56.27 |
| 26 | 83.33 | 77.1 | 56.97 | 87.2 | 60.56 | 80.6 | 58.10 |
| 27 | 87.50 | 82.1 | 58.98 | 90.6 | 62.25 | 85.1 | 59.93 |
| 28 | 91.67 | 88.1 | 61.00 | 94.9 | 63.94 | 90.4 | 61.76 |
| 29 | 95.83 | 93.1 | 63.02 | 95.7 | 65.63 | 94.0 | 63.59 |
| 30 | 100.00 | 100.0 | 65.03 | 100.0 | 67.32 | 100.0 | 65.41 |

| DCSM-AsM-S WORRY SELF-REPORT | | Total sample 8-12 (n = 230) | | Total sample 13-16 (n = 121) | | Total sample Overall (n = 351) | |
|---|---|---|---|---|---|---|---|
| RS | TRS | PR | TS | PR | TS | PR | TS |
| 5 | 0.00 | - | - | - | - | - | - |
| 6 | 5.00 | - | - | .8 | 17.82 | .3 | 14.77 |
| 7 | 10.00 | .9 | 15.36 | .8 | 17.82 | .9 | 17.13 |
| 8 | 15.00 | 1.7 | 17.82 | .8 | 17.82 | 1.4 | 19.50 |
| 9 | 20.00 | 1.7 | 17.82 | 1.7 | 24.44 | 1.7 | 21.86 |
| 10 | 25.00 | 2.2 | 22.75 | 2.5 | 26.64 | 2.3 | 24.22 |
| 11 | 30.00 | 3.0 | 25.21 | 5.0 | 28.85 | 3.7 | 26.59 |
| 12 | 35.00 | 3.5 | 27.68 | 8.3 | 31.05 | 5.1 | 28.95 |
| 13 | 40.00 | 7.0 | 30.14 | 11.6 | 33.26 | 8.5 | 31.32 |
| 14 | 45.00 | 9.1 | 32.61 | 12.4 | 35.46 | 10.3 | 33.68 |
| 15 | 50.00 | 11.7 | 35.07 | 13.2 | 37.67 | 12.3 | 36.05 |
| 16 | 55.00 | 13.9 | 37.53 | 19.0 | 39.87 | 15.7 | 38.41 |
| 17 | 60.00 | 18.7 | 40.00 | 25.6 | 42.07 | 21.1 | 40.78 |
| 18 | 65.00 | 21.7 | 42.46 | 29.8 | 44.28 | 24.5 | 43.14 |
| 19 | 70.00 | 26.5 | 44.92 | 33.1 | 46.48 | 28.8 | 45.51 |
| 20 | 75.00 | 34.3 | 47.39 | 38.0 | 48.69 | 35.6 | 47.87 |
| 21 | 80.00 | 45.2 | 49.85 | 46.3 | 50.89 | 45.6 | 50.24 |
| 22 | 85.00 | 52.2 | 52.31 | 52.9 | 53.10 | 52.4 | 52.60 |
| 23 | 90.00 | 62.6 | 54.78 | 62.8 | 55.30 | 62.7 | 54.97 |
| 24 | 95.00 | 77.8 | 57.24 | 76.0 | 57.51 | 77.2 | 57.33 |
| 25 | 100.00 | 100.0 | 59.70 | 100.0 | 59.71 | 100.0 | 59.69 |

Note: Calculation of scores was restricted to complete cases. RS = raw score; TRS = transformed raw score (range 0-100); PR = percentile; TS = T-score; TS = T-score (M = 50, SD = 10).

**Table 14 DISABKIDS condition specific module arthritis, sub-scales "impact" and "understanding" (self-report) – DCSM-ArM-S**

**DCSM-ArM-S IMPACT SELF-REPORT**

| RS | TRS | Total sample 8-12 (n = 68) | | Total sample 13-16 (n = 64) | | Total sample Overall (n = 132) | |
|----|------|------|-------|------|-------|------|-------|
| | | PR | TS | PR | TS | PR | TS |
| 9 | 0.00 | - | - | - | - | - | - |
| 10 | 2.78 | 1.5 | 18.37 | - | - | .8 | 22.81 |
| 11 | 5.56 | 1.5 | 18.37 | - | - | .8 | 22.81 |
| 12 | 8.33 | 1.5 | 18.37 | - | - | .8 | 22.81 |
| 13 | 11.11 | 1.5 | 18.37 | - | - | .8 | 22.81 |
| 14 | 13.89 | 1.5 | 18.37 | 1.6 | 30.78 | 1.5 | 27.75 |
| 15 | 16.67 | 1.5 | 18.37 | 3.1 | 31.92 | 2.3 | 28.98 |
| 16 | 19.44 | 1.5 | 18.37 | 4.7 | 33.06 | 3.0 | 30.21 |
| 17 | 22.22 | 1.5 | 18.37 | 7.8 | 34.19 | 4.5 | 31.45 |
| 18 | 25.00 | 1.5 | 18.37 | 9.4 | 35.33 | 5.3 | 32.68 |
| 19 | 27.78 | 2.9 | 30.67 | 10.9 | 36.47 | 6.8 | 33.91 |
| 20 | 30.56 | 2.9 | 30.67 | 12.5 | 37.61 | 7.6 | 35.15 |
| 21 | 33.33 | 2.9 | 30.67 | 15.6 | 38.75 | 9.1 | 36.38 |
| 22 | 36.11 | 5.9 | 34.77 | 18.8 | 39.89 | 12.1 | 37.61 |
| 23 | 38.89 | 7.4 | 36.14 | 21.9 | 41.03 | 14.4 | 38.84 |
| 24 | 41.67 | 10.3 | 37.50 | 28.1 | 42.17 | 18.9 | 40.08 |
| 25 | 44.44 | 19.1 | 38.87 | 31.3 | 43.31 | 25.0 | 41.31 |
| 26 | 47.22 | 22.1 | 40.23 | 35.9 | 44.45 | 28.8 | 42.54 |
| 27 | 50.00 | 25.0 | 41.60 | 40.6 | 45.59 | 32.6 | 43.78 |
| 28 | 52.78 | 26.5 | 42.97 | 43.8 | 46.72 | 34.8 | 45.01 |
| 29 | 55.56 | 30.9 | 44.33 | 48.4 | 47.86 | 39.4 | 46.24 |
| 30 | 58.33 | 36.8 | 45.70 | 51.6 | 49.00 | 43.9 | 47.48 |
| 31 | 61.11 | 39.7 | 47.07 | 53.1 | 50.14 | 46.2 | 48.71 |
| 32 | 63.89 | 44.1 | 48.43 | 53.1 | 50.14 | 48.5 | 49.94 |
| 33 | 66.67 | 50.0 | 49.80 | 56.3 | 52.42 | 53.0 | 51.18 |
| 34 | 69.44 | 54.4 | 51.17 | 64.1 | 53.56 | 59.1 | 52.41 |
| 35 | 72.22 | 61.8 | 52.53 | 64.1 | 53.56 | 62.9 | 53.64 |
| 36 | 75.00 | 64.7 | 53.90 | 70.3 | 55.84 | 67.4 | 54.88 |
| 37 | 77.78 | 70.6 | 55.26 | 71.9 | 56.98 | 71.2 | 56.11 |
| 38 | 80.56 | 73.5 | 56.63 | 75.0 | 58.12 | 74.2 | 57.34 |
| 39 | 83.33 | 77.9 | 58.00 | 75.0 | 58.12 | 76.5 | 58.58 |
| 40 | 86.11 | 80.9 | 59.36 | 78.1 | 60.39 | 79.5 | 59.81 |
| 41 | 88.89 | 83.8 | 60.73 | 82.8 | 61.53 | 83.3 | 61.04 |
| 42 | 91.67 | 89.7 | 62.10 | 90.6 | 62.67 | 90.2 | 62.28 |
| 43 | 94.44 | 92.6 | 63.46 | 95.3 | 63.81 | 93.9 | 63.51 |
| 44 | 97.22 | 95.6 | 64.83 | 96.9 | 64.95 | 96.2 | 64.74 |
| 45 | 100.00 | 100.0 | 66.20 | 100.0 | 66.09 | 100.0 | 65.98 |

**DCSM-ArM-S UNDERSTANDING SELF-REPORT**

| RS | TRS | Total sample 8-12 (n = 70) | | Total sample 13-16 (n = 65) | | Total sample Overall (n = 135) | |
|----|------|------|-------|------|-------|------|-------|
| | | PR | TS | PR | TS | PR | TS |
| 3 | 0.00 | 2.9 | 20.55 | 3.1 | 27.70 | 3.0 | 24.59 |
| 4 | 8.33 | 4.3 | 23.96 | 6.2 | 30.65 | 5.2 | 27.72 |
| 5 | 16.67 | 4.3 | 23.96 | 9.2 | 33.60 | 6.7 | 30.86 |
| 6 | 25.00 | 4.3 | 23.96 | 13.8 | 36.55 | 8.9 | 33.99 |
| 7 | 33.33 | 7.1 | 34.20 | 20.0 | 39.51 | 13.3 | 37.12 |
| 8 | 41.67 | 12.9 | 37.62 | 27.7 | 42.46 | 20.0 | 40.25 |
| 9 | 50.00 | 21.4 | 41.03 | 35.4 | 45.41 | 28.1 | 43.39 |
| 10 | 58.33 | 28.6 | 44.44 | 46.2 | 48.36 | 37.0 | 46.52 |
| 11 | 66.67 | 47.1 | 47.85 | 55.4 | 51.32 | 51.1 | 49.65 |
| 12 | 75.00 | 57.1 | 51.27 | 66.2 | 54.27 | 61.5 | 52.78 |
| 13 | 83.33 | 71.4 | 54.68 | 75.4 | 57.22 | 73.3 | 55.92 |
| 14 | 91.67 | 75.7 | 58.09 | 86.2 | 60.18 | 80.7 | 59.05 |
| 15 | 100.00 | 100.0 | 61.51 | 100.0 | 63.13 | 100.0 | 62.18 |

*Note: Calculation of scores was restricted to complete cases. RS = raw score; TRS = transformed raw score (range 0-100); PR = percentile; TS = T-score (M = 50, SD = 10).*

**Table 15  DISABKIDS condition specific module dermatitis, sub-scales "impact" and "stigma" (self-report) – DCSM-ADM-S**

| DCSM-ADM-S IMPACT SELF-REPORT | | Total sample 8-12 (n = 10) | | Total sample 13-16 (n = 26) | | Total sample Overall (n = 36) | |
|---|---|---|---|---|---|---|---|
| RS | TRS | PR | TS | PR | TS | PR | TS |
| 8 | 0.00 | - | - | - | - | - | - |
| 9 | 3.13 | - | - | - | - | - | - |
| 10 | 6.25 | - | - | - | - | - | - |
| 11 | 9.38 | - | - | - | - | - | - |
| 12 | 12.5 | - | - | 3.8 | 31,46 | 2.8 | 29,48 |
| 13 | 15.63 | - | - | 3.8 | 31,46 | 2.8 | 29,48 |
| 14 | 18.75 | 10.0 | 25,67 | 7.7 | 34,74 | 8.3 | 32,86 |
| 15 | 21.88 | 10.0 | 25,67 | 11.5 | 36,38 | 11.1 | 34,55 |
| 16 | 25.00 | 10.0 | 25,67 | 11.5 | 36,38 | 11.1 | 34,55 |
| 17 | 28.13 | 10.0 | 25,67 | 23.1 | 39,66 | 19.4 | 37,93 |
| 18 | 31.25 | 10.0 | 25,67 | 26.9 | 41,30 | 22.2 | 39,62 |
| 19 | 34.38 | 10.0 | 25,67 | 26.9 | 44,58 | 22.2 | 39,62 |
| 20 | 37.50 | 10.0 | 25,67 | 34.6 | 46,22 | 27.8 | 43,00 |
| 21 | 40.63 | 10.0 | 25,67 | 42.3 | 47,86 | 33.3 | 44,69 |
| 22 | 43.75 | 10.0 | 25,67 | 50.0 | 49,50 | 38.9 | 46,38 |
| 23 | 46.88 | 10.0 | 25,67 | 53.8 | 52,78 | 41.7 | 48,07 |
| 24 | 50.00 | 30.0 | 45,45 | 53.8 | 52,78 | 47.2 | 49,77 |
| 25 | 53.13 | 30.0 | 45,45 | 61.5 | 54,42 | 52.8 | 51,46 |
| 26 | 56.25 | 50.0 | 49,41 | 65.4 | 56,06 | 61.1 | 53,15 |
| 27 | 59.38 | 50.0 | 49,41 | 69.2 | 56,06 | 63.9 | 54,84 |
| 28 | 62.5 | 60.0 | 53,36 | 69.2 | 56,06 | 66.7 | 56,53 |
| 29 | 65.63 | 70.0 | 55,34 | 80.8 | 59,34 | 77.8 | 58,22 |
| 30 | 68.75 | 80.0 | 57,32 | 88.5 | 60,98 | 86.1 | 59,91 |
| 31 | 71.88 | 100.0 | 59,30 | 92.3 | 62,62 | 94.4 | 61,60 |
| 32 | 75.00 | 100.0 | 59,30 | 96.2 | 64,26 | 97.2 | 63,29 |
| 33 | 78.13 | 100.0 | 59,30 | 96.2 | 64,26 | 97.2 | 63,29 |
| 34 | 81.25 | 100.0 | 59,30 | 100.0 | 67,54 | 100.0 | 66,67 |
| 35 | 84.38 | 100.0 | 59,30 | 100.0 | 67,54 | 100.0 | 66,67 |
| 36 | 87.50 | 100.0 | 59,30 | 100.0 | 67,54 | 100.0 | 66,67 |
| 37 | 90.63 | 100.0 | 59,30 | 100.0 | 67,54 | 100.0 | 66,67 |
| 38 | 93.75 | 100.0 | 59,30 | 100.0 | 67,54 | 100.0 | 66,67 |
| 39 | 96.88 | 100.0 | 59,30 | 100.0 | 67,54 | 100.0 | 66,67 |
| 40 | 100.00 | 100.0 | 59,30 | 100.0 | 67,54 | 100.0 | 66,67 |

| DCSM-ADM-S STIGMA SELF-REPORT | | Total sample 8-12 (n = 10) | | Total sample 13-16 (n = 38) | | Total sample Overall (n = 48) | |
|---|---|---|---|---|---|---|---|
| RS | TRS | PR | TS | PR | TS | PR | TS |
| 4 | 0.00 | - | - | - | - | - | - |
| 5 | 6.25 | - | - | - | - | - | - |
| 6 | 12.50 | - | - | - | - | - | - |
| 7 | 18.75 | - | - | - | - | - | - |
| 8 | 25.00 | - | - | - | - | - | - |
| 9 | 31.25 | - | - | 5.3 | 31,55 | 4.2 | 29,66 |
| 10 | 37.50 | - | - | 7.9 | 34,72 | 6.3 | 32,83 |
| 11 | 43.75 | - | - | 15.8 | 37,90 | 12.5 | 36,00 |
| 12 | 50.00 | - | - | 28.9 | 41,07 | 22.9 | 39,17 |
| 13 | 56.25 | 10.0 | 25,85 | 36.8 | 44,24 | 31.3 | 42,34 |
| 14 | 62.50 | 10.0 | 25,85 | 50.0 | 47,41 | 41.7 | 45,51 |
| 15 | 68.75 | 10.0 | 25,85 | 55.3 | 50,58 | 45.8 | 48,68 |
| 16 | 75.00 | 10.0 | 25,85 | 65.8 | 53,76 | 54.2 | 51,85 |
| 17 | 81.25 | 40.0 | 46,40 | 71.1 | 56,93 | 64.6 | 55,02 |
| 18 | 87.50 | 60.0 | 51,54 | 84.2 | 60,10 | 79.2 | 58,19 |
| 19 | 93.75 | 90.0 | 56,68 | 97.4 | 63,27 | 95.8 | 61,36 |
| 20 | 100.00 | 100.0 | 61,82 | 100.0 | 66,44 | 100.0 | 64,53 |

*Note: Calculation of z-scores was restricted to complete cases. RS = raw score; TRS = transformed raw score (range 0-100); PR = percentile; TS = T-score (M = 50, SD = 10).*

187

**Table 16  DISABKIDS condition specific module diabetes, sub-scales "impact" and "treatment" (self-report) – DCSM-DM-S**

**DCSM-DM-S IMPACT SELF-REPORT**

| RS | TRS | Total sample 8-12 (n=94) | | Total sample 13-16 (n=92) | | Total sample Overall (n=186) | |
|---|---|---|---|---|---|---|---|
| | | PR | TS | PR | TS | PR | TS |
| 6 | 0.00 | - | - | - | - | - | - |
| 7 | 4.17 | - | - | - | - | - | - |
| 8 | 8.33 | - | - | - | - | - | - |
| 9 | 12.50 | - | - | - | - | - | - |
| 10 | 16.67 | 2.1 | 28.96 | 3.3 | 30.48 | 2.7 | 29.69 |
| 11 | 20.83 | 4.3 | 30.87 | 5.4 | 32.29 | 4.8 | 31.55 |
| 12 | 25.00 | 6.4 | 32.78 | 6.5 | 34.10 | 6.5 | 33.42 |
| 13 | 29.17 | 9.6 | 34.69 | 15.2 | 35.91 | 12.4 | 35.28 |
| 14 | 33.33 | 14.9 | 36.60 | 17.4 | 37.73 | 16.1 | 37.14 |
| 15 | 37.50 | 18.1 | 38.51 | 20.7 | 39.54 | 19.4 | 39.01 |
| 16 | 41.67 | 24.5 | 40.41 | 25.0 | 41.35 | 24.7 | 40.87 |
| 17 | 45.83 | 25.5 | 42.32 | 28.3 | 43.16 | 26.9 | 42.73 |
| 18 | 50.00 | 31.9 | 44.23 | 31.5 | 44.98 | 31.7 | 44.60 |
| 19 | 54.17 | 38.3 | 46.14 | 43.5 | 46.79 | 40.9 | 46.46 |
| 20 | 58.33 | 44.7 | 48.05 | 47.8 | 48.60 | 46.2 | 48.33 |
| 21 | 62.50 | 48.9 | 49.96 | 53.3 | 50.41 | 51.1 | 50.19 |
| 22 | 66.67 | 55.3 | 51.87 | 56.5 | 52.23 | 55.9 | 52.05 |
| 23 | 70.83 | 58.5 | 53.78 | 63.0 | 54.04 | 60.8 | 53.92 |
| 24 | 75.00 | 68.1 | 55.69 | 68.5 | 55.85 | 68.3 | 55.78 |
| 25 | 79.17 | 79.8 | 57.60 | 72.8 | 57.66 | 76.3 | 57.65 |
| 26 | 83.33 | 87.2 | 59.50 | 85.9 | 59.48 | 86.6 | 59.51 |
| 27 | 87.50 | 89.4 | 61.41 | 89.1 | 61.29 | 89.2 | 61.37 |
| 28 | 91.67 | 93.6 | 63.32 | 92.4 | 63.10 | 93.0 | 63.24 |
| 29 | 95.83 | 96.8 | 65.23 | 96.7 | 64.91 | 96.8 | 65.10 |
| 30 | 100.00 | 100.0 | 67.14 | 100.0 | 66.73 | 100.0 | 66.97 |

**DCSM-DM-S TREATMENT SELF-REPORT**

| RS | TRS | Total sample 8-12 (n = 95) | | Total sample 13-16 (n =93) | | Total sample Overall (n =188.) | |
|---|---|---|---|---|---|---|---|
| | | PR | TS | PR | TS | PR | TS |
| 4 | 0.00 | 3.2 | 27.65 | 2.2 | 29.31 | 2.7 | 28.55 |
| 5 | 6.25 | 6.3 | 29.99 | 7.5 | 31.73 | 6.9 | 30.92 |
| 6 | 12.50 | 8.4 | 32.34 | 11.8 | 34.15 | 10.1 | 33.29 |
| 7 | 18.75 | 9.5 | 34.68 | 11.8 | 34.15 | 10.6 | 35.67 |
| 8 | 25.00 | 12.6 | 37.02 | 17.2 | 38.99 | 14.9 | 38.04 |
| 9 | 31.25 | 16.8 | 39.37 | 26.9 | 41.41 | 21.8 | 40.41 |
| 10 | 37.50 | 22.1 | 41.71 | 32.3 | 43.83 | 27.1 | 42.78 |
| 11 | 43.75 | 28.4 | 44.05 | 34.4 | 46.25 | 31.4 | 45.15 |
| 12 | 50.00 | 36.8 | 46.40 | 43.0 | 48.67 | 39.9 | 47.52 |
| 13 | 56.25 | 47.4 | 48.74 | 59.1 | 51.09 | 53.2 | 49.89 |
| 14 | 62.50 | 57.9 | 51.09 | 63.4 | 53.51 | 60.6 | 52.26 |
| 15 | 68.75 | 68.4 | 53.43 | 75.3 | 55.93 | 71.8 | 54.63 |
| 16 | 75.00 | 75.8 | 55.77 | 81.7 | 58.35 | 78.7 | 57.00 |
| 17 | 81.25 | 77.9 | 58.12 | 89.2 | 60.77 | 83.5 | 59.37 |
| 18 | 87.50 | 85.3 | 60.46 | 93.5 | 63.19 | 89.4 | 61.74 |
| 19 | 93.75 | 89.5 | 62.80 | 95.7 | 65.61 | 92.6 | 64.11 |
| 20 | 100.00 | 100.0 | 65.15 | 100.0 | 68.03 | 100.0 | 66.48 |

*Note: Calculation of scores was restricted to complete cases. RS = raw score; TRS = transformed raw score (range 0-100); PR = percentile; TS = T-score (M = 50, SD = 10).*

**Table 17   DISABKIDS condition specific module cerebral palsy, sub-scales "impact" and "communication" (self-report) – DCSM-CPM-S**

| DCSM-CPM-S IMPACT SELF-REPORT | | Total sample 8-12 (n = 36) | | Total sample 13-16 (n = 27) | | Total sample Overall (n = 63) | |
|---|---|---|---|---|---|---|---|
| RS | TRS | PR | TS | PR | TS | PR | PR |
| 10 | 0.00 | - | - | - | - | - | - |
| 11 | 2.50 | - | - | - | - | - | - |
| 12 | 5.00 | - | - | - | - | - | - |
| 13 | 7.50 | - | - | - | - | - | - |
| 14 | 10.00 | - | - | - | - | - | - |
| 15 | 12.50 | - | - | - | - | - | - |
| 16 | 15.00 | - | - | - | - | - | - |
| 17 | 17.50 | - | - | - | - | - | - |
| 18 | 20.00 | 2.8 | 30,26 | - | - | 1.6 | 26,86 |
| 19 | 22.50 | 8.3 | 31,50 | - | - | 4.8 | 28,21 |
| 20 | 25.00 | 8.3 | 31,50 | - | - | 4.8 | 28,21 |
| 21 | 27.50 | 8.3 | 31,50 | - | - | 4.8 | 28,21 |
| 22 | 30.00 | 11.1 | 35,23 | - | - | 6.3 | 32,25 |
| 23 | 32.50 | 11.1 | 35,23 | - | - | 6.3 | 32,25 |
| 24 | 35.00 | 16.7 | 37,71 | 3.7 | 29,33 | 11.1 | 34,95 |
| 25 | 37.50 | 16.7 | 37,71 | 3.7 | 29,33 | 11.1 | 34,95 |
| 26 | 40.00 | 16.7 | 37,71 | 3.7 | 29,33 | 11.1 | 34,95 |
| 27 | 42.50 | 16.7 | 37,71 | 3.7 | 29,33 | 11.1 | 34,95 |
| 28 | 45.00 | 19.4 | 42,68 | 7.4 | 35,77 | 14.3 | 40,34 |
| 29 | 47.50 | 27.8 | 43,93 | 11.1 | 37,37 | 20.6 | 41,69 |
| 30 | 50.00 | 30.6 | 45,17 | 18.5 | 38,98 | 25.4 | 43,04 |
| 31 | 52.50 | 33.3 | 46,41 | 25.9 | 40,59 | 30.2 | 44,39 |
| 32 | 55.00 | 41.7 | 47,65 | 33.3 | 42,20 | 38.1 | 45,74 |
| 33 | 57.50 | 50.0 | 48,90 | 33.3 | 42,20 | 42.9 | 47,09 |
| 34 | 60.00 | 50.0 | 48,90 | 33.3 | 42,20 | 42.9 | 47,09 |
| 35 | 62.50 | 55.6 | 51,38 | 33.3 | 42,20 | 46.0 | 49,79 |
| 36 | 65.00 | 61.1 | 52,62 | 51.9 | 48,63 | 57.1 | 51,13 |
| 37 | 67.50 | 69.4 | 53,87 | 59.3 | 50,24 | 65.1 | 52,48 |
| 38 | 70.00 | 75.0 | 55,11 | 59.3 | 50,24 | 68.3 | 53,83 |

| DCSM-CPM-S IMPACT SELF-REPORT | | Total sample 8-12 (n = 36) | | Total sample 13-16 (n = 27) | | Total sample Overall (n = 63) | |
|---|---|---|---|---|---|---|---|
| RS | TRS | PR | TS | PR | TS | PR | PR |
| 39 | 72.50 | 77.8 | 56,35 | 63.0 | 53,45 | 71.4 | 55,18 |
| 40 | 75.00 | 83.3 | 57,59 | 66.7 | 55,06 | 76.2 | 56,53 |
| 41 | 77.50 | 83.3 | 57,59 | 66.7 | 55,06 | 76.2 | 56,53 |
| 42 | 80.00 | 86.1 | 60,08 | 77.8 | 58,28 | 82.5 | 59,23 |
| 43 | 82.50 | 88.9 | 61,32 | 85.2 | 59,89 | 87.3 | 60,58 |
| 44 | 85.00 | 91.7 | 62,56 | 85.2 | 59,89 | 88.9 | 61,92 |
| 45 | 87.50 | 91.7 | 62,56 | 88.9 | 63,10 | 90.5 | 63,27 |
| 46 | 90.00 | 94.4 | 65,05 | 100.0 | 64,71 | 96.8 | 64,62 |
| 47 | 92.50 | 94.4 | 65,05 | 100.0 | 64,71 | 96.8 | 64,62 |
| 48 | 95.00 | 94.4 | 65,05 | 100.0 | 64,71 | 96.8 | 64,62 |
| 49 | 97.50 | 94.4 | 65,05 | 100.0 | 64,71 | 96.8 | 64,62 |
| 50 | 100.00 | 100.0 | 70,02 | 100.0 | 64,71 | 100.0 | 70,02 |

| DCSM-CPM-S COMMUNICATION SELF-REPORT | | Total sample 8-12 (n = 39) | | Total sample 13-16 (n = 33) | | Total sample Overall (n = 72) | |
|---|---|---|---|---|---|---|---|
| RS | TRS | PR | TS | PR | TS | PR | PR |
| 2 | 0.00 | - | - | - | - | - | - |
| 3 | 12.50 | 5.1 | 23,44 | 3.0 | 19,06 | 4.2 | 21,45 |
| 4 | 25.00 | 7.7 | 28,26 | 3.0 | 19,06 | 5.6 | 26,56 |
| 5 | 37.50 | 10.3 | 33,08 | 6.1 | 29,98 | 8.3 | 31,68 |
| 6 | 50.00 | 15.4 | 37,89 | 15.2 | 35,44 | 15.3 | 36,79 |
| 7 | 62.50 | 28.2 | 42,71 | 24.2 | 40,90 | 26.4 | 41,90 |
| 8 | 75.00 | 33.3 | 47,53 | 33.3 | 46,36 | 33.3 | 47,02 |
| 9 | 87.50 | 48.7 | 52,35 | 48.5 | 51,82 | 48.6 | 52,13 |
| 10 | 10.00 | 100.0 | 57,16 | 100.0 | 57,28 | 100.0 | 57,24 |

*Note: Calculation of z-scores was restricted to complete cases. RS = raw score; TRS = transformed raw score (range 0-100); PR = percentile; TS = T-score (M = 50, SD = 10).*

189

**Table 18  DISABKIDS condition specific module cystic fibrosis, sub-scales "imapct" and "treatment" (self-report) – DCSM-CFM-S**

DCSM-CFM-S TREATMENT SELF-REPORT

| RS | TRS | Total sample 8-12 (n = 12) | | Total sample 13-16 (n = 12) | | Total sample Overall (n = 24) | |
|---|---|---|---|---|---|---|---|
| | | PR | TS | PR | TS | PR | TS |
| 6 | 0.00 | - | - | 8.3 | 27,14 | 4.2 | 27,26 |
| 7 | 4.17 | 8.3 | 29,07 | 8.3 | 27,14 | 8.3 | 29,02 |
| 8 | 8.33 | 8.3 | 29,07 | 8.3 | 27,14 | 8.3 | 29,02 |
| 9 | 12.50 | 8.3 | 29,07 | 8.3 | 27,14 | 8.3 | 29,02 |
| 10 | 16.67 | 8.3 | 29,07 | 8.3 | 27,14 | 8.3 | 29,02 |
| 11 | 20.83 | 8.3 | 29,07 | 8.3 | 27,14 | 8.3 | 29,02 |
| 12 | 25.00 | 8.3 | 29,07 | 8.3 | 27,14 | 8.3 | 29,02 |
| 13 | 29.17 | 16.7 | 38,79 | 16.7 | 40,57 | 16.7 | 39,58 |
| 14 | 33.33 | 16.7 | 38,79 | 16.7 | 40,57 | 16.7 | 39,58 |
| 15 | 37.50 | 16.7 | 38,79 | 25.0 | 44,40 | 20.8 | 43,10 |
| 16 | 41.67 | 16.7 | 38,79 | 25.0 | 44,40 | 20.8 | 43,10 |
| 17 | 45.83 | 25.0 | 45,27 | 41.7 | 48,24 | 33.3 | 46,63 |
| 18 | 50.00 | 41.7 | 46,89 | 50.0 | 50,16 | 45.8 | 48,39 |
| 19 | 54.17 | 58.3 | 48,51 | 75.0 | 52,08 | 66.7 | 50,15 |
| 20 | 58.33 | 58.3 | 48,51 | 75.0 | 52,08 | 66.7 | 50,15 |
| 21 | 62.50 | 58.3 | 48,51 | 75.0 | 52,08 | 66.7 | 50,15 |
| 22 | 66.67 | 58.3 | 48,51 | 83.3 | 57,83 | 70.8 | 55,43 |
| 23 | 70.83 | 75.0 | 55,00 | 83.3 | 57,83 | 79.2 | 57,19 |
| 24 | 75.00 | 75.0 | 55,00 | 91.7 | 61,67 | 83.3 | 58,95 |
| 25 | 79.17 | 75.0 | 55,00 | 91.7 | 61,67 | 83.3 | 58,95 |
| 26 | 83.33 | 83.3 | 59,86 | 100.0 | 65,51 | 91.7 | 62,47 |
| 27 | 87.50 | 83.3 | 59,86 | 100.0 | 65,51 | 91.7 | 62,47 |
| 28 | 91.67 | 100.0 | 63,10 | 100.0 | 65,51 | 100.0 | 65,99 |
| 29 | 95.83 | 100.0 | 63,10 | 100.0 | 65,51 | 100.0 | 65,99 |
| 30 | 100.00 | 100.0 | 63,10 | 100.0 | 65,51 | 100.0 | 65,99 |

DCSM-CFM-S IMPACT SELF-REPORT

| RS | TRS | Total sample 8-12 (n = 13) | | Total sample 13-16 (n = 10) | | Total sample Overall (n = 23) | |
|---|---|---|---|---|---|---|---|
| | | PR | TS | PR | TS | PR | TS |
| 4 | 0.00 | - | - | - | - | - | - |
| 5 | 6.25 | - | - | - | - | - | - |
| 6 | 12.50 | - | - | - | - | - | - |
| 7 | 18.75 | - | - | - | - | - | - |
| 8 | 25.00 | - | - | - | - | - | - |
| 9 | 31.25 | - | - | - | - | - | - |
| 10 | 37.50 | - | - | - | - | - | - |
| 11 | 43.75 | 15.4 | 37,17 | 20.0 | 38,17 | 17.4 | 37,41 |
| 12 | 50.00 | 30.8 | 40,26 | 30.0 | 41,65 | 30.4 | 40,70 |
| 13 | 56.25 | 46.2 | 43,34 | 50.0 | 45,13 | 47.8 | 43,99 |
| 14 | 62.50 | 46.2 | 43,34 | 50.0 | 45,13 | 47.8 | 43,99 |
| 15 | 68.75 | 46.2 | 43,34 | 70.0 | 52,09 | 56.5 | 50,57 |
| 16 | 75.00 | 53.8 | 52,61 | 70.0 | 52,09 | 60.9 | 53,86 |
| 17 | 81.25 | 69.2 | 55,70 | 80.0 | 59,04 | 73.9 | 57,15 |
| 18 | 87.50 | 84.6 | 58,79 | 90.0 | 62,52 | 87.0 | 60,44 |
| 19 | 93.75 | 92.3 | 61,88 | 100.0 | 66,00 | 95.7 | 63,73 |
| 20 | 100.00 | 100.0 | 64,97 | 100.0 | 66,00 | 100.0 | 67,02 |

*Note: Calculation of scores was restricted to complete cases. RS = raw score; TRS = transformed raw score (range 0-100); PR = percentile; TS = T-score (M = 50, SD = 10).*

**Table 21 DISABKIDS condition specific module epilepsy, sub-scales "impact" and "social" (self-report) – DCSM-EM-S**

| DCSM-EM-S IMPACT SELF-REPORT | | Total sample 8-12 (n = 73) | | Total sample 13-16 (n = 74) | | Total sample Overall (n = 147) | |
|---|---|---|---|---|---|---|---|
| RS | TRS | PR | TS | PR | TS | PR | TS |
| 5 | 0.00 | 4.1 | 25,16 | 4.1 | 28,48 | 4.1 | 26,89 |
| 6 | 5.00 | 4.1 | 25,16 | 6.8 | 30,08 | 5.4 | 28,57 |
| 7 | 10.00 | 4.1 | 25,16 | 9.5 | 31,69 | 6.8 | 30,24 |
| 8 | 15.00 | 5.5 | 30,40 | 10.8 | 33,29 | 8.2 | 31,91 |
| 9 | 20.00 | 5.5 | 30,40 | 13.5 | 34,90 | 9.5 | 33,59 |
| 10 | 25.00 | 9.6 | 33,89 | 16.2 | 36,50 | 12.9 | 35,26 |
| 11 | 30.00 | 13.7 | 35,64 | 17.6 | 38,11 | 15.6 | 36,93 |
| 12 | 35.00 | 16.4 | 37,39 | 18.9 | 39,72 | 17.7 | 38,61 |
| 13 | 40.00 | 20.5 | 39,13 | 20.3 | 41,32 | 20.4 | 40,28 |
| 14 | 45.00 | 21.9 | 40,88 | 23.0 | 42,93 | 22.4 | 41,95 |
| 15 | 50.00 | 21.9 | 40,88 | 28.4 | 44,53 | 25.2 | 43,63 |
| 16 | 55.00 | 24.7 | 44,38 | 33.8 | 46,14 | 29.3 | 45,30 |
| 17 | 60.00 | 32.9 | 46,12 | 35.1 | 47,74 | 34.0 | 46,97 |
| 18 | 65.00 | 41.1 | 47,87 | 44.6 | 49,35 | 42.9 | 48,65 |
| 19 | 70.00 | 45.2 | 49,62 | 51.4 | 50,95 | 48.3 | 50,32 |
| 20 | 75.00 | 49.3 | 51,36 | 54.1 | 52,56 | 51.7 | 51,99 |
| 21 | 80.00 | 54.8 | 53,11 | 58.1 | 54,17 | 56.5 | 53,67 |
| 22 | 85.00 | 61.6 | 54,86 | 64.9 | 55,77 | 63.3 | 55,34 |
| 23 | 90.00 | 68.5 | 56,61 | 71.6 | 57,38 | 70.1 | 57,01 |
| 24 | 95.00 | 72.6 | 58,35 | 77.0 | 58,98 | 74.8 | 58,69 |
| 25 | 100.00 | 100.0 | 60,10 | 100.0 | 60,59 | 100.0 | 60,36 |

| DCSM-EM-S SOCIAL SELF-REPORT | | Total sample 8-12 (n = 71) | | Total sample 13-16 (n = 74) | | Total sample Overall (n = 145) | |
|---|---|---|---|---|---|---|---|
| RS | TRS | PR | TS | PR | TS | PR | TS |
| 5 | 0.00 | - | - | 1.4 | 23,38 | .7 | 19,80 |
| 6 | 5.00 | 1.4 | 16,84 | 1.4 | 23,38 | 1.4 | 21,75 |
| 7 | 10.00 | 1.4 | 16,84 | 4.1 | 26,94 | 2.8 | 23,71 |
| 8 | 15.00 | 1.4 | 16,84 | 4.1 | 26,94 | 2.8 | 23,71 |
| 9 | 20.00 | 1.4 | 16,84 | 6.8 | 30,51 | 4.1 | 27,61 |
| 10 | 25.00 | 1.4 | 16,84 | 10.8 | 32,29 | 6.2 | 29,56 |
| 11 | 30.00 | 4.2 | 27,87 | 10.8 | 32,29 | 7.6 | 31,51 |
| 12 | 35.00 | 7.0 | 30,07 | 12.2 | 35,86 | 9.7 | 33,46 |
| 13 | 40.00 | 8.5 | 32,27 | 14.9 | 37,64 | 11.7 | 35,41 |
| 14 | 45.00 | 9.9 | 34,48 | 21.6 | 39,42 | 15.9 | 37,36 |
| 15 | 50.00 | 14.1 | 36,68 | 24.3 | 41,21 | 19.3 | 39,32 |
| 16 | 55.00 | 18.3 | 38,89 | 27.0 | 42,99 | 22.8 | 41,27 |
| 17 | 60.00 | 19.7 | 41,09 | 28.4 | 44,77 | 24.1 | 43,22 |
| 18 | 65.00 | 28.2 | 43,29 | 32.4 | 46,55 | 30.3 | 45,17 |
| 19 | 70.00 | 32.4 | 45,50 | 37.8 | 48,34 | 35.2 | 47,12 |
| 20 | 75.00 | 35.2 | 47,70 | 40.5 | 50,12 | 37.9 | 49,07 |
| 21 | 80.00 | 40.8 | 49,91 | 47.3 | 51,90 | 44.1 | 51,02 |
| 22 | 85.00 | 46.5 | 52,11 | 50.0 | 53,69 | 48.3 | 52,97 |
| 23 | 90.00 | 57.7 | 54,32 | 58.1 | 55,47 | 57.9 | 54,93 |
| 24 | 95.00 | 66.2 | 56,52 | 73.0 | 57,25 | 69.7 | 56,88 |
| 25 | 100.00 | 100.0 | 58,72 | 100.0 | 59,03 | 100.0 | 58,83 |

*Note: Calculation of scores was restricted to complete cases. RS = raw score; TRS = transformed raw score (range 0-100); PR = percentile; TS = T-score; TRS = T-score (M = 50, SD = 10).*

**Table 22  DISABKIDS chronic generic module, sub-scale "independence" (proxy-report) – DCGM-37-P**

| DCGM-37-P INDEPENDENCE PROXY-REPORT | | Total sample 8-12 (n = 494) | | Total sample 13-16 (n = 363) | | Total sample Overall (n = 857) | | Females 8-12 (n = 224) | | Females 13-16 (n = 177) | | Females Overall (n = 401) | | Males 8-12 (n = 268) | | Males 13-16 (n = 184) | | Males Overall (n = 452) | |
|---|---|---|---|---|---|---|---|---|---|---|---|---|---|---|---|---|---|---|---|
| RS | TRS | PR | TS | PR | TS | PR | TS | PR | TS | PR | TS | PR | TS | PR | TS | PR | TS | PR | TS |
| 6 | 0.00 | - | - | - | - | - | - | - | - | - | - | - | - | - | - | - | - | - | - |
| 7 | 4.17 | .2 | 7,49 | .3 | 8,93 | .2 | 8,15 | - | - | - | - | - | - | .4 | 8,44 | .5 | 10,95 | .4 | 9,48 |
| 8 | 8.33 | .2 | 7,49 | .3 | 8,93 | .2 | 8,15 | - | - | - | - | - | - | .4 | 8,44 | .5 | 10,95 | .4 | 9,48 |
| 9 | 12.50 | .2 | 7,49 | .3 | 8,93 | .2 | 8,15 | - | - | - | - | - | - | .4 | 8,44 | .5 | 10,95 | .4 | 9,48 |
| 10 | 16.67 | .4 | 14,73 | .3 | 8,93 | .4 | 15,36 | .4 | 13,83 | - | - | .2 | 13,46 | .4 | 8,44 | .5 | 10,95 | .4 | 9,48 |
| 11 | 20.83 | .4 | 14,73 | .6 | 18,53 | .5 | 17,77 | .4 | 13,83 | - | - | .2 | 13,46 | .4 | 8,44 | .5 | 10,95 | .4 | 9,48 |
| 12 | 25.00 | 1.4 | 19,57 | 1.4 | 20,93 | 1.4 | 20,18 | 1.3 | 18,74 | - | - | .7 | 18,50 | 1.5 | 20,34 | 2.2 | 22,34 | 1.8 | 21,17 |
| 13 | 29.17 | 1.8 | 21,98 | 1.4 | 20,93 | 1.6 | 22,58 | 2.2 | 21,19 | - | - | 1.2 | 21,02 | 1.5 | 20,34 | 2.2 | 22,34 | 1.8 | 21,17 |
| 14 | 33.33 | 3.0 | 24,40 | 3.3 | 25,73 | 3.2 | 24,99 | 3.6 | 23,64 | 2.3 | 23,29 | 3.0 | 23,54 | 2.6 | 25,09 | 3.8 | 26,90 | 3.1 | 25,84 |
| 15 | 37.50 | 4.0 | 26,81 | 4.4 | 28,13 | 4.2 | 27,40 | 4.0 | 26,10 | 4.0 | 25,91 | 4.0 | 26,06 | 4.1 | 27,47 | 4.3 | 29,18 | 4.2 | 28,18 |
| 16 | 41.67 | 5.3 | 29,23 | 6.6 | 30,53 | 5.8 | 29,80 | 4.0 | 26,10 | 5.1 | 28,53 | 4.5 | 28,58 | 6.3 | 29,85 | 7.6 | 31,45 | 6.9 | 30,52 |
| 17 | 45.83 | 6.5 | 31,64 | 8.5 | 32,93 | 7.4 | 32,21 | 5.4 | 31,00 | 7.9 | 31,16 | 6.5 | 31,10 | 7.5 | 32,23 | 8.7 | 33,73 | 8.0 | 32,85 |
| 18 | 50.00 | 8.9 | 34,06 | 11.6 | 35,33 | 10.0 | 34,62 | 7.6 | 33,45 | 10.7 | 33,78 | 9.0 | 33,62 | 10.1 | 34,61 | 12.0 | 36,01 | 10.8 | 35,19 |
| 19 | 54.17 | 11.3 | 36,47 | 14.0 | 37,73 | 12.5 | 37,02 | 9.4 | 35,91 | 13.6 | 36,41 | 11.2 | 36,14 | 13.1 | 36,99 | 13.6 | 38,29 | 13.3 | 37,53 |
| 20 | 58.33 | 15.0 | 38,89 | 17.4 | 40,13 | 16.0 | 39,43 | 15.2 | 38,36 | 16.9 | 39,03 | 16.0 | 38,67 | 14.9 | 39,37 | 16.8 | 40,57 | 15.7 | 39,87 |
| 21 | 62.50 | 19.4 | 41,31 | 23.4 | 42,53 | 21.1 | 41,84 | 19.2 | 40,81 | 22.0 | 41,65 | 20.4 | 41,19 | 19.8 | 41,75 | 23.9 | 42,84 | 21.5 | 42,20 |
| 22 | 66.67 | 24.9 | 43,72 | 29.8 | 44,93 | 27.0 | 44,24 | 24.6 | 43,27 | 26.6 | 44,28 | 25.4 | 43,71 | 25.4 | 44,12 | 32.1 | 45,12 | 28.1 | 44,54 |
| 23 | 70.83 | 32.0 | 46,14 | 35.8 | 47,33 | 33.6 | 46,65 | 32.1 | 45,72 | 32.8 | 46,90 | 32.4 | 46,23 | 31.7 | 46,50 | 38.0 | 47,40 | 34.3 | 46,88 |
| 24 | 75.00 | 43.1 | 48,55 | 43.8 | 49,74 | 43.4 | 49,06 | 40.6 | 48,17 | 42.4 | 49,53 | 41.4 | 48,75 | 45.1 | 48,88 | 44.6 | 49,68 | 44.9 | 49,21 |
| 25 | 79.17 | 54.0 | 50,97 | 55.6 | 52,14 | 54.7 | 51,46 | 50.4 | 50,62 | 56.5 | 52,15 | 53.1 | 51,27 | 57.1 | 51,26 | 54.3 | 51,96 | 56.0 | 51,55 |
| 26 | 83.33 | 63.4 | 53,38 | 68.9 | 54,54 | 65.7 | 53,87 | 61.2 | 53,08 | 71.8 | 54,77 | 65.8 | 53,79 | 65.3 | 53,64 | 65.8 | 54,23 | 65.5 | 53,89 |
| 27 | 87.50 | 71.5 | 55,80 | 78.5 | 56,94 | 74.4 | 56,28 | 71.0 | 55,53 | 83.1 | 57,40 | 76.3 | 56,31 | 72.0 | 56,02 | 73.9 | 56,51 | 72.8 | 56,23 |
| 28 | 91.67 | 81.6 | 58,22 | 87.9 | 59,34 | 84.2 | 58,68 | 81.3 | 57,98 | 89.8 | 60,02 | 85.0 | 58,83 | 81.7 | 58,40 | 85.9 | 58,79 | 83.4 | 58,56 |
| 29 | 95.83 | 91.5 | 60,63 | 95.0 | 61,74 | 93.0 | 61,09 | 91.5 | 60,44 | 96.6 | 62,65 | 93.8 | 61,35 | 91.4 | 60,78 | 93.5 | 61,07 | 92.3 | 60,90 |
| 30 | 100.00 | 100.0 | 63,05 | 100.0 | 64,14 | 100.0 | 63,50 | 100.0 | 62,89 | 100.0 | 65,27 | 100.0 | 63,87 | 100.0 | 63,15 | 100.0 | 63,35 | 100.0 | 63,24 |

*Note: Calculation of scores was restricted to complete cases. RS = raw score; TRS = transformed raw score (range 0-100); PR = percentile; TS = T-score (M = 50, SD = 10).*

Table 23   DISABKIDS chronic generic module, sub-scale "emotion" (proxy-report) – DCGM-37-P

| DCGM-37-P EMOTION PROXY-REPORT | | Total sample 8-12 (n = 500) | | Total sample 13-16 (n = 368) | | Total sample Overall (n = 868) | | Females 8-12 (n = 229) | | Females 13-16 (n = 177) | | Females Overall (n = 406) | | Males 8-12 (n = 269) | | Males 13-16 (n = 189) | | Males Overall (n = 458) | |
|---|---|---|---|---|---|---|---|---|---|---|---|---|---|---|---|---|---|---|---|
| RS | TRS | PR | TS | PR | TS | PR | TS | PR | TS | PR | TS | PR | TS | PR | TS | PR | TS | PR | TS |
| 7 | 0.00 | - | - | - | - | - | - | - | - | - | - | - | - | - | - | - | - | - | - |
| 8 | 3.57 | - | - | - | - | - | - | - | - | - | - | - | - | - | - | - | - | - | - |
| 9 | 7.14 | - | - | - | - | - | - | - | - | - | - | - | - | - | - | - | - | - | - |
| 10 | 10.71 | .2 | 18.31 | - | - | .1 | 19.41 | - | - | - | - | - | - | .4 | 18.37 | - | - | .2 | 19.10 |
| 11 | 14.29 | .6 | 20.10 | .3 | 22.35 | .5 | 21.18 | .4 | 20.16 | - | - | .2 | 21.35 | .7 | 20.14 | .5 | 21.81 | .7 | 20.86 |
| 12 | 17.86 | 1.2 | 21.88 | .5 | 24.13 | .9 | 22.96 | .9 | 21.97 | .6 | 24.27 | .7 | 23.16 | 1.5 | 21.91 | .5 | 21.81 | 1.1 | 22.61 |
| 13 | 21.43 | 1.2 | 21.88 | 1.4 | 25.90 | 1.3 | 24.73 | .9 | 21.97 | 1.7 | 26.10 | 1.2 | 24.96 | 1.5 | 21.91 | 1.1 | 25.30 | 1.3 | 24.37 |
| 14 | 25.00 | 2.2 | 25.46 | 1.9 | 27.67 | 2.1 | 26.51 | 1.7 | 25.59 | 2.3 | 27.93 | 2.0 | 26.77 | 2.6 | 25.44 | 1.6 | 27.04 | 2.2 | 26.13 |
| 15 | 28.57 | 3.0 | 27.25 | 2.7 | 29.45 | 2.9 | 28.28 | 2.6 | 27.40 | 2.3 | 27.93 | 2.5 | 28.58 | 3.3 | 27.21 | 2.6 | 28.78 | 3.1 | 27.89 |
| 16 | 32.14 | 4.8 | 29.04 | 6.0 | 31.22 | 5.3 | 30.05 | 4.4 | 29.21 | 5.6 | 31.60 | 4.9 | 30.39 | 5.2 | 28.98 | 5.8 | 30.53 | 5.5 | 29.64 |
| 17 | 35.71 | 6.4 | 30.83 | 8.2 | 32.99 | 7.1 | 31.83 | 6.1 | 31.02 | 9.0 | 33.43 | 7.4 | 32.19 | 6.7 | 30.75 | 6.9 | 32.27 | 6.8 | 31.40 |
| 18 | 39.29 | 8.6 | 32.62 | 9.8 | 34.76 | 9.1 | 33.60 | 8.3 | 32.84 | 10.2 | 35.26 | 9.1 | 34.00 | 8.9 | 32.52 | 9.0 | 34.02 | 9.0 | 33.16 |
| 19 | 42.86 | 10.0 | 34.41 | 12.0 | 36.54 | 10.8 | 35.38 | 10.0 | 34.65 | 11.9 | 37.09 | 10.8 | 35.81 | 10.0 | 34.29 | 11.6 | 35.76 | 10.7 | 34.91 |
| 20 | 46.43 | 10.6 | 36.20 | 14.9 | 38.31 | 12.4 | 37.15 | 10.9 | 36.46 | 15.8 | 38.92 | 13.1 | 37.61 | 10.4 | 36.06 | 13.8 | 37.50 | 11.8 | 36.67 |
| 21 | 50.00 | 13.2 | 37.99 | 18.8 | 40.08 | 15.6 | 38.93 | 14.0 | 38.27 | 20.3 | 40.76 | 16.7 | 39.42 | 12.6 | 37.83 | 16.9 | 39.25 | 14.4 | 38.43 |
| 22 | 53.57 | 16.6 | 39.77 | 23.6 | 41.86 | 19.6 | 40.70 | 17.9 | 40.08 | 26.0 | 42.59 | 21.4 | 41.23 | 15.6 | 39.60 | 21.2 | 40.99 | 17.9 | 40.19 |
| 23 | 57.14 | 20.2 | 41.56 | 30.2 | 43.63 | 24.4 | 42.48 | 22.3 | 41.89 | 32.8 | 44.42 | 26.8 | 43.04 | 18.6 | 41.37 | 27.5 | 42.74 | 22.3 | 41.94 |
| 24 | 60.71 | 24.0 | 43.35 | 35.6 | 45.40 | 28.9 | 44.25 | 26.6 | 43.70 | 38.4 | 46.25 | 31.8 | 44.84 | 21.9 | 43.13 | 32.8 | 44.48 | 26.4 | 43.70 |
| 25 | 64.29 | 31.0 | 45.14 | 40.5 | 47.18 | 35.0 | 46.03 | 33.2 | 45.52 | 44.6 | 48.09 | 38.2 | 46.65 | 29.4 | 44.90 | 36.5 | 46.23 | 32.3 | 45.46 |
| 26 | 67.86 | 38.2 | 46.93 | 47.3 | 48.95 | 42.1 | 47.80 | 41.0 | 47.33 | 49.7 | 49.92 | 44.8 | 48.46 | 36.1 | 46.67 | 45.0 | 47.97 | 39.7 | 47.21 |
| 27 | 71.43 | 45.6 | 48.72 | 53.5 | 50.72 | 49.0 | 49.57 | 47.6 | 49.14 | 58.2 | 51.75 | 52.2 | 50.27 | 44.2 | 48.44 | 48.7 | 49.71 | 46.1 | 48.97 |
| 28 | 75.00 | 53.2 | 50.51 | 59.5 | 52.50 | 55.9 | 51.35 | 54.6 | 50.95 | 65.5 | 53.58 | 59.4 | 52.07 | 52.4 | 50.21 | 53.4 | 51.46 | 52.8 | 50.73 |
| 29 | 78.57 | 58.2 | 52.30 | 65.5 | 54.27 | 61.3 | 53.12 | 61.1 | 52.76 | 71.8 | 55.41 | 65.8 | 53.88 | 56.1 | 51.98 | 59.3 | 53.20 | 57.4 | 52.49 |
| 30 | 82.14 | 64.6 | 54.09 | 68.8 | 56.04 | 66.4 | 54.90 | 65.9 | 54.57 | 74.6 | 57.25 | 69.7 | 55.69 | 63.9 | 53.75 | 63.0 | 54.95 | 63.5 | 54.24 |
| 31 | 85.71 | 69.2 | 55.87 | 76.1 | 57.82 | 72.1 | 56.67 | 72.1 | 56.38 | 82.5 | 59.08 | 76.6 | 57.50 | 67.3 | 55.52 | 69.8 | 56.69 | 68.3 | 56.00 |
| 32 | 89.29 | 75.4 | 57.66 | 81.3 | 59.59 | 77.9 | 58.45 | 77.3 | 58.19 | 85.9 | 60.91 | 81.0 | 59.30 | 74.0 | 57.29 | 76.7 | 58.43 | 75.1 | 57.76 |
| 33 | 92.86 | 81.6 | 59.45 | 89.4 | 61.36 | 84.9 | 60.22 | 84.7 | 60.01 | 92.1 | 62.74 | 87.9 | 61.11 | 79.2 | 59.06 | 86.8 | 60.18 | 82.3 | 59.51 |
| 34 | 96.43 | 88.6 | 61.24 | 93.2 | 63.13 | 90.6 | 62.00 | 87.8 | 61.82 | 93.8 | 64.57 | 90.4 | 62.92 | 89.2 | 60.82 | 92.6 | 61.92 | 90.6 | 61.27 |
| 35 | 100.00 | 100.0 | 63.03 | 100.0 | 64.91 | 100.0 | 63.77 | 100.0 | 63.63 | 100.0 | 66.41 | 100.0 | 64.73 | 100.0 | 62.59 | 100.0 | 63.67 | 100.0 | 63.03 |

Note: Calculation of scores was restricted to complete cases. RS = raw score; TRS = transformed raw score (range 0-100); PR = percentile; TS = T-score (M = 50, SD = 10).

**Table 24  DISABKIDS chronic generic module, sub-scale "social inclusion" (proxy-report) – DCGM-37-P**

| RS | TRS | Total sample 8-12 (n=490) PR | TS | Total sample 13-16 (n=368) PR | TS | Total sample Overall (n=858) PR | TS | Females 8-12 (n=227) PR | TS | Females 13-16 (n=176) PR | TS | Females Overall (n=403) PR | TS | Males 8-12 (n=261) PR | TS | Males 13-16 (n=190) PR | TS | Males Overall (n=451) PR | TS |
|---|---|---|---|---|---|---|---|---|---|---|---|---|---|---|---|---|---|---|---|
| 6 | 0.00 | .2 | 5,68 | - | - | .1 | 7,48 | - | - | - | - | - | - | .4 | 6,72 | - | - | .2 | 8,50 |
| 7 | 4.17 | .2 | 5,68 | - | - | .1 | 7,48 | - | - | - | - | - | - | .4 | 6,72 | - | - | .2 | 8,50 |
| 8 | 8.33 | .2 | 5,68 | - | - | .1 | 7,48 | - | - | - | - | - | - | .4 | 6,72 | - | - | .2 | 8,50 |
| 9 | 12.50 | .2 | 5,68 | .3 | 16,51 | .2 | 14,66 | - | - | - | - | .2 | 13,23 | .4 | 6,72 | - | - | .2 | 8,50 |
| 10 | 16.67 | .4 | 15,57 | .8 | 18,81 | .6 | 17,05 | .4 | 14,57 | .6 | 14,66 | .7 | 15,72 | .4 | 6,72 | .5 | 19,62 | .4 | 17,84 |
| 11 | 20.83 | .6 | 18,04 | 1.4 | 21,11 | .9 | 19,44 | .9 | 17,10 | 1.1 | 17,09 | 1.2 | 18,20 | .4 | 6,72 | .5 | 19,62 | .4 | 17,84 |
| 12 | 25.00 | .8 | 20,52 | 2.2 | 23,40 | 1.4 | 21,83 | .9 | 17,10 | 1.7 | 19,53 | 1.2 | 18,20 | .8 | 21,28 | 2.1 | 24,06 | 1.3 | 22,51 |
| 13 | 29.17 | 1.4 | 22,99 | 3.0 | 25,70 | 2.1 | 24,22 | 1.3 | 22,17 | 1.7 | 19,53 | 1.5 | 23,18 | 1.5 | 23,71 | 3.7 | 26,28 | 2.4 | 24,85 |
| 14 | 33.33 | 2.7 | 25,46 | 3.8 | 28,00 | 3.1 | 26,62 | 3.1 | 24,71 | 2.3 | 26,82 | 2.7 | 25,66 | 2.3 | 26,13 | 4.7 | 28,50 | 3.3 | 27,18 |
| 15 | 37.50 | 4.1 | 27,93 | 5.2 | 30,29 | 4.5 | 29,01 | 4.8 | 27,24 | 2.8 | 29,26 | 4.0 | 28,15 | 3.4 | 28,56 | 6.8 | 30,72 | 4.9 | 29,52 |
| 16 | 41.67 | 5.3 | 30,40 | 7.6 | 32,59 | 6.3 | 31,40 | 5.3 | 29,77 | 6.3 | 31,69 | 5.7 | 30,64 | 5.4 | 30,99 | 8.4 | 32,94 | 6.7 | 31,85 |
| 17 | 45.83 | 6.7 | 32,88 | 11.4 | 34,89 | 8.7 | 33,79 | 7.0 | 32,31 | 10.8 | 34,12 | 8.7 | 33,13 | 6.5 | 33,41 | 11.6 | 35,16 | 8.6 | 34,19 |
| 18 | 50.00 | 10.0 | 35,35 | 13.0 | 37,19 | 11.3 | 36,18 | 8.4 | 34,84 | 13.1 | 36,55 | 10.4 | 35,61 | 11.5 | 35,84 | 12.6 | 37,38 | 12.0 | 36,52 |
| 19 | 54.17 | 13.5 | 37,82 | 16.6 | 39,48 | 14.8 | 38,57 | 12.3 | 37,38 | 17.0 | 38,99 | 14.4 | 38,10 | 14.6 | 38,27 | 15.8 | 39,60 | 15.1 | 38,86 |
| 20 | 58.33 | 17.6 | 40,29 | 21.2 | 41,78 | 19.1 | 40,97 | 15.9 | 39,91 | 21.6 | 41,42 | 18.4 | 40,59 | 19.2 | 40,69 | 20.5 | 41,82 | 19.7 | 41,19 |
| 21 | 62.50 | 24.7 | 42,77 | 26.6 | 44,08 | 25.5 | 43,36 | 22.9 | 42,44 | 26.1 | 43,85 | 24.3 | 43,08 | 26.4 | 43,12 | 26.8 | 44,04 | 26.6 | 43,53 |
| 22 | 66.67 | 33.1 | 45,24 | 33.2 | 46,37 | 33.1 | 45,75 | 33.0 | 44,98 | 31.8 | 46,28 | 32.5 | 45,56 | 33.3 | 45,55 | 34.2 | 46,26 | 33.7 | 45,86 |
| 23 | 70.83 | 40.8 | 47,71 | 42.4 | 48,67 | 41.5 | 48,14 | 38.3 | 47,51 | 40.9 | 48,71 | 39.5 | 48,05 | 43.3 | 47,97 | 43.7 | 48,48 | 43.5 | 48,20 |
| 24 | 75.00 | 50.6 | 50,18 | 51.1 | 50,97 | 50.8 | 50,53 | 48.5 | 50,04 | 51.1 | 51,15 | 49.6 | 50,54 | 52.9 | 50,40 | 51.1 | 50,70 | 52.1 | 50,53 |
| 25 | 79.17 | 61.6 | 52,65 | 66.0 | 53,26 | 63.5 | 52,92 | 61.2 | 52,58 | 67.0 | 53,58 | 63.8 | 53,02 | 62.5 | 52,83 | 64.7 | 52,92 | 63.4 | 52,87 |
| 26 | 83.33 | 70.6 | 55,13 | 73.6 | 55,56 | 71.9 | 55,32 | 71.4 | 55,11 | 79.0 | 56,01 | 74.7 | 55,51 | 70.5 | 55,25 | 68.4 | 55,14 | 69.6 | 55,20 |
| 27 | 87.50 | 80.8 | 57,60 | 81.3 | 57,86 | 81.0 | 57,71 | 81.9 | 57,65 | 84.7 | 58,44 | 83.1 | 58,00 | 80.5 | 57,68 | 77.9 | 57,36 | 79.4 | 57,54 |
| 28 | 91.67 | 87.8 | 60,07 | 87.8 | 60,16 | 87.8 | 60,10 | 89.4 | 60,18 | 90.3 | 60,88 | 89.8 | 60,49 | 87.0 | 60,11 | 85.3 | 59,58 | 86.3 | 59,87 |
| 29 | 95.83 | 93.5 | 62,54 | 93.8 | 62,45 | 93.6 | 62,49 | 94.7 | 62,71 | 95.5 | 63,31 | 95.0 | 62,97 | 92.7 | 62,53 | 92.1 | 61,80 | 92.5 | 62,21 |
| 30 | 100.00 | 100.0 | 65,01 | 100.0 | 64,75 | 100.0 | 64,88 | 100.0 | 65,25 | 100.0 | 65,74 | 100.0 | 65,46 | 100.0 | 64,96 | 100.0 | 64,02 | 100.0 | 64,54 |

*Note: Calculation of scores was restricted to complete cases. RS = raw score; TRS = transformed raw score (range 0-100); PR = percentile; TS = T-score (M = 50, SD = 10).*

Table 25  DISABKIDS chronic generic module, sub-scale "social exclusion" (proxy-report) – DCGM-37-P

| DCGM-37-P EXCLUSION PROXY-REPORT | | Total sample 8-12 (n = 495) | | Total sample 13-16 (n = 371) | | Total sample Overall (n = 866) | | Females 8-12 (n = 226) | | Females 13-16 (n =177) | | Females Overall (n = 403) | | Males 8-12 (n = 267) | | Males 13-16 (n = 192) | | Males Overall (n = 459) | |
|---|---|---|---|---|---|---|---|---|---|---|---|---|---|---|---|---|---|---|---|
| RS | TRS | PR | TS | PR | TS | PR | TS | PR | TS | PR | TS | PR | TS | PR | TS | PR | TS | PR | TS |
| 6 | 0.00 | - | - | - | - | - | - | - | - | - | - | - | - | - | - | - | - | - | - |
| 7 | 4.17 | - | - | - | 8,19 | - | 7,02 | - | - | - | - | - | - | - | - | - | - | - | 6,69 |
| 8 | 8.33 | - | - | .3 | 8,19 | .1 | 7,02 | - | - | - | - | - | - | - | - | - | 7,60 | .2 | 6,69 |
| 9 | 12.50 | - | - | .3 | 8,19 | .1 | 7,02 | - | - | - | - | - | - | - | - | .5 | 7,60 | .2 | 6,69 |
| 10 | 16.67 | - | - | .3 | 15,53 | .1 | 14,44 | - | - | - | 16,13 | - | 14,88 | - | - | .5 | 7,60 | .2 | 6,69 |
| 11 | 20.83 | - | - | .8 | 15,53 | .3 | 14,44 | - | - | 1.1 | 16,13 | .5 | 14,88 | - | - | .5 | 7,60 | .2 | 6,69 |
| 12 | 25.00 | - | 18,54 | .8 | 15,53 | .3 | 19,39 | - | - | 1.1 | 16,13 | .5 | 14,88 | - | 18,52 | .5 | 7,60 | .2 | 19,05 |
| 13 | 29.17 | .4 | 21,04 | .8 | 22,87 | .6 | 21,87 | - | 21,26 | 1.1 | 23,46 | .5 | 22,30 | .7 | 21,01 | .5 | 22,27 | .7 | 21,53 |
| 14 | 33.33 | 1.2 | 23,54 | 1.6 | 25,31 | 1.4 | 24,34 | 1.3 | 23,76 | 2.3 | 25,91 | 1.7 | 24,77 | 1.1 | 23,50 | 1.0 | 24,71 | 1.1 | 24,00 |
| 15 | 37.50 | 2.4 | 26,04 | 2.7 | 27,76 | 2.5 | 26,81 | 2.2 | 26,26 | 2.8 | 28,35 | 2.5 | 27,24 | 2.6 | 25,99 | 2.6 | 27,16 | 2.6 | 26,47 |
| 16 | 41.67 | 3.4 | 28,54 | 3.8 | 30,20 | 3.6 | 29,29 | 4.0 | 28,76 | 4.5 | 30,80 | 4.2 | 29,71 | 3.0 | 28,48 | 3.1 | 29,60 | 3.1 | 28,94 |
| 17 | 45.83 | 5.3 | 31,04 | 5.4 | 32,65 | 5.3 | 31,76 | 6.2 | 31,26 | 5.6 | 33,24 | 6.0 | 32,18 | 4.5 | 30,97 | 5.2 | 32,05 | 4.8 | 31,42 |
| 18 | 50.00 | 5.9 | 33,54 | 7.5 | 35,09 | 6.6 | 34,23 | 6.2 | 33,76 | 7.9 | 35,69 | 6.9 | 34,65 | 5.6 | 33,46 | 7.3 | 34,49 | 6.3 | 33,89 |
| 19 | 54.17 | 8.5 | 36,04 | 10.2 | 37,54 | 9.2 | 36,71 | 9.3 | 36,26 | 9.6 | 38,13 | 9.4 | 37,12 | 7.9 | 35,95 | 10.9 | 36,94 | 9.2 | 36,36 |
| 20 | 58.33 | 11.7 | 38,55 | 13.2 | 39,98 | 12.4 | 39,18 | 12.8 | 38,76 | 13.6 | 40,58 | 13.2 | 39,59 | 10.9 | 38,44 | 12.5 | 39,38 | 11.5 | 38,83 |
| 21 | 62.50 | 16.4 | 41,05 | 17.5 | 42,43 | 16.9 | 41,66 | 16.8 | 41,26 | 18.6 | 43,02 | 17.6 | 42,06 | 16.1 | 40,93 | 16.1 | 41,82 | 16.1 | 41,31 |
| 22 | 66.67 | 22.0 | 43,55 | 22.9 | 44,87 | 22.4 | 44,13 | 21.7 | 43,76 | 25.4 | 45,47 | 23.3 | 44,53 | 22.5 | 43,42 | 20.3 | 44,27 | 21.6 | 43,78 |
| 23 | 70.83 | 27.9 | 46,05 | 30.5 | 47,32 | 29.0 | 46,60 | 28.3 | 46,26 | 31.6 | 47,91 | 29.8 | 47,00 | 27.7 | 45,91 | 29.2 | 46,71 | 28.3 | 46,25 |
| 24 | 75.00 | 35.8 | 48,55 | 40.7 | 49,76 | 37.9 | 49,08 | 33.6 | 48,76 | 45.2 | 50,36 | 38.7 | 49,47 | 37.8 | 48,40 | 36.5 | 49,16 | 37.3 | 48,72 |
| 25 | 79.17 | 41.2 | 51,05 | 47.4 | 52,21 | 43.9 | 51,55 | 41.6 | 51,26 | 49.2 | 52,80 | 44.9 | 51,94 | 41.2 | 50,90 | 45.8 | 51,60 | 43.1 | 51,20 |
| 26 | 83.33 | 49.5 | 53,55 | 58.0 | 54,65 | 53.1 | 54,02 | 49.6 | 53,76 | 60.5 | 55,25 | 54.3 | 54,41 | 49.4 | 53,39 | 55.2 | 54,05 | 51.9 | 53,67 |
| 27 | 87.50 | 58.8 | 56,05 | 64.4 | 57,10 | 61.2 | 56,50 | 59.7 | 56,26 | 68.9 | 57,69 | 63.8 | 56,88 | 58.1 | 55,88 | 59.9 | 56,49 | 58.8 | 56,14 |
| 28 | 91.67 | 70.5 | 58,55 | 74.1 | 59,54 | 72.1 | 58,97 | 73.5 | 58,76 | 77.4 | 60,14 | 75.2 | 56,88 | 67.8 | 58,37 | 70.8 | 58,94 | 69.1 | 58,61 |
| 29 | 95.83 | 81.2 | 61,06 | 87.1 | 61,99 | 83.7 | 61,45 | 83.6 | 61,26 | 88.1 | 62,58 | 85.6 | 59,36 | 79.0 | 60,86 | 85.9 | 61,38 | 81.9 | 61,09 |
| 30 | 100.00 | 100.0 | - | 100.0 | - | 100.0 | - | 100.0 | - | 100.0 | - | 100.0 | 61,83 | 100.0 | - | 100.0 | - | 100.0 | - |

Note: Calculation of scores was restricted to complete cases. RS = raw score; TRS = transformed raw score (range 0-100); PR = percentile; TS = T-score (M = 50, SD = 10).

195

**Table 26  DISABKIDS chronic generic module, sub-scale "physical limitation" (proxy-report) – DCGM-37-P**

| DCGM-37-P LIMITATION PROXY-REPORT | | Total sample 8-12 (n=501) | | Total sample 13-16 (n=374) | | Total sample Overall (n=875) | | Females 8-12 (n=232) | | Females 13-16 (n=178) | | Females Overall (n=410) | | Males 8-12 (n=267) | | Males 13-16 (n=194) | | Males Overall (n=461) | |
|---|---|---|---|---|---|---|---|---|---|---|---|---|---|---|---|---|---|---|---|
| RS | TRS | PR | TS | PR | TS | PR | TS | PR | TS | PR | TS | PR | TS | PR | TS | PR | TS | PR | TS |
| 6 | 0.00 | - | - | - | - | - | - | - | - | - | - | - | - | - | - | - | - | - | - |
| 7 | 4.17 | .2 | 12,57 | - | - | .1 | 13,51 | - | - | - | - | - | - | - | - | - | - | .2 | 13,85 |
| 8 | 8.33 | .4 | 14,87 | - | - | .2 | 15,79 | - | - | - | - | - | - | .4 | 13,43 | - | - | .4 | 16,08 |
| 9 | 12.50 | .6 | 17,18 | .3 | 19,12 | .5 | 18,07 | .4 | 16,43 | - | - | .2 | 17,49 | .7 | 15,67 | .5 | 18,91 | .7 | 18,31 |
| 10 | 16.67 | .6 | 17,18 | .3 | 19,12 | .5 | 18,07 | .4 | 16,43 | - | - | .2 | 17,49 | .7 | 15,67 | .5 | 18,91 | .7 | 18,31 |
| 11 | 20.83 | 1.0 | 21,78 | 1.1 | 23,64 | 1.0 | 22,63 | 1.3 | 21,17 | .6 | 23,26 | 1.0 | 22,21 | .7 | 15,67 | 1.0 | 23,33 | .9 | 22,77 |
| 12 | 25.00 | 1.8 | 24,08 | 2.7 | 25,91 | 2.2 | 24,91 | 1.7 | 23,53 | 2.2 | 25,64 | 2.0 | 24,57 | 1.9 | 24,63 | 2.6 | 25,54 | 2.2 | 25,00 |
| 13 | 29.17 | 2.4 | 26,38 | 4.0 | 28,17 | 3.1 | 27,19 | 2.2 | 25,90 | 4.5 | 28,02 | 3.2 | 26,93 | 2.6 | 26,88 | 3.1 | 27,75 | 2.8 | 27,23 |
| 14 | 33.33 | 3.0 | 28,68 | 4.8 | 30,43 | 3.8 | 29,47 | 3.0 | 28,27 | 6.2 | 30,39 | 4.4 | 29,29 | 3.0 | 29,12 | 3.1 | 29,96 | 3.0 | 29,46 |
| 15 | 37.50 | 4.6 | 30,98 | 6.1 | 32,69 | 5.3 | 31,75 | 5.2 | 30,63 | 7.3 | 32,77 | 6.1 | 31,65 | 4.1 | 31,36 | 4.6 | 32,18 | 4.3 | 31,69 |
| 16 | 41.67 | 7.8 | 33,28 | 9.9 | 34,96 | 8.7 | 34,03 | 7.3 | 33,00 | 10.7 | 35,14 | 8.8 | 34,01 | 8.2 | 33,60 | 8.8 | 34,39 | 8.5 | 33,92 |
| 17 | 45.83 | 10.0 | 35,58 | 13.6 | 37,22 | 11.5 | 36,31 | 10.3 | 35,37 | 14.0 | 37,52 | 12.0 | 36,37 | 9.7 | 35,84 | 12.9 | 36,60 | 11.1 | 36,15 |
| 18 | 50.00 | 13.6 | 37,88 | 16.8 | 39,48 | 15.0 | 38,59 | 13.8 | 37,74 | 16.9 | 39,90 | 15.1 | 38,72 | 13.5 | 38,08 | 16.5 | 38,81 | 14.8 | 38,38 |
| 19 | 54.17 | 18.4 | 40,18 | 23.0 | 41,74 | 20.3 | 40,87 | 18.1 | 40,10 | 23.0 | 42,27 | 20.2 | 41,08 | 18.7 | 40,32 | 22.7 | 41,03 | 20.4 | 40,61 |
| 20 | 58.33 | 24.2 | 42,48 | 28.3 | 44,01 | 25.9 | 43,15 | 23.7 | 42,47 | 28.7 | 44,65 | 25.9 | 43,44 | 24.7 | 42,56 | 27.8 | 43,24 | 26.0 | 42,84 |
| 21 | 62.50 | 33.3 | 44,78 | 38.0 | 46,27 | 35.3 | 45,43 | 32.8 | 44,84 | 39.9 | 47,02 | 35.9 | 45,80 | 34.1 | 44,80 | 36.1 | 45,45 | 34.9 | 45,08 |
| 22 | 66.67 | 40.7 | 47,08 | 45.2 | 48,53 | 42.6 | 47,71 | 40.1 | 47,20 | 50.0 | 49,40 | 44.4 | 48,16 | 41.6 | 47,05 | 40.7 | 47,66 | 41.2 | 47,31 |
| 23 | 70.83 | 48.5 | 49,38 | 54.3 | 50,79 | 51.0 | 49,99 | 48.7 | 49,57 | 58.4 | 51,78 | 52.9 | 50,52 | 48.7 | 49,29 | 50.5 | 49,87 | 49.5 | 49,54 |
| 24 | 75.00 | 56.9 | 51,69 | 63.1 | 53,05 | 59.5 | 52,27 | 57.8 | 51,94 | 68.0 | 54,15 | 62.2 | 52,88 | 56.6 | 51,53 | 58.8 | 52,09 | 57.5 | 51,77 |
| 25 | 79.17 | 66.5 | 53,99 | 70.9 | 55,32 | 68.3 | 54,55 | 68.5 | 54,31 | 76.4 | 56,53 | 72.0 | 55,24 | 64.8 | 53,77 | 66.0 | 54,30 | 65.3 | 54,00 |
| 26 | 83.33 | 75.0 | 56,29 | 78.6 | 57,58 | 76.6 | 56,83 | 76.7 | 56,67 | 84.3 | 58,90 | 80.0 | 57,60 | 73.8 | 56,01 | 73.2 | 56,51 | 73.5 | 56,23 |
| 27 | 87.50 | 81.6 | 58,59 | 87.7 | 59,84 | 84.2 | 59,11 | 83.2 | 59,04 | 92.7 | 61,28 | 87.3 | 59,96 | 80.5 | 58,25 | 83.0 | 58,72 | 81.6 | 58,46 |
| 28 | 91.67 | 87.6 | 60,89 | 92.0 | 62,10 | 89.5 | 61,39 | 90.9 | 61,41 | 94.9 | 63,65 | 92.7 | 62,32 | 84.6 | 60,49 | 89.2 | 60,93 | 86.6 | 60,69 |
| 29 | 95.83 | 94.6 | 63,19 | 94.4 | 64,37 | 94.5 | 63,67 | 95.7 | 63,77 | 96.1 | 66,03 | 95.9 | 64,68 | 93.6 | 62,73 | 92.8 | 63,15 | 93.3 | 62,92 |
| 30 | 100.00 | 100.0 | 65,49 | 100.0 | 66,63 | 100.0 | 65,95 | 100.0 | 66,14 | 100.0 | 68,41 | 100.0 | 67,04 | 100.0 | 64,97 | 100.0 | 65,36 | 100.0 | 65,15 |

*Note: Calculation of scores was restricted to complete cases. RS = raw score; TRS = transformed raw score (range 0-100); PR = percentile; TS = T-score (M = 50, SD = 10).*

196

Table 27  DISABKIDS chronic generic module, sub-scale "treatment/ medication" (proxy-report) – DCGM-37-P

| DCGM-37-P TREATMENT PROXY-REPORT | | Total sample 8-12 (n = 445) | | Total sample 13-16 (n = 328) | | Total sample Overall (n = 773) | | Females 8-12 (n = 200) | | Females 13-16 (n = 164) | | Females Overall (n = 364) | | Males 8-12 (n = 243) | | Males 13-16 (n = 161) | | Males Overall (n = 404) | |
|---|---|---|---|---|---|---|---|---|---|---|---|---|---|---|---|---|---|---|---|
| RS | TRS | PR | TS | PR | TS | PR | TS | PR | TS | PR | TS | PR | TS | PR | TS | PR | TS | PR | TS |
| 6 | 0.00 | - | - | - | - | - | - | - | - | - | - | - | - | - | - | - | - | - | - |
| 7 | 4.17 | .2 | 18,43 | .3 | 21,52 | .3 | 19,83 | .5 | 18,41 | .6 | 20,51 | .5 | 19,39 | - | - | - | - | - | - |
| 8 | 8.33 | .2 | 20,42 | .6 | 23,33 | .4 | 21,73 | .5 | 20,44 | 1.2 | 22,39 | .8 | 21,34 | - | - | - | - | - | - |
| 9 | 12.50 | .9 | 22,40 | 1.5 | 25,14 | 1.2 | 23,64 | 1.5 | 22,47 | 1.2 | 24,26 | 1.4 | 23,30 | .4 | 22,43 | 1.9 | 26,14 | 1.0 | 24,04 |
| 10 | 16.67 | 1.8 | 24,39 | 2.4 | 26,95 | 2.1 | 25,55 | 1.5 | 24,50 | 1.8 | 26,13 | 1.6 | 25,26 | 2.1 | 24,38 | 3.1 | 27,88 | 2.5 | 25,90 |
| 11 | 20.83 | 2.5 | 26,37 | 4.0 | 28,75 | 3.1 | 27,45 | 3.0 | 26,53 | 3.0 | 28,01 | 3.0 | 27,21 | 2.1 | 26,33 | 5.0 | 29,61 | 3.2 | 27,75 |
| 12 | 25.00 | 4.3 | 28,36 | 4.9 | 30,56 | 4.5 | 29,36 | 3.5 | 28,56 | 4.3 | 29,88 | 3.8 | 29,17 | 4.9 | 28,28 | 5.6 | 31,35 | 5.2 | 29,61 |
| 13 | 29.17 | 5.6 | 30,35 | 7.9 | 32,37 | 6.6 | 31,26 | 5.5 | 30,58 | 7.9 | 31,75 | 6.6 | 31,12 | 5.8 | 30,23 | 8.1 | 33,09 | 6.7 | 31,47 |
| 14 | 33.33 | 7.4 | 32,33 | 9.8 | 34,18 | 8.4 | 33,17 | 7.0 | 32,61 | 9.1 | 33,62 | 8.0 | 33,08 | 7.8 | 32,18 | 10.6 | 34,82 | 8.9 | 33,32 |
| 15 | 37.50 | 9.7 | 34,32 | 13.4 | 35,98 | 11.3 | 35,07 | 9.0 | 34,64 | 12.8 | 35,50 | 10.7 | 35,04 | 10.3 | 34,13 | 14.3 | 36,56 | 11.9 | 35,18 |
| 16 | 41.67 | 12.1 | 36,30 | 15.5 | 37,79 | 13.6 | 36,98 | 11.5 | 36,67 | 14.6 | 37,37 | 12.9 | 36,99 | 12.8 | 36,08 | 16.8 | 38,30 | 14.4 | 37,04 |
| 17 | 45.83 | 14.4 | 38,29 | 19.5 | 39,60 | 16.6 | 38,88 | 15.5 | 38,70 | 18.3 | 39,24 | 16.8 | 38,95 | 13.6 | 38,03 | 21.1 | 40,03 | 16.6 | 38,90 |
| 18 | 50.00 | 18.7 | 40,28 | 22.9 | 41,41 | 20.4 | 40,79 | 20.5 | 40,73 | 20.7 | 41,12 | 20.6 | 40,91 | 17.3 | 39,98 | 25.5 | 41,77 | 20.5 | 40,75 |
| 19 | 54.17 | 22.2 | 42,26 | 26.8 | 43,22 | 24.2 | 42,69 | 24.5 | 42,76 | 25.0 | 42,99 | 24.7 | 42,86 | 20.6 | 41,93 | 28.6 | 43,51 | 23.8 | 42,61 |
| 20 | 58.33 | 28.5 | 44,25 | 29.9 | 45,02 | 29.1 | 44,60 | 31.0 | 44,79 | 28.7 | 44,86 | 29.9 | 44,82 | 26.7 | 43,88 | 31.1 | 45,24 | 28.5 | 44,47 |
| 21 | 62.50 | 34.4 | 46,23 | 36.3 | 46,83 | 35.2 | 46,50 | 36.5 | 46,81 | 38.4 | 46,73 | 37.4 | 46,78 | 32.9 | 45,83 | 34.2 | 46,98 | 33.4 | 46,32 |
| 22 | 66.67 | 42.0 | 48,22 | 43.0 | 48,64 | 42.4 | 48,41 | 43.5 | 48,84 | 42.1 | 48,61 | 42.9 | 48,73 | 41.2 | 47,78 | 44.1 | 48,72 | 42.3 | 48,18 |
| 23 | 70.83 | 50.1 | 50,21 | 48.5 | 50,45 | 49.4 | 50,31 | 52.0 | 50,87 | 47.0 | 50,48 | 49.7 | 50,69 | 49.0 | 49,73 | 50.3 | 50,45 | 49.5 | 50,04 |
| 24 | 75.00 | 59.1 | 52,19 | 54.3 | 52,25 | 57.1 | 52,22 | 62.0 | 52,90 | 53.0 | 52,35 | 58.0 | 52,64 | 57.2 | 51,68 | 55.3 | 52,19 | 56.4 | 51,89 |
| 25 | 79.17 | 66.7 | 54,18 | 63.1 | 54,06 | 65.2 | 54,12 | 71.5 | 54,93 | 64.0 | 54,23 | 68.1 | 54,60 | 63.4 | 53,63 | 62.1 | 53,93 | 62.9 | 53,75 |
| 26 | 83.33 | 74.8 | 56,16 | 69.2 | 55,87 | 72.4 | 56,03 | 79.5 | 56,96 | 72.6 | 56,10 | 76.4 | 56,56 | 70.8 | 55,58 | 65.8 | 55,66 | 68.8 | 55,61 |
| 27 | 87.50 | 80.4 | 58,15 | 77.4 | 57,68 | 79.2 | 57,93 | 84.5 | 58,99 | 81.1 | 57,97 | 83.0 | 58,51 | 77.0 | 57,53 | 73.9 | 57,40 | 75.7 | 57,46 |
| 28 | 91.67 | 84.7 | 60,14 | 84.1 | 59,48 | 84.5 | 59,84 | 88.0 | 61,02 | 87.2 | 59,84 | 87.6 | 60,47 | 81.9 | 59,47 | 81.4 | 59,14 | 81.7 | 59,32 |
| 29 | 95.83 | 89.4 | 62,12 | 89.3 | 61,29 | 89.4 | 61,74 | 90.5 | 63,04 | 90.9 | 61,72 | 90.7 | 62,43 | 88.5 | 61,42 | 87.6 | 60,87 | 88.1 | 61,18 |
| 30 | 100.00 | 100.0 | 64,11 | 100.0 | 63,10 | 100.0 | 63,65 | 100.0 | 65,07 | 100.0 | 63,59 | 100.0 | 64,38 | 100.0 | 63,37 | 100.0 | 62,61 | 100.0 | 63,03 |

Note: Calculation of z-scores was restricted to complete cases. RS = raw score; TRS = transformed raw score (range 0-100); PR = percentile; TS = T-score (M = 50, SD = 10).

197

**Table 28 DISABKIDS chronic generic module, total score including items from the treatment scale\* (proxy-report) – DCGM-37-P**

| RS | TRS | Total sample 8-12 (n = 407) PR | TS | Total sample 13-16 (n = 295) PR | TS | Total sample Overall (n = 702) PR | TS | Females 8-12 (n = 185) PR | TS | Females 13-16 (n = 146) PR | TS | Females Overall (n = 331) PR | TS | Males 8-12 (n = 220) PR | TS | Males 13-16 (n = 147) PR | TS | Males Overall (n = 367) PR | TS |
|---|---|---|---|---|---|---|---|---|---|---|---|---|---|---|---|---|---|---|---|
| <= 90 | 35.81 | .7 | 20.84 | 1.4 | 23.80 | 1.0 | 22.93 | - | | 1.4 | 22.48 | .3 | 17.71 | 1.4 | 22.71 | .7 | 9.71 | 1.1 | 23.36 |
| 91 | 36.49 | .7 | 20.84 | 1.4 | 23.80 | 1.1 | 24.32 | - | | 2.1 | 24.90 | .6 | 21.10 | 1.4 | 22.71 | .7 | 9.71 | 1.1 | 23.36 |
| 92 | 37.16 | 1.2 | 21.78 | 1.7 | 25.63 | 1.6 | 24.78 | .5 | 22.66 | 2.1 | 24.90 | .9 | 23.53 | 1.8 | 24.51 | 1.4 | 26.08 | 1.6 | 25.15 |
| 93 | 37.84 | 1.5 | 23.65 | 2.0 | 26.09 | 1.9 | 25.24 | .5 | 22.66 | 2.7 | 25.87 | 1.2 | 24.01 | 2.3 | 24.96 | 1.4 | 26.08 | 1.9 | 25.60 |
| 94 | 38.51 | 1.7 | 24.12 | 2.4 | 26.55 | 2.0 | 25.24 | .5 | 22.66 | 2.7 | 25.87 | 1.5 | 24.50 | 2.7 | 25.41 | 1.4 | 26.08 | 2.2 | 26.04 |
| 95 | 39.19 | 1.7 | 24.12 | 2.4 | 26.55 | 2.0 | 25.70 | .5 | 22.66 | 2.7 | 25.87 | 1.5 | 24.50 | 2.7 | 25.41 | 1.4 | 26.08 | 2.2 | 26.04 |
| 96 | 39.86 | 2.0 | 24.59 | 2.4 | 26.55 | 2.1 | 26.63 | .5 | 22.66 | 2.7 | 25.87 | 1.5 | 24.50 | 3.2 | 26.31 | 1.4 | 26.08 | 2.5 | 26.94 |
| 97 | 40.54 | 2.2 | 25.52 | 2.4 | 26.55 | 2.3 | 27.09 | .5 | 22.66 | 2.7 | 25.87 | 1.5 | 24.50 | 3.6 | 26.76 | 1.4 | 26.08 | 2.7 | 27.38 |
| 98 | 41.22 | 2.7 | 25.99 | 3.4 | 28.83 | 3.0 | 27.55 | 1.1 | 25.60 | 3.4 | 28.29 | 2.1 | 26.93 | 4.1 | 27.21 | 2.7 | 28.73 | 3.5 | 27.83 |
| 99 | 41.90 | 3.2 | 26.46 | 3.4 | 28.83 | 3.3 | 28.01 | 2.2 | 26.09 | 3.4 | 28.29 | 2.7 | 27.41 | 4.1 | 27.21 | 2.7 | 28.73 | 3.5 | 27.83 |
| 100 | 42.57 | 3.2 | 26.46 | 4.1 | 29.75 | 3.6 | 28.47 | 2.2 | 26.09 | 4.1 | 29.26 | 3.0 | 27.90 | 4.1 | 27.21 | 3.4 | 29.61 | 3.8 | 28.72 |
| 101 | 43.24 | 3.7 | 26.93 | 4.1 | 29.75 | 3.8 | 28.94 | 2.2 | 26.09 | 4.1 | 29.26 | 3.0 | 27.90 | 5.0 | 28.56 | 3.4 | 29.61 | 4.4 | 29.17 |
| 102 | 43.92 | 3.7 | 26.93 | 4.1 | 29.75 | 3.8 | 28.94 | 2.2 | 26.09 | 4.1 | 29.26 | 3.0 | 27.90 | 5.0 | 28.56 | 3.4 | 29.61 | 4.4 | 29.17 |
| 103 | 44.60 | 4.2 | 27.86 | 4.1 | 29.75 | 4.1 | 29.86 | 3.2 | 26.09 | 4.1 | 29.26 | 3.0 | 27.90 | 5.0 | 28.56 | 3.4 | 29.61 | 4.4 | 29.17 |
| 104 | 45.27 | 4.4 | 28.80 | 4.4 | 31.58 | 4.4 | 30.32 | 3.8 | 28.05 | 4.8 | 31.20 | 3.6 | 29.35 | 5.0 | 28.56 | 3.4 | 29.61 | 4.4 | 29.17 |
| 105 | 45.94 | 4.7 | 29.27 | 5.1 | 32.04 | 4.8 | 30.78 | 4.3 | 28.54 | 5.5 | 31.68 | 4.2 | 29.84 | 5.0 | 28.56 | 4.1 | 31.82 | 4.6 | 30.96 |
| 106 | 46.62 | 5.2 | 29.73 | 5.1 | 32.04 | 5.1 | 31.25 | 4.9 | 29.04 | 5.5 | 31.68 | 4.8 | 30.32 | 5.5 | 30.82 | 4.1 | 31.82 | 4.9 | 31.41 |
| 107 | 47.30 | 5.2 | 29.73 | 5.4 | 32.95 | 5.3 | 31.71 | 4.9 | 29.04 | 6.2 | 32.65 | 5.1 | 30.81 | 5.5 | 30.82 | 4.1 | 31.82 | 4.9 | 31.41 |
| 108 | 47.97 | 5.2 | 29.73 | 5.8 | 33.41 | 5.4 | 32.17 | 4.9 | 29.04 | 6.8 | 33.14 | 5.4 | 31.29 | 5.5 | 30.82 | 4.1 | 31.82 | 4.9 | 31.41 |
| 109 | 48.65 | 5.2 | 29.73 | 6.1 | 33.87 | 5.6 | 32.63 | 4.9 | 29.04 | 6.8 | 33.14 | 5.7 | 31.78 | 5.5 | 30.82 | 4.8 | 33.59 | 5.2 | 32.75 |
| 110 | 49.32 | 5.9 | 30.20 | 6.4 | 34.32 | 6.1 | 33.09 | 4.9 | 29.04 | 6.8 | 33.14 | 5.7 | 31.78 | 6.8 | 32.62 | 5.4 | 34.04 | 6.3 | 33.19 |
| 111 | 50.00 | 6.1 | 32.07 | 8.1 | 34.78 | 7.0 | 33.55 | 4.9 | 29.04 | 8.2 | 34.59 | 5.7 | 31.78 | 7.3 | 33.07 | 7.5 | 34.48 | 7.4 | 33.64 |
| 112 | 50.67 | 7.6 | 32.54 | 8.8 | 35.24 | 8.1 | 34.02 | 5.9 | 29.53 | 8.9 | 35.07 | 6.3 | 33.23 | 9.1 | 33.52 | 8.2 | 34.92 | 8.7 | 34.09 |
| 113 | 51.35 | 8.1 | 33.01 | 9.2 | 35.69 | 8.5 | 34.48 | 7.0 | 32.47 | 9.6 | 35.56 | 7.3 | 33.72 | 9.1 | 33.52 | 8.2 | 34.92 | 8.7 | 34.09 |
| 114 | 52.02 | 8.6 | 33.48 | 9.2 | 35.69 | 8.8 | 34.94 | 8.1 | 32.96 | 9.6 | 35.56 | 8.2 | 34.20 | 9.1 | 33.52 | 8.2 | 34.92 | 8.7 | 34.09 |
| 115 | 52.70 | 9.1 | 33.95 | 9.5 | 36.61 | 9.3 | 35.40 | 9.2 | 33.45 | 10.3 | 36.53 | 8.8 | 34.69 | 9.1 | 33.52 | 8.2 | 34.92 | 9.3 | 35.88 |
| 116 | 53.38 | 9.8 | 34.42 | 10.2 | 37.07 | 10.0 | 35.86 | 9.7 | 33.94 | 11.6 | 37.01 | 9.7 | 35.17 | 10.0 | 35.32 | 8.2 | 34.92 | 9.3 | 35.88 |
| 117 | 54.05 | 9.8 | 34.88 | 11.2 | 37.52 | 10.4 | 36.33 | 9.7 | 33.94 | 13.7 | 37.49 | 10.6 | 35.66 | 10.0 | 35.32 | 8.2 | 34.92 | 9.3 | 35.88 |
| 118 | 54.73 | 10.3 | 35.82 | 11.2 | 37.52 | 10.7 | 36.79 | 10.8 | 34.43 | 13.7 | 37.49 | 11.5 | 36.14 | 10.0 | 35.32 | 10.2 | 38.46 | 10.1 | 37.22 |
| 119 | 55.40 | 10.8 | 36.29 | 12.2 | 38.44 | 11.4 | 37.25 | 11.9 | 35.41 | 13.7 | 37.49 | 12.1 | 36.63 | 10.0 | 35.32 | 11.6 | 38.90 | 10.6 | 37.66 |
| 120 | 56.08 | 11.1 | 36.76 | 13.6 | 38.90 | 12.1 | 37.71 | 12.4 | 35.90 | 15.1 | 38.95 | 12.7 | 37.11 | 10.0 | 35.32 | 13.6 | 38.46 | 12.5 | 38.11 |
| 121 | 56.76 | 12.3 | 37.22 | 14.6 | 39.35 | 13.2 | 38.17 | 13.0 | 36.40 | 15.1 | 38.95 | 13.9 | 37.60 | 11.8 | 37.57 | 13.6 | 38.90 | 12.5 | 38.11 |
| 122 | 57.43 | 12.5 | 37.69 | 16.3 | 39.81 | 14.1 | 38.63 | 13.0 | 36.40 | 16.4 | 39.92 | 13.9 | 38.08 | 12.3 | 38.02 | 15.6 | 39.34 | 13.6 | 38.56 |
| 123 | 58.10 | 13.3 | 38.16 | 16.6 | 40.27 | 14.7 | 39.10 | 13.5 | 36.89 | 16.4 | 39.92 | 14.5 | 38.57 | 13.2 | 38.47 | 16.3 | 39.78 | 14.4 | 39.00 |
| 124 | 58.78 | 14.0 | 38.63 | 18.0 | 40.72 | 15.7 | 39.56 | 14.6 | 37.87 | 18.5 | 40.88 | 14.8 | 39.05 | 13.6 | 38.92 | 17.0 | 40.23 | 15.0 | 39.45 |
| 125 | 59.46 | 14.7 | 39.10 | 19.7 | 41.18 | 16.8 | 40.02 | 15.7 | 38.36 | 19.2 | 41.37 | 16.3 | 39.54 | 14.1 | 39.37 | 19.7 | 40.67 | 16.3 | 39.90 |
| 126 | 60.13 | 15.2 | 39.56 | 20.7 | 41.64 | 17.5 | 40.48 | 16.2 | 38.85 | 19.9 | 41.85 | 17.2 | 40.02 | 14.5 | 39.82 | 21.1 | 41.11 | 17.2 | 40.35 |
| 127 | 60.81 | 16.5 | 40.03 | 21.4 | 42.10 | 18.5 | 40.94 | 17.8 | 39.34 | 20.5 | 42.34 | 17.8 | 40.51 | 15.5 | 40.27 | 21.8 | 41.55 | 18.0 | 40.79 |
| 128 | 61.49 | 17.2 | 40.50 | 22.4 | 42.55 | 19.4 | 41.41 | 18.9 | 39.83 | 21.9 | 42.82 | 19.0 | 40.99 | 15.9 | 40.72 | 22.4 | 42.00 | 18.5 | 41.24 |
| 129 | 62.16 | 18.4 | 40.97 | 23.7 | 43.01 | 20.7 | 41.87 | 20.0 | 40.32 | 23.3 | 43.31 | 20.2 | 41.48 | 17.3 | 41.17 | 23.8 | 42.44 | 19.9 | 41.69 |

**Table 28   continued**

| DCGM-3-P TOTAL SCORE PROXY-REPORT | | Total sample 8-12 (n = 407) | | Total sample 13-16 (n = 295) | | Total sample Overall (n = 702) | | Females 8-12 (n = 185) | | Females 13-16 (n = 146) | | Females Overall (n = 331) | | Males 8-12 (n = 220) | | Males 13-16 (n = 147) | | Males Overall (n = 367) | |
|---|---|---|---|---|---|---|---|---|---|---|---|---|---|---|---|---|---|---|---|
| RS | TRS | PR | TS | PR | TS | PR | TS | PR | TS | RS | TRS | PR | TS | PR | TS | PR | TS | PR | TS |
| 130 | 62.83 | 18.9 | 41,44 | 25.8 | 43,47 | 21.8 | 42,33 | 21.1 | 40,81 | 27.4 | 43,79 | 21.5 | 41,96 | 17.3 | 41,17 | 23.8 | 42,44 | 19.9 | 41,69 |
| 131 | 63.51 | 19.9 | 41,90 | 26.8 | 43,93 | 22.8 | 42,79 | 21.6 | 41,30 | 28.8 | 44,27 | 23.9 | 42,45 | 18.6 | 42,07 | 24.5 | 43,32 | 21.0 | 42,58 |
| 132 | 64.19 | 20.9 | 42,37 | 28.5 | 44,38 | 24.1 | 43,25 | 23.2 | 41,79 | 30.8 | 44,76 | 24.8 | 42,93 | 19.1 | 42,52 | 25.9 | 43,76 | 21.8 | 43,03 |
| 133 | 64.86 | 21.9 | 42,84 | 29.8 | 44,84 | 25.2 | 43,71 | 24.3 | 42,28 | 30.8 | 44,76 | 26.6 | 43,42 | 20.0 | 42,97 | 28.6 | 44,21 | 23.4 | 43,47 |
| 134 | 65.54 | 23.3 | 43,31 | 31.5 | 45,30 | 26.8 | 44,18 | 24.9 | 42,77 | 31.5 | 45,73 | 27.2 | 43,90 | 22.3 | 43,43 | 31.3 | 44,65 | 25.9 | 43,92 |
| 135 | 66.22 | 24.1 | 43,78 | 32.5 | 45,76 | 27.6 | 44,64 | 24.9 | 43,26 | 31.5 | 45,73 | 27.8 | 44,39 | 23.6 | 43,88 | 33.3 | 45,09 | 27.5 | 44,37 |
| 136 | 66.89 | 25.3 | 44,24 | 33.2 | 46,21 | 28.6 | 45,10 | 25.4 | 44,25 | 33.6 | 47,18 | 28.1 | 45,36 | 25.5 | 44,33 | 34.7 | 45,53 | 29.2 | 44,82 |
| 137 | 67.57 | 26.3 | 44,71 | 35.6 | 46,67 | 30.2 | 45,56 | 25.9 | 44,74 | 34.2 | 47,66 | 29.3 | 45,85 | 26.8 | 44,78 | 37.4 | 45,98 | 31.1 | 45,26 |
| 138 | 68.24 | 28.5 | 45,18 | 36.3 | 47,13 | 31.8 | 46,02 | 27.0 | 45,23 | 37.7 | 48,15 | 30.2 | 46,33 | 30.0 | 45,23 | 38.1 | 46,42 | 33.2 | 45,71 |
| 139 | 68.92 | 30.2 | 45,65 | 38.3 | 47,58 | 33.6 | 46,49 | 28.6 | 45,72 | 42.5 | 48,63 | 32.6 | 46,82 | 31.8 | 45,68 | 38.8 | 46,86 | 34.6 | 46,16 |
| 140 | 69.59 | 31.9 | 46,12 | 42.0 | 48,04 | 36.2 | 46,95 | 29.7 | 46,21 | 44.5 | 49,12 | 35.3 | 47,30 | 34.1 | 46,13 | 41.5 | 47,30 | 37.1 | 46,60 |
| 141 | 70.27 | 32.9 | 46,58 | 44.1 | 48,50 | 37.6 | 47,41 | 30.3 | 46,70 | 45.2 | 49,60 | 36.6 | 47,79 | 35.5 | 46,58 | 43.5 | 47,74 | 38.7 | 47,05 |
| 142 | 70.94 | 34.2 | 47,05 | 44.4 | 48,96 | 38.5 | 47,87 | 31.4 | 47,19 | 45.9 | 50,09 | 37.5 | 48,27 | 36.8 | 47,03 | 43.5 | 47,74 | 39.5 | 47,50 |
| 143 | 71.62 | 36.4 | 47,52 | 45.1 | 49,41 | 40.0 | 48,33 | 35.7 | 47,68 | 47.9 | 50,57 | 40.2 | 48,76 | 37.3 | 47,48 | 44.2 | 48,63 | 40.1 | 47,94 |
| 144 | 72.23 | 38.1 | 47,99 | 47.1 | 49,87 | 41.9 | 48,79 | 37.8 | 48,17 | 47.9 | 50,57 | 42.3 | 49,24 | 38.6 | 47,93 | 46.3 | 49,07 | 41.7 | 48,39 |
| 145 | 72.98 | 40.5 | 48,46 | 48.8 | 50,33 | 44.0 | 49,26 | 41.1 | 48,66 | 49.3 | 51,05 | 44.7 | 49,73 | 40.5 | 48,38 | 48.3 | 49,51 | 43.6 | 48,84 |
| 146 | 73.65 | 42.8 | 48,92 | 50.2 | 50,79 | 45.9 | 49,72 | 43.8 | 49,15 | 50.7 | 51,54 | 46.8 | 50,21 | 42.3 | 48,83 | 49.7 | 49,95 | 45.2 | 49,29 |
| 147 | 74.32 | 45.7 | 49,39 | 52.2 | 51,24 | 48.4 | 50,18 | 46.5 | 49,64 | 52.7 | 52,02 | 49.2 | 50,70 | 45.5 | 49,28 | 51.0 | 50,40 | 47.7 | 49,73 |
| 148 | 75.00 | 47.2 | 49,86 | 53.6 | 51,70 | 49.9 | 50,64 | 47.6 | 50,13 | 55.5 | 52,51 | 51.1 | 51,18 | 47.3 | 49,73 | 51.0 | 50,40 | 48.8 | 50,18 |
| 149 | 75.67 | 48.6 | 50,33 | 55.6 | 52,16 | 51.6 | 51,10 | 48.6 | 50,62 | 58.2 | 52,99 | 52.9 | 51,67 | 49.1 | 50,18 | 52.4 | 51,28 | 50.4 | 50,63 |
| 150 | 76.35 | 50.6 | 50,80 | 56.6 | 52,62 | 53.1 | 51,57 | 51.9 | 51,11 | 58.9 | 53,48 | 55.0 | 52,15 | 50.0 | 50,63 | 53.7 | 51,72 | 51.5 | 51,07 |
| 151 | 77.03 | 51.6 | 51,27 | 58.3 | 53,07 | 54.4 | 52,03 | 53.5 | 51,60 | 61.6 | 53,96 | 57.1 | 52,64 | 50.5 | 51,08 | 54.4 | 52,17 | 52.0 | 51,52 |
| 152 | 77.70 | 53.3 | 51,73 | 61.7 | 53,53 | 56.8 | 52,49 | 55.7 | 52,10 | 67.1 | 54,44 | 60.7 | 53,12 | 51.8 | 51,53 | 55.8 | 52,61 | 53.4 | 51,97 |
| 153 | 78.38 | 54.8 | 52,20 | 63.1 | 53,99 | 58.3 | 52,95 | 58.4 | 52,59 | 67.1 | 54,44 | 62.2 | 53,61 | 52.3 | 51,98 | 58.5 | 53,05 | 54.8 | 52,41 |
| 154 | 79.05 | 57.7 | 52,67 | 64.1 | 54,44 | 60.4 | 53,41 | 61.6 | 53,08 | 68.5 | 55,41 | 64.7 | 54,09 | 55.0 | 52,43 | 59.2 | 53,49 | 56.7 | 52,86 |
| 155 | 79.73 | 59.7 | 53,14 | 65.4 | 54,90 | 62.1 | 53,87 | 63.2 | 53,57 | 71.2 | 55,90 | 66.8 | 54,58 | 57.3 | 52,88 | 59.2 | 54,38 | 58.0 | 53,31 |
| 156 | 80.40 | 62.2 | 53,61 | 66.8 | 55,33 | 64.1 | 54,34 | 65.4 | 54,06 | 72.6 | 56,38 | 68.6 | 55,06 | 60.0 | 53,33 | 60.5 | 54,82 | 60.2 | 53,75 |
| 157 | 81.08 | 64.1 | 54,07 | 68.5 | 55,82 | 66.0 | 54,80 | 67.0 | 54,55 | 72.6 | 56,38 | 69.5 | 55,55 | 62.3 | 53,78 | 63.9 | 55,26 | 62.9 | 54,20 |
| 158 | 81.76 | 64.6 | 54,54 | 69.8 | 56,27 | 66.8 | 55,26 | 67.6 | 55,04 | 74.0 | 57,35 | 70.4 | 56,03 | 62.7 | 54,23 | 65.3 | 55,70 | 63.8 | 54,65 |
| 159 | 82.43 | 66.8 | 55,01 | 72.5 | 56,73 | 69.2 | 55,72 | 68.1 | 55,53 | 77.4 | 57,84 | 72.2 | 56,52 | 66.4 | 54,68 | 67.3 | 56,15 | 66.8 | 55,10 |
| 160 | 83.10 | 68.6 | 55,48 | 74.2 | 57,19 | 70.9 | 56,18 | 70.3 | 56,02 | 79.5 | 58,32 | 74.3 | 57,00 | 67.7 | 55,13 | 68.7 | 56,59 | 68.1 | 55,54 |
| 161 | 83.78 | 70.3 | 55,95 | 76.6 | 57,65 | 72.9 | 56,65 | 70.8 | 56,51 | 82.2 | 58,80 | 75.8 | 57,49 | 70.0 | 55,58 | 70.7 | 57,03 | 70.3 | 55,99 |
| 162 | 84.46 | 71.7 | 56,41 | 78.0 | 58,10 | 74.4 | 57,11 | 73.0 | 57,00 | 83.6 | 59,29 | 77.6 | 57,97 | 70.9 | 56,03 | 72.1 | 57,47 | 71.4 | 56,44 |
| 163 | 85.13 | 73.0 | 56,88 | 80.0 | 58,56 | 75.9 | 57,57 | 74.1 | 57,49 | 85.6 | 59,77 | 79.2 | 58,46 | 72.3 | 56,48 | 74.1 | 57,91 | 73.0 | 56,88 |
| 164 | 85.81 | 73.7 | 57,35 | 81.0 | 59,02 | 76.8 | 58,03 | 74.6 | 57,98 | 87.0 | 60,26 | 80.1 | 58,94 | 73.2 | 56,94 | 74.8 | 58,36 | 73.8 | 57,33 |
| 165 | 86.49 | 74.7 | 57,82 | 82.4 | 59,48 | 77.9 | 58,49 | 75.7 | 58,47 | 88.4 | 60,74 | 81.3 | 59,43 | 74.1 | 57,39 | 76.2 | 58,80 | 74.9 | 57,78 |
| 166 | 87.16 | 78.1 | 58,29 | 84.7 | 59,93 | 80.9 | 58,96 | 80.5 | 58,96 | 91.1 | 61,23 | 85.2 | 59,91 | 76.4 | 57,84 | 78.2 | 59,24 | 77.1 | 58,22 |
| 167 | 87.84 | 80.1 | 58,75 | 86.1 | 60,39 | 82.6 | 59,42 | 83.2 | 59,45 | 91.1 | 61,23 | 86.7 | 60,40 | 77.7 | 58,29 | 81.0 | 59,68 | 79.0 | 58,67 |
| 168 | 88.51 | 81.1 | 59,22 | 87.5 | 60,85 | 83.8 | 59,88 | 83.8 | 59,95 | 92.5 | 62,19 | 87.6 | 60,88 | 79.1 | 58,74 | 82.3 | 60,13 | 80.4 | 59,12 |
| 169 | 89.19 | 83.0 | 59,69 | 88.5 | 61,30 | 85.3 | 60,34 | 85.4 | 60,44 | 93.2 | 62,68 | 88.8 | 61,37 | 81.4 | 59,19 | 83.7 | 60,57 | 82.3 | 59,57 |

**Table 28** continued

| DCGM-37-P TOTAL SCORE PROXY-REPORT | | Total sample 8-12 (n = 407) | | Total sample 13-16 (n = 295) | | Total sample Overall (n = 702) | | Females 8-12 (n = 185) | | Females 13-16 (n = 146) | | Females Overall (n = 331) | | Males 8-12 (n = 220) | | Males 13-16 (n = 147) | | Males Overall (n = 367) | |
|---|---|---|---|---|---|---|---|---|---|---|---|---|---|---|---|---|---|---|---|
| RS | TRS | PR | TS | PR | TS | PR | TS | PR | TS | RS | TRS | PR | TS | PR | TS | PR | TS | PR | TS |
| 170 | 89.87 | 84.0 | 60.16 | 89.5 | 61.76 | 86.3 | 60.80 | 86.5 | 60.93 | 93.8 | 63.16 | 89.7 | 61.85 | 82.3 | 59.64 | 85.0 | 61.01 | 83.4 | 60.01 |
| 171 | 90.54 | 85.3 | 60.63 | 90.2 | 62.22 | 87.3 | 61.26 | 87.6 | 61.42 | 94.5 | 63.65 | 90.6 | 62.34 | 83.6 | 60.09 | 85.7 | 61.45 | 84.5 | 60.46 |
| 172 | 91.22 | 86.7 | 61.09 | 91.5 | 62.68 | 88.7 | 61.73 | 89.2 | 61.91 | 95.2 | 64.13 | 91.8 | 62.82 | 85.0 | 60.54 | 87.8 | 61.89 | 86.1 | 60.91 |
| 173 | 91.89 | 87.7 | 61.56 | 92.5 | 63.13 | 89.7 | 62.19 | 90.3 | 62.40 | 96.6 | 64.62 | 93.1 | 63.31 | 85.9 | 60.99 | 88.4 | 62.34 | 86.9 | 61.35 |
| 174 | 92.57 | 89.4 | 62.03 | 93.9 | 63.59 | 91.3 | 62.65 | 91.9 | 62.89 | 96.6 | 64.62 | 94.0 | 63.79 | 87.3 | 61.44 | 91.2 | 63.22 | 88.8 | 61.80 |
| 175 | 93.24 | 90.9 | 62.50 | 93.9 | 63.59 | 92.2 | 63.11 | 94.1 | 63.38 | 96.6 | 64.62 | 95.2 | 64.28 | 88.2 | 61.89 | 91.2 | 63.22 | 89.4 | 62.25 |
| 176 | 93.92 | 92.4 | 62.97 | 94.9 | 64.51 | 93.4 | 63.57 | 95.1 | 63.87 | 97.3 | 66.07 | 96.1 | 64.76 | 90.0 | 62.34 | 92.5 | 63.66 | 91.0 | 62.69 |
| 177 | 94.59 | 94.8 | 63.43 | 96.3 | 64.96 | 95.4 | 64.04 | 97.3 | 64.36 | 97.9 | 66.55 | 97.6 | 65.25 | 92.7 | 62.79 | 94.6 | 64.11 | 93.5 | 63.14 |
| 178 | 95.27 | 95.6 | 63.90 | 97.3 | 65.42 | 96.3 | 64.50 | 97.3 | 64.36 | 98.6 | 67.04 | 97.9 | 65.73 | 94.1 | 63.24 | 95.9 | 64.55 | 94.8 | 63.59 |
| 179 | 95.94 | 96.6 | 64.37 | 97.6 | 65.88 | 97.0 | 64.96 | 97.3 | 64.36 | 98.6 | 67.04 | 98.2 | 66.22 | 95.5 | 63.69 | 98.0 | 64.99 | 95.9 | 64.04 |
| 180 | 96.62 | 97.1 | 64.84 | 98.3 | 66.33 | 97.6 | 65.42 | 97.8 | 65.34 | 98.6 | 67.04 | 98.2 | 66.22 | 96.4 | 64.14 | 98.0 | 64.99 | 97.0 | 64.48 |
| 181 | 97.23 | 98.0 | 65.31 | 98.6 | 66.79 | 98.3 | 65.88 | 98.4 | 66.32 | 99.3 | 68.49 | 98.8 | 67.19 | 97.7 | 64.59 | 98.0 | 64.99 | 97.8 | 64.93 |
| 182 | 97.97 | 99.0 | 65.77 | 98.6 | 66.79 | 98.9 | 66.34 | 99.5 | 66.81 | 99.3 | 68.49 | 99.4 | 67.68 | 98.6 | 65.04 | 98.0 | 64.99 | 98.4 | 65.38 |
| 183 | 98.65 | 99.5 | 66.24 | 99.3 | 67.71 | 99.4 | 66.81 | 100.0 | 67.30 | 99.3 | 68.49 | 99.7 | 68.16 | 99.1 | 65.49 | 99.3 | 66.32 | 99.2 | 65.82 |
| 184 | 99.32 | 99.8 | 66.71 | 99.7 | 68.16 | 99.7 | 67.27 | 100.0 | 67.30 | 99.3 | 68.49 | 99.7 | 68.16 | 99.5 | 65.94 | 100.0 | 66.76 | 99.7 | 66.27 |
| 185 | 100.00 | 100.0 | 67.18 | 100.0 | 68.62 | 100.0 | 67.73 | 100.0 | 67.30 | 100.0 | 70.43 | 100.0 | 69.13 | 100.0 | 66.39 | 100.0 | 66.76 | 100.0 | 66.72 |

*Note: Calculation of scores was restricted to complete cases. RS = raw score; TRS = transformed raw score (range 0-100); PR = percentile; TS = T-score (M = 50, SD = 10).*
*These reference values should be selected when children receive medication/treatment and the respective scale is applicable.*

**Table 29 DISABKIDS chronic generic module, total score (if the "treatment" is not applicable; proxy-report) – DCGM-37-P (V-31)**

| DCGM-37-P (V-31) TOTAL SCORE (V-31) PROXY-REPORT | | Total sample 8-12 (n =458) | | Total sample 13-16 (n =339) | | Total sample Overall (n =797) | | Females 8-12 (n =212) | | Females 13-16 (n =161) | | Females Overall (n =373) | | Males 8-12 (n =244) | | Males 13-16 (n =176) | | Males Overall (n =420) | |
|---|---|---|---|---|---|---|---|---|---|---|---|---|---|---|---|---|---|---|---|
| RS | TRS | PR | TS | PR | TS | PR | TS | PR | TS | PR | TS | PR | TS | PR | TS | PR | TS | PR | TS |
| <= 75 | 35,48 | 1,3 | 22,54 | 2,1 | 25,35 | 1,6 | 24,16 | 1,4 | 20,52 | 2,5 | 24,66 | 1,9 | 23,75 | 1,2 | 22,99 | 1,1 | 25,18 | 1,2 | 24,23 |
| 76 | 36,29 | 1,5 | 23,61 | 2,1 | 25,35 | 1,8 | 24,69 | 1,4 | 20,52 | 2,5 | 24,66 | 1,9 | 23,75 | 1,6 | 24,04 | 1,1 | 25,18 | 1,4 | 24,75 |
| 77 | 37,10 | 1,5 | 23,61 | 2,1 | 25,35 | 1,8 | 24,69 | 1,4 | 20,52 | 2,5 | 24,66 | 1,9 | 23,75 | 1,6 | 24,04 | 1,1 | 25,18 | 1,4 | 24,75 |
| 78 | 37,90 | 2,0 | 24,68 | 2,1 | 25,35 | 2,0 | 25,75 | 1,4 | 20,52 | 2,5 | 24,66 | 1,9 | 23,75 | 2,5 | 25,09 | 1,1 | 25,18 | 1,9 | 25,78 |
| 79 | 38,71 | 2,2 | 25,75 | 2,4 | 27,47 | 2,1 | 26,28 | 1,4 | 20,52 | 3,1 | 26,91 | 2,1 | 25,94 | 2,5 | 25,09 | 1,1 | 25,18 | 1,9 | 25,78 |
| 80 | 39,52 | 2,2 | 25,75 | 2,4 | 27,47 | 2,3 | 26,81 | 1,9 | 25,43 | 3,1 | 26,91 | 2,4 | 26,49 | 2,5 | 25,09 | 1,1 | 25,18 | 1,9 | 25,78 |
| 81 | 40,32 | 2,6 | 26,29 | 2,9 | 28,52 | 2,8 | 27,34 | 1,9 | 25,43 | 3,7 | 28,04 | 2,7 | 27,04 | 3,3 | 26,66 | 1,7 | 28,25 | 2,6 | 27,34 |
| 82 | 41,13 | 2,6 | 26,29 | 3,2 | 29,05 | 2,9 | 27,87 | 1,9 | 25,43 | 3,7 | 28,04 | 2,7 | 27,04 | 3,3 | 26,66 | 2,3 | 28,76 | 2,9 | 27,86 |
| 83 | 41,94 | 2,6 | 26,29 | 3,2 | 29,05 | 2,9 | 27,87 | 1,9 | 25,43 | 3,7 | 28,04 | 2,7 | 27,04 | 3,3 | 26,66 | 2,3 | 28,76 | 2,9 | 27,86 |
| 84 | 42,74 | 2,6 | 26,29 | 3,2 | 29,05 | 2,9 | 27,87 | 1,9 | 25,43 | 3,7 | 28,04 | 2,7 | 27,04 | 3,3 | 26,66 | 2,3 | 28,76 | 2,9 | 27,86 |
| 85 | 43,55 | 3,3 | 28,43 | 3,5 | 30,64 | 3,4 | 29,46 | 2,8 | 28,16 | 3,7 | 28,04 | 3,2 | 29,24 | 3,7 | 28,76 | 2,8 | 30,30 | 3,3 | 29,42 |
| 86 | 44,35 | 3,9 | 28,96 | 4,4 | 31,16 | 4,1 | 29,99 | 3,3 | 28,71 | 5,6 | 30,86 | 4,3 | 29,79 | 4,5 | 29,29 | 2,8 | 30,30 | 3,8 | 29,94 |
| 87 | 45,16 | 4,1 | 29,50 | 5,6 | 31,69 | 4,8 | 30,52 | 3,8 | 29,26 | 6,8 | 31,42 | 5,1 | 30,34 | 4,5 | 29,29 | 4,0 | 31,32 | 4,3 | 30,46 |
| 88 | 45,97 | 4,4 | 30,03 | 5,6 | 31,69 | 4,9 | 31,05 | 3,8 | 29,26 | 6,8 | 31,42 | 5,1 | 30,34 | 4,9 | 30,34 | 4,0 | 31,32 | 4,5 | 30,98 |
| 89 | 46,77 | 5,2 | 30,57 | 6,2 | 32,75 | 5,6 | 31,58 | 4,2 | 30,35 | 7,5 | 32,55 | 5,6 | 31,43 | 6,1 | 30,86 | 4,5 | 32,34 | 5,5 | 31,49 |
| 90 | 47,58 | 5,5 | 31,10 | 6,2 | 32,75 | 5,8 | 32,11 | 4,2 | 30,35 | 7,5 | 32,55 | 5,6 | 31,43 | 6,6 | 31,38 | 4,5 | 32,34 | 5,7 | 32,01 |
| 91 | 48,39 | 5,9 | 31,64 | 6,2 | 32,75 | 6,0 | 32,64 | 4,2 | 30,35 | 7,5 | 32,55 | 5,6 | 31,43 | 7,4 | 31,91 | 4,5 | 32,34 | 6,2 | 32,53 |
| 92 | 49,19 | 6,8 | 32,17 | 7,1 | 34,33 | 6,9 | 33,17 | 6,1 | 31,99 | 8,7 | 34,24 | 7,2 | 33,08 | 7,4 | 31,91 | 5,1 | 33,88 | 6,4 | 33,05 |
| 93 | 50,00 | 6,8 | 32,17 | 7,4 | 34,86 | 7,0 | 33,70 | 6,1 | 31,99 | 8,7 | 34,24 | 7,2 | 33,08 | 7,4 | 31,91 | 5,7 | 34,39 | 6,7 | 33,57 |
| 94 | 50,81 | 7,2 | 33,24 | 8,6 | 35,39 | 7,8 | 34,23 | 6,6 | 33,08 | 9,9 | 35,37 | 8,0 | 34,18 | 7,8 | 33,48 | 6,8 | 34,91 | 7,4 | 34,09 |
| 95 | 51,61 | 8,3 | 33,78 | 9,7 | 35,92 | 8,9 | 34,76 | 8,5 | 33,63 | 11,2 | 35,93 | 9,7 | 34,73 | 8,2 | 34,01 | 8,0 | 35,42 | 8,1 | 34,61 |
| 96 | 52,42 | 8,7 | 34,31 | 10,6 | 36,45 | 9,5 | 35,29 | 9,0 | 34,17 | 11,2 | 35,93 | 9,9 | 35,28 | 8,6 | 34,53 | 9,7 | 35,93 | 9,0 | 35,13 |
| 97 | 53,23 | 8,7 | 34,31 | 12,4 | 36,98 | 10,3 | 35,82 | 9,0 | 34,17 | 11,8 | 37,06 | 10,2 | 35,83 | 8,6 | 34,53 | 12,5 | 36,44 | 10,2 | 35,65 |
| 98 | 54,03 | 9,4 | 35,38 | 13,0 | 37,51 | 10,9 | 36,35 | 9,4 | 35,26 | 13,0 | 37,62 | 11,0 | 36,38 | 9,4 | 35,58 | 12,5 | 36,44 | 10,7 | 36,17 |
| 99 | 54,84 | 9,4 | 35,38 | 14,5 | 38,03 | 11,5 | 36,88 | 9,4 | 35,26 | 14,9 | 38,18 | 11,8 | 36,92 | 9,4 | 35,58 | 13,6 | 37,47 | 11,2 | 36,69 |
| 100 | 55,65 | 10,3 | 36,45 | 15,3 | 38,56 | 12,4 | 37,41 | 10,8 | 36,36 | 15,5 | 38,75 | 12,9 | 37,47 | 9,8 | 36,63 | 14,8 | 37,98 | 11,9 | 37,20 |
| 101 | 56,45 | 11,6 | 36,99 | 15,9 | 39,09 | 13,4 | 37,94 | 11,8 | 36,90 | 16,1 | 39,31 | 13,7 | 38,02 | 11,5 | 37,15 | 15,3 | 38,49 | 13,1 | 37,72 |
| 102 | 57,26 | 12,2 | 37,52 | 17,1 | 39,62 | 14,3 | 38,47 | 11,8 | 36,90 | 16,8 | 39,87 | 13,9 | 38,57 | 12,7 | 37,68 | 17,0 | 39,00 | 14,5 | 38,24 |
| 103 | 58,06 | 12,7 | 38,06 | 18,3 | 40,15 | 15,1 | 39,00 | 11,8 | 36,90 | 18,0 | 40,44 | 14,5 | 39,12 | 13,5 | 38,20 | 18,2 | 39,51 | 15,5 | 38,76 |
| 104 | 58,87 | 13,8 | 38,59 | 18,6 | 40,68 | 15,8 | 39,53 | 13,7 | 38,54 | 18,6 | 41,00 | 15,8 | 39,67 | 13,9 | 38,73 | 18,2 | 39,51 | 15,7 | 39,28 |
| 105 | 59,68 | 14,6 | 39,13 | 19,8 | 41,20 | 16,8 | 40,06 | 15,6 | 39,09 | 19,9 | 41,57 | 17,4 | 40,22 | 13,9 | 38,73 | 19,3 | 40,54 | 16,2 | 39,80 |
| 106 | 60,48 | 16,2 | 39,66 | 20,4 | 41,73 | 17,9 | 40,59 | 17,5 | 39,63 | 20,5 | 42,13 | 18,8 | 40,77 | 15,2 | 39,77 | 19,9 | 41,05 | 17,1 | 40,32 |
| 107 | 61,29 | 17,0 | 40,20 | 21,5 | 42,26 | 18,9 | 41,12 | 18,4 | 40,18 | 22,4 | 42,69 | 20,1 | 41,32 | 16,0 | 40,30 | 20,5 | 41,56 | 17,9 | 40,84 |
| 108 | 62,10 | 18,1 | 40,73 | 23,3 | 42,79 | 20,3 | 41,65 | 19,3 | 40,73 | 24,2 | 43,26 | 21,4 | 41,87 | 17,2 | 40,82 | 22,2 | 42,07 | 19,3 | 41,36 |
| 109 | 62,90 | 19,4 | 41,27 | 24,5 | 43,32 | 21,6 | 42,18 | 20,8 | 41,27 | 26,1 | 43,82 | 23,1 | 42,41 | 18,4 | 41,35 | 22,7 | 42,59 | 20,2 | 41,88 |
| 110 | 63,71 | 20,3 | 41,80 | 26,0 | 43,85 | 22,7 | 42,71 | 21,7 | 41,82 | 26,7 | 44,38 | 23,9 | 42,96 | 19,3 | 41,87 | 25,0 | 43,10 | 21,7 | 42,39 |
| 111 | 64,52 | 21,2 | 42,34 | 28,3 | 44,37 | 24,2 | 43,24 | 22,6 | 42,37 | 29,2 | 44,95 | 25,5 | 43,51 | 20,1 | 42,40 | 27,3 | 43,61 | 23,1 | 42,91 |
| 112 | 65,32 | 21,8 | 42,87 | 30,7 | 44,90 | 25,6 | 43,77 | 23,6 | 42,91 | 31,1 | 45,51 | 26,8 | 44,06 | 20,5 | 42,92 | 30,1 | 44,12 | 24,5 | 43,43 |
| 113 | 66,13 | 22,9 | 43,41 | 31,6 | 45,43 | 26,6 | 44,30 | 24,5 | 43,46 | 32,3 | 46,07 | 27,9 | 44,61 | 21,7 | 43,45 | 30,7 | 44,63 | 25,5 | 43,95 |
| 114 | 66,94 | 26,0 | 43,94 | 32,7 | 45,96 | 28,9 | 44,83 | 26,9 | 44,00 | 33,5 | 46,64 | 29,8 | 45,16 | 25,4 | 43,97 | 31,8 | 45,15 | 28,1 | 44,47 |
| 115 | 67,74 | 26,9 | 44,48 | 34,5 | 46,49 | 30,1 | 45,36 | 27,4 | 44,55 | 35,4 | 47,20 | 30,8 | 45,71 | 26,6 | 44,49 | 33,5 | 45,66 | 29,5 | 44,99 |

**Table 29   continued**

| DCGM-37-P (V-31) TOTAL SCORE (V-31) PROXY-REPORT | | Total sample 8-12 (n=458) | | Total sample 13-16 (n=339) | | Total sample Overall (n=797) | | Females 8-12 (n=212) | | Females 13-16 (n=161) | | Females Overall (n=373) | | Males 8-12 (n=244) | | Males 13-16 (n=176) | | Males Overall (n=420) | |
|---|---|---|---|---|---|---|---|---|---|---|---|---|---|---|---|---|---|---|---|
| RS | TRS | PR | TS | PR | TS | PR | TS | PR | TS | RS | TRS | PR | TS | PR | TS | PR | TS | PR | TS |
| 116 | 68,55 | 28,8 | 45,01 | 36,0 | 47,02 | 31,9 | 45,89 | 29,2 | 45,10 | 36,6 | 47,76 | 32,4 | 46,26 | 28,7 | 45,02 | 35,2 | 46,17 | 31,4 | 45,51 |
| 117 | 69,35 | 30,3 | 45,55 | 37,8 | 47,54 | 33,5 | 46,42 | 31,1 | 45,64 | 38,5 | 48,33 | 34,3 | 46,81 | 29,9 | 45,54 | 36,9 | 46,68 | 32,9 | 46,03 |
| 118 | 70,16 | 31,7 | 46,08 | 39,2 | 48,07 | 34,9 | 46,95 | 31,6 | 46,19 | 39,8 | 48,89 | 35,1 | 47,36 | 32,0 | 46,07 | 38,6 | 47,20 | 34,8 | 46,55 |
| 119 | 70,97 | 33,8 | 46,62 | 41,0 | 48,60 | 36,9 | 47,48 | 33,5 | 46,74 | 41,6 | 49,45 | 37,0 | 47,91 | 34,4 | 46,59 | 40,3 | 47,71 | 36,9 | 47,07 |
| 120 | 71,77 | 36,2 | 47,15 | 42,8 | 49,13 | 39,0 | 48,01 | 35,4 | 47,28 | 43,5 | 50,02 | 38,9 | 48,45 | 37,3 | 47,12 | 42,0 | 48,22 | 39,3 | 47,59 |
| 121 | 72,58 | 37,3 | 47,69 | 44,8 | 49,66 | 40,5 | 48,54 | 37,3 | 47,83 | 44,7 | 50,58 | 40,5 | 49,00 | 37,7 | 47,64 | 44,9 | 48,73 | 40,7 | 48,10 |
| 122 | 73,39 | 38,6 | 48,22 | 46,9 | 50,19 | 42,2 | 49,07 | 37,7 | 48,37 | 46,6 | 51,14 | 41,6 | 49,55 | 39,8 | 48,16 | 47,2 | 49,24 | 42,9 | 48,62 |
| 123 | 74,19 | 41,0 | 48,76 | 50,4 | 50,72 | 45,0 | 49,60 | 41,0 | 48,92 | 52,2 | 51,71 | 45,8 | 50,10 | 41,4 | 48,69 | 48,3 | 49,76 | 44,3 | 49,14 |
| 124 | 75,00 | 43,4 | 49,29 | 51,6 | 51,24 | 46,9 | 50,13 | 44,3 | 49,47 | 54,0 | 52,27 | 48,5 | 50,65 | 43,0 | 49,21 | 48,9 | 50,27 | 45,5 | 49,66 |
| 125 | 75,81 | 44,8 | 49,82 | 54,0 | 51,77 | 48,7 | 50,66 | 46,2 | 50,01 | 57,8 | 52,83 | 51,2 | 51,20 | 43,9 | 49,74 | 50,0 | 50,78 | 46,4 | 50,18 |
| 126 | 76,61 | 47,2 | 50,36 | 56,9 | 52,30 | 51,3 | 51,19 | 49,1 | 50,56 | 62,1 | 53,40 | 54,7 | 51,75 | 45,9 | 50,26 | 51,7 | 51,29 | 48,3 | 50,70 |
| 127 | 77,42 | 50,2 | 50,89 | 58,1 | 52,83 | 53,6 | 51,72 | 50,5 | 51,11 | 63,4 | 53,96 | 56,0 | 52,30 | 50,4 | 50,79 | 52,8 | 51,80 | 51,4 | 51,22 |
| 128 | 78,23 | 51,5 | 51,43 | 59,0 | 53,36 | 54,7 | 52,25 | 51,9 | 51,65 | 64,6 | 54,53 | 57,4 | 52,85 | 51,6 | 51,31 | 53,4 | 52,32 | 52,4 | 51,74 |
| 129 | 79,03 | 53,7 | 51,96 | 61,4 | 53,89 | 57,0 | 52,78 | 53,3 | 52,20 | 66,5 | 55,09 | 59,0 | 53,40 | 54,5 | 51,84 | 56,3 | 52,83 | 55,2 | 52,26 |
| 130 | 79,84 | 56,6 | 52,50 | 63,4 | 54,41 | 59,5 | 53,31 | 56,6 | 52,74 | 67,7 | 55,65 | 61,4 | 53,94 | 57,0 | 52,36 | 59,1 | 53,34 | 57,9 | 52,78 |
| 131 | 80,65 | 57,4 | 53,03 | 65,2 | 54,94 | 60,7 | 53,84 | 58,0 | 53,29 | 69,6 | 56,22 | 63,0 | 54,49 | 57,4 | 52,88 | 60,8 | 53,85 | 58,8 | 53,29 |
| 132 | 81,45 | 59,2 | 53,57 | 66,4 | 55,47 | 62,2 | 54,37 | 59,4 | 53,84 | 70,8 | 56,78 | 64,3 | 55,04 | 59,4 | 53,41 | 61,9 | 54,36 | 60,5 | 53,81 |
| 133 | 82,26 | 62,7 | 54,10 | 68,4 | 56,00 | 65,1 | 54,90 | 62,7 | 54,38 | 73,3 | 57,34 | 67,3 | 55,59 | 63,1 | 53,93 | 63,6 | 54,88 | 63,3 | 54,33 |
| 134 | 83,06 | 65,5 | 54,64 | 70,5 | 56,53 | 67,6 | 55,43 | 65,6 | 54,93 | 76,4 | 57,91 | 70,2 | 56,14 | 66,0 | 54,46 | 64,8 | 55,39 | 65,5 | 54,85 |
| 135 | 83,87 | 67,7 | 55,17 | 73,5 | 57,06 | 70,1 | 55,96 | 67,0 | 55,48 | 80,7 | 58,47 | 72,9 | 56,69 | 68,4 | 54,98 | 66,5 | 55,90 | 67,6 | 55,37 |
| 136 | 84,68 | 69,4 | 55,71 | 75,2 | 57,58 | 71,9 | 56,49 | 68,9 | 56,02 | 83,2 | 59,03 | 75,1 | 57,24 | 70,1 | 55,51 | 67,6 | 56,41 | 69,0 | 55,89 |
| 137 | 85,48 | 71,4 | 56,24 | 76,4 | 58,11 | 73,5 | 57,02 | 71,2 | 56,57 | 85,1 | 59,60 | 77,2 | 57,79 | 71,7 | 56,03 | 68,2 | 56,92 | 70,2 | 56,41 |
| 138 | 86,29 | 73,4 | 56,78 | 79,1 | 58,64 | 75,8 | 57,55 | 73,6 | 57,11 | 87,6 | 60,16 | 79,6 | 58,34 | 73,4 | 56,55 | 71,0 | 57,44 | 72,4 | 56,93 |
| 139 | 87,10 | 74,5 | 57,31 | 81,7 | 59,17 | 77,5 | 58,08 | 75,5 | 57,66 | 90,1 | 60,72 | 81,8 | 58,89 | 73,8 | 57,08 | 73,9 | 57,95 | 73,8 | 57,45 |
| 140 | 87,90 | 74,9 | 57,85 | 83,8 | 59,70 | 78,7 | 58,61 | 75,5 | 58,21 | 91,3 | 61,29 | 82,3 | 59,44 | 74,6 | 57,60 | 76,7 | 58,46 | 75,5 | 57,97 |
| 141 | 88,71 | 77,7 | 58,38 | 85,3 | 60,23 | 80,9 | 59,14 | 78,8 | 58,75 | 93,2 | 61,85 | 85,0 | 59,98 | 77,0 | 58,13 | 77,8 | 58,97 | 77,4 | 58,49 |
| 142 | 89,52 | 79,3 | 58,92 | 85,8 | 60,76 | 82,1 | 59,67 | 79,7 | 59,30 | 93,8 | 62,41 | 85,8 | 60,53 | 79,1 | 58,65 | 78,4 | 59,49 | 78,8 | 59,00 |
| 143 | 90,32 | 81,9 | 59,45 | 88,8 | 61,28 | 84,8 | 60,20 | 82,5 | 59,85 | 95,0 | 62,98 | 87,9 | 61,08 | 81,6 | 59,18 | 83,0 | 60,00 | 82,1 | 59,52 |
| 144 | 91,13 | 83,8 | 59,99 | 90,9 | 61,81 | 86,8 | 60,73 | 85,8 | 60,39 | 95,7 | 63,54 | 90,1 | 61,63 | 82,4 | 59,70 | 86,4 | 60,51 | 84,0 | 60,04 |
| 145 | 91,94 | 85,6 | 60,52 | 92,3 | 62,34 | 88,5 | 61,26 | 88,7 | 60,94 | 96,3 | 64,10 | 92,0 | 62,18 | 83,2 | 60,23 | 88,6 | 61,02 | 85,5 | 60,56 |
| 146 | 92,74 | 87,3 | 61,06 | 92,9 | 62,87 | 89,7 | 61,79 | 91,0 | 61,48 | 96,3 | 64,66 | 93,3 | 62,73 | 84,4 | 60,75 | 89,8 | 61,53 | 86,7 | 61,08 |
| 147 | 93,55 | 88,9 | 61,59 | 94,4 | 63,40 | 91,2 | 62,32 | 92,5 | 62,03 | 97,5 | 65,23 | 94,6 | 63,28 | 86,1 | 61,27 | 91,5 | 62,05 | 88,3 | 61,60 |
| 148 | 94,35 | 90,4 | 62,13 | 95,3 | 63,93 | 92,5 | 62,85 | 93,4 | 62,58 | 98,1 | 65,80 | 95,4 | 63,83 | 87,7 | 61,80 | 92,6 | 62,56 | 89,8 | 62,12 |
| 149 | 95,16 | 92,4 | 62,66 | 95,9 | 64,45 | 93,9 | 63,38 | 94,8 | 63,12 | 98,1 | 66,36 | 96,2 | 64,38 | 90,2 | 62,32 | 93,8 | 63,07 | 91,7 | 62,64 |
| 150 | 95,97 | 93,4 | 63,20 | 97,1 | 64,98 | 95,0 | 63,91 | 95,8 | 63,67 | 98,1 | 66,93 | 96,8 | 64,93 | 91,4 | 62,85 | 96,0 | 63,58 | 93,3 | 63,16 |
| 151 | 96,77 | 96,1 | 63,73 | 97,6 | 65,51 | 96,7 | 64,44 | 98,1 | 64,21 | 98,1 | 67,49 | 98,4 | 65,47 | 94,3 | 63,37 | 96,6 | 64,09 | 95,2 | 63,68 |
| 152 | 97,58 | 98,3 | 64,27 | 98,5 | 66,04 | 98,4 | 64,97 | 99,5 | 64,76 | 99,4 | 68,05 | 99,5 | 66,02 | 97,1 | 63,90 | 97,7 | 64,61 | 97,4 | 64,19 |
| 153 | 98,39 | 99,3 | 64,80 | 99,4 | 66,57 | 99,4 | 65,50 | 100,0 | 65,31 | 100,0 | 68,62 | 99,7 | 66,57 | 98,8 | 64,42 | 99,4 | 65,12 | 99,0 | 64,71 |
| 154 | 99,19 | 99,8 | 65,34 | 99,7 | 67,10 | 99,7 | 66,03 | 100,0 | 65,86 | 100,0 | 69,18 | 99,7 | 67,12 | 99,6 | 64,95 | 100,0 | 65,63 | 99,8 | 65,23 |
| 155 | 100,00 | 100,0 | 65,87 | 100,0 | 67,62 | 100,0 | 66,56 | 100,0 | 66,41 | 100,0 | 69,74 | 100,0 | 67,67 | 100,0 | 65,47 | 100,0 | 66,14 | 100,0 | 65,75 |

*Note: Calculation of scores was restricted to complete cases. RS = raw score; TRS = transformed raw score (range 0-100); PR = percentile; TS = T-score (M = 50, SD = 10). \*These reference values should be selected when children **do not** receive medication/treatment and the respective scale is **not** applicable.*

**Table 30    DISABKIDS chronic generic short-form score including treatment items (proxy-report) – DCGM-12-P**

| DCGM-2-P SCORE PROXY-REPORT | | Total sample 8-12 (n = 446) | | Total sample 13-16 (n = 326) | | Total sample Overall (n = 772) | | Females 8-12 (n = 202) | | Females 13-16 (n = 160) | | Females Overall (n = 362) | | Males 8-12 (n = 242) | | Males 13-16 (n = 164) | | Males Overall (n = 406) | |
|---|---|---|---|---|---|---|---|---|---|---|---|---|---|---|---|---|---|---|---|
| RS | TRS | PR | TS | PR | TS | PR | TS | PR | TS | PR | TS | PR | TS | PR | TS | PR | TS | PR | TS |
| <= 25 | 27.08 | .4 | 20.76 | 1.5 | 23.73 | .9 | 22.13 | - | - | 1.9 | 23.48 | .8 | 22.03 | .8 | 20.93 | .6 | 10.09 | .7 | 21.87 |
| 26 | 29.17 | .4 | 20.76 | 1.8 | 24.94 | 1.0 | 23.36 | - | - | 2.5 | 24.74 | 1.1 | 23.30 | .8 | 20.93 | .6 | 10.09 | .7 | 21.87 |
| 27 | 31.25 | .9 | 23.29 | 2.5 | 26.14 | 1.6 | 24.60 | .5 | 23.24 | 3.8 | 25.99 | 1.9 | 24.57 | 1.2 | 23.43 | .6 | 10.09 | 1.0 | 24.32 |
| 28 | 33.33 | 1.3 | 24.56 | 2.8 | 27.35 | 1.9 | 25.84 | 1.5 | 24.53 | 3.8 | 25.99 | 2.5 | 25.84 | 1.2 | 23.43 | 1.2 | 26.75 | 1.2 | 25.54 |
| 29 | 35.42 | 2.5 | 25.83 | 3.4 | 28.55 | 2.8 | 27.07 | 2.0 | 25.82 | 4.4 | 28.50 | 3.0 | 27.11 | 2.9 | 25.92 | 1.8 | 27.94 | 2.5 | 26.76 |
| 30 | 37.50 | 3.4 | 27.09 | 3.7 | 29.76 | 3.5 | 28.31 | 3.0 | 27.11 | 4.4 | 28.50 | 3.6 | 28.38 | 3.7 | 27.17 | 2.4 | 29.13 | 3.2 | 27.98 |
| 31 | 39.58 | 3.8 | 28.36 | 4.6 | 30.97 | 4.1 | 29.55 | 3.0 | 27.11 | 4.4 | 28.50 | 3.6 | 28.38 | 4.5 | 28.41 | 4.3 | 30.32 | 4.4 | 29.21 |
| 32 | 41.67 | 4.5 | 29.63 | 5.8 | 32.17 | 5.1 | 30.79 | 3.0 | 27.11 | 5.0 | 32.26 | 3.9 | 30.92 | 5.8 | 29.66 | 6.1 | 31.51 | 5.9 | 30.43 |
| 33 | 43.75 | 5.2 | 30.90 | 6.7 | 33.38 | 5.8 | 32.02 | 4.0 | 30.99 | 5.6 | 33.51 | 4.7 | 32.19 | 6.2 | 30.90 | 7.3 | 32.70 | 6.7 | 31.65 |
| 34 | 45.83 | 6.7 | 32.16 | 7.7 | 34.58 | 7.1 | 33.26 | 6.4 | 32.28 | 6.9 | 34.77 | 6.6 | 33.46 | 7.0 | 32.15 | 7.9 | 33.89 | 7.4 | 32.87 |
| 35 | 47.92 | 7.6 | 33.43 | 9.5 | 35.79 | 8.4 | 34.50 | 7.9 | 33.57 | 8.8 | 36.02 | 8.3 | 34.73 | 7.4 | 33.40 | 9.8 | 35.08 | 8.4 | 34.10 |
| 36 | 50.00 | 8.7 | 34.70 | 11.0 | 36.99 | 9.7 | 35.74 | 9.4 | 34.86 | 10.0 | 37.28 | 9.7 | 36.00 | 8.3 | 34.64 | 11.6 | 36.27 | 9.6 | 35.32 |
| 37 | 52.08 | 10.1 | 35.97 | 13.2 | 38.20 | 11.4 | 36.97 | 10.9 | 36.15 | 13.1 | 38.53 | 11.9 | 37.27 | 9.5 | 35.89 | 12.8 | 37.46 | 10.8 | 36.54 |
| 38 | 54.17 | 11.9 | 37.23 | 15.3 | 39.41 | 13.3 | 38.21 | 13.4 | 37.45 | 15.0 | 39.79 | 14.1 | 38.54 | 10.7 | 37.14 | 15.2 | 38.65 | 12.6 | 37.77 |
| 39 | 56.25 | 14.8 | 38.50 | 18.7 | 40.61 | 16.5 | 39.45 | 16.8 | 38.74 | 19.4 | 41.04 | 18.0 | 39.81 | 13.2 | 38.38 | 17.7 | 39.84 | 15.0 | 38.99 |
| 40 | 58.33 | 17.5 | 39.77 | 21.2 | 41.82 | 19.0 | 40.68 | 20.3 | 40.03 | 21.9 | 42.29 | 21.0 | 41.08 | 15.3 | 39.63 | 20.1 | 41.03 | 17.2 | 40.21 |
| 41 | 60.42 | 20.0 | 41.03 | 23.3 | 43.02 | 21.4 | 41.92 | 22.3 | 41.32 | 25.0 | 43.55 | 23.5 | 42.35 | 18.2 | 40.87 | 21.3 | 42.22 | 19.5 | 41.43 |
| 42 | 62.50 | 24.0 | 42.30 | 26.4 | 44.23 | 25.0 | 43.16 | 25.7 | 42.61 | 30.0 | 44.80 | 27.6 | 43.62 | 22.7 | 42.12 | 22.6 | 43.41 | 22.7 | 42.66 |
| 43 | 64.58 | 25.8 | 43.57 | 31.9 | 45.44 | 28.4 | 44.40 | 26.7 | 43.91 | 33.1 | 46.06 | 29.6 | 44.89 | 25.2 | 43.37 | 30.5 | 44.60 | 27.3 | 43.88 |
| 44 | 66.67 | 29.6 | 44.84 | 33.1 | 46.64 | 31.1 | 45.63 | 31.2 | 45.20 | 35.0 | 47.31 | 32.9 | 46.16 | 28.5 | 44.61 | 31.1 | 45.79 | 29.6 | 45.10 |
| 45 | 68.75 | 34.3 | 46.10 | 39.6 | 47.85 | 36.5 | 46.87 | 37.1 | 46.49 | 43.8 | 48.57 | 40.1 | 47.43 | 32.2 | 45.86 | 35.4 | 46.98 | 33.5 | 46.33 |
| 46 | 70.83 | 38.8 | 47.37 | 44.5 | 49.05 | 41.2 | 48.11 | 41.1 | 47.78 | 46.3 | 49.82 | 43.4 | 48.70 | 37.2 | 47.11 | 42.7 | 48.17 | 39.4 | 47.55 |
| 47 | 72.92 | 43.0 | 48.64 | 48.8 | 50.26 | 45.5 | 49.34 | 43.1 | 49.07 | 50.6 | 51.07 | 46.4 | 49.97 | 43.4 | 48.35 | 47.0 | 49.36 | 44.8 | 48.77 |
| 48 | 75.00 | 47.8 | 49.91 | 54.9 | 51.46 | 50.8 | 50.58 | 50.0 | 50.36 | 58.8 | 52.33 | 53.9 | 51.24 | 46.3 | 49.60 | 51.2 | 50.55 | 48.3 | 49.99 |
| 49 | 77.08 | 52.7 | 51.17 | 58.9 | 52.67 | 55.3 | 51.82 | 55.0 | 51.66 | 63.1 | 53.58 | 58.6 | 52.51 | 51.2 | 50.84 | 54.9 | 51.74 | 52.7 | 51.22 |
| 50 | 79.17 | 57.6 | 52.44 | 64.4 | 53.88 | 60.5 | 53.06 | 58.4 | 52.95 | 68.1 | 54.84 | 62.7 | 53.78 | 57.0 | 52.09 | 60.4 | 52.93 | 58.4 | 52.44 |
| 51 | 81.25 | 62.3 | 53.71 | 70.6 | 55.08 | 65.8 | 54.29 | 64.9 | 54.24 | 76.3 | 56.09 | 69.9 | 55.05 | 60.3 | 53.34 | 64.6 | 54.12 | 62.1 | 53.66 |
| 52 | 83.33 | 69.1 | 54.98 | 73.9 | 56.29 | 71.1 | 55.53 | 70.3 | 55.53 | 79.4 | 57.35 | 74.3 | 56.32 | 68.2 | 54.58 | 68.3 | 55.31 | 68.2 | 54.89 |
| 53 | 85.42 | 72.9 | 56.24 | 77.9 | 57.49 | 75.0 | 56.77 | 73.8 | 56.82 | 83.8 | 58.60 | 78.2 | 57.59 | 72.3 | 55.83 | 72.0 | 56.50 | 72.2 | 56.11 |
| 54 | 87.50 | 77.1 | 57.51 | 81.6 | 58.70 | 79.0 | 58.01 | 76.7 | 58.12 | 85.6 | 59.85 | 80.7 | 58.86 | 77.7 | 57.08 | 77.7 | 57.69 | 77.6 | 57.33 |
| 55 | 89.58 | 79.1 | 58.78 | 85.6 | 59.91 | 81.9 | 59.24 | 80.2 | 59.41 | 89.4 | 61.11 | 84.3 | 60.13 | 78.5 | 58.32 | 81.7 | 58.88 | 79.8 | 58.55 |
| 56 | 91.67 | 84.3 | 60.05 | 88.0 | 61.11 | 85.9 | 60.48 | 87.6 | 60.70 | 91.9 | 62.36 | 89.5 | 61.40 | 81.8 | 59.57 | 84.1 | 60.07 | 82.8 | 59.78 |
| 57 | 93.75 | 87.0 | 61.31 | 90.2 | 62.32 | 88.3 | 61.72 | 90.6 | 61.99 | 93.1 | 63.62 | 91.7 | 62.67 | 84.3 | 60.81 | 87.2 | 61.26 | 85.5 | 61.00 |
| 58 | 95.83 | 91.3 | 62.58 | 93.6 | 63.52 | 92.2 | 62.95 | 94.1 | 63.28 | 96.3 | 64.87 | 95.0 | 63.94 | 88.8 | 62.06 | 90.9 | 62.45 | 89.7 | 62.22 |
| 59 | 97.92 | 96.2 | 63.85 | 97.5 | 64.73 | 96.8 | 64.19 | 97.5 | 64.57 | 98.8 | 66.12 | 98.1 | 65.21 | 95.0 | 63.31 | 96.3 | 63.64 | 95.6 | 63.44 |
| 60 | 100.00 | 100.0 | 65.11 | 100.0 | 65.93 | 100.0 | 65.43 | 100.0 | 65.87 | 100.0 | 67.38 | 100.0 | 66.48 | 100.0 | 64.55 | 100.0 | 64.83 | 100.0 | 64.67 |

Note: Calculation of scores was restricted to complete cases. RS = raw score; TRS = transformed raw score (range 0-100); PR = percentile; TS = T-score (M = 50, SD = 10).

*These reference values should be selected when children receive medication/treatment and the respective scale is applicable.

Table 31  DISABKIDS chronic generic short-form score excluding treatment/medication items* (proxy-report) – DCGM-12-P (V-10)

| DCGM-12-P (V-10) SCORE (V-10) PROXY-REPORT | | Total sample 8-12 (n = 494) | | Total sample 13-16 (n = 366) | | Total sample Overall (n = 860) | | Females 8-12 (n = 228) | | Females 13-16 (n = 173) | | Females Overall (n = 401) | | Males 8-12 (n = 264) | | Males 13-16 (n = 191) | | Males Overall (n = 455) | |
|---|---|---|---|---|---|---|---|---|---|---|---|---|---|---|---|---|---|---|---|
| RS | TRS | PR | TS | PR | TS | PR | TS | PR | TS | PR | TS | PR | TS | PR | TS | PR | TS | PR | TS |
| <= 20 | <= 25.00 | ,6 | 19,78 | 1,1 | 20,39 | ,8 | 20,72 | ,9 | 19,71 | 1,2 | 19,62 | 1,0 | 20,46 | ,4 | 18,53 | ,5 | 10,32 | ,4 | 19,18 |
| 21 | 27.50 | 1,2 | 21,22 | 1,1 | 20,39 | 1,2 | 22,15 | 1,3 | 21,18 | 1,2 | 19,62 | 1,2 | 21,94 | 1,1 | 21,39 | ,5 | 10,32 | ,9 | 22,01 |
| 22 | 30.00 | 1,2 | 21,22 | 1,1 | 20,39 | 1,2 | 22,15 | 1,3 | 21,18 | 1,2 | 19,62 | 1,2 | 21,94 | 1,1 | 21,39 | ,5 | 10,32 | ,9 | 22,01 |
| 23 | 32.50 | 2,2 | 24,12 | 1,4 | 26,08 | 1,9 | 25,02 | 1,3 | 21,18 | 1,7 | 25,65 | 1,5 | 24,89 | 3,0 | 24,25 | 2,6 | 27,06 | 2,0 | 24,84 |
| 24 | 35.00 | 2,4 | 25,57 | 3,0 | 27,51 | 2,7 | 26,46 | 1,8 | 27,04 | 2,9 | 27,16 | 2,0 | 26,36 | 3,4 | 25,68 | 3,1 | 28,45 | 3,1 | 26,26 |
| 25 | 37.50 | 3,0 | 27,02 | 4,1 | 28,93 | 3,5 | 27,89 | 3,1 | 28,50 | 4,6 | 28,66 | 3,0 | 27,84 | 4,2 | 27,11 | 3,7 | 29,84 | 3,7 | 27,67 |
| 26 | 40.00 | 3,8 | 28,46 | 4,6 | 30,36 | 4,2 | 29,33 | 3,9 | 29,91 | 5,2 | 30,17 | 4,0 | 29,31 | 4,5 | 28,54 | 4,2 | 31,24 | 4,2 | 29,09 |
| 27 | 42.50 | 4,9 | 29,91 | 6,3 | 31,78 | 5,5 | 30,76 | 5,3 | 31,43 | 6,4 | 31,67 | 5,0 | 30,79 | 5,7 | 29,97 | 5,8 | 32,63 | 5,7 | 30,50 |
| 28 | 45.00 | 6,1 | 31,36 | 7,9 | 33,20 | 6,9 | 32,19 | 6,6 | 32,90 | 7,5 | 33,18 | 6,2 | 32,26 | 6,8 | 31,40 | 7,9 | 34,03 | 7,3 | 31,92 |
| 29 | 47.50 | 6,9 | 32,81 | 9,3 | 34,63 | 7,9 | 33,63 | 7,9 | 34,37 | 8,7 | 34,69 | 7,5 | 33,74 | 7,2 | 32,83 | 9,4 | 35,42 | 8,1 | 33,33 |
| 30 | 50.00 | 8,3 | 34,25 | 11,7 | 36,05 | 9,8 | 35,06 | 11,0 | 35,83 | 11,6 | 36,19 | 9,5 | 35,21 | 8,7 | 34,25 | 11,5 | 36,82 | 9,9 | 34,75 |
| 31 | 52.50 | 10,3 | 35,70 | 12,8 | 37,48 | 11,4 | 36,50 | 12,3 | 37,30 | 12,1 | 37,70 | 11,5 | 36,69 | 9,8 | 35,68 | 13,1 | 38,21 | 11,2 | 36,16 |
| 32 | 55.00 | 12,3 | 37,15 | 14,8 | 38,90 | 13,4 | 37,93 | 14,9 | 38,76 | 13,3 | 39,20 | 12,7 | 38,16 | 12,5 | 37,11 | 15,7 | 39,60 | 13,8 | 37,58 |
| 33 | 57.50 | 14,2 | 38,60 | 17,5 | 40,33 | 15,6 | 39,37 | 20,6 | 40,23 | 16,8 | 40,71 | 15,7 | 39,64 | 13,6 | 38,54 | 17,8 | 41,00 | 15,4 | 38,99 |
| 34 | 60.00 | 18,6 | 40,05 | 20,2 | 41,75 | 19,3 | 40,80 | 22,8 | 41,69 | 22,0 | 42,22 | 21,2 | 41,12 | 17,0 | 39,97 | 18,3 | 42,39 | 17,6 | 40,41 |
| 35 | 62.50 | 21,1 | 41,49 | 23,5 | 43,17 | 22,1 | 42,23 | 26,3 | 43,16 | 26,0 | 43,72 | 24,2 | 42,59 | 19,7 | 41,40 | 20,9 | 43,79 | 20,2 | 41,82 |
| 36 | 65.00 | 24,9 | 42,94 | 27,6 | 44,60 | 26,0 | 43,67 | 29,4 | 44,62 | 30,1 | 45,23 | 27,9 | 44,07 | 23,9 | 42,83 | 25,1 | 45,18 | 24,4 | 43,24 |
| 37 | 67.50 | 27,9 | 44,39 | 31,7 | 46,02 | 29,5 | 45,10 | 35,1 | 46,09 | 32,9 | 46,74 | 30,9 | 45,54 | 26,9 | 44,26 | 30,4 | 46,58 | 28,4 | 44,65 |
| 38 | 70.00 | 32,4 | 45,84 | 38,8 | 47,45 | 35,1 | 46,54 | 39,0 | 47,55 | 41,6 | 48,24 | 37,9 | 47,02 | 30,3 | 45,69 | 36,1 | 47,97 | 32,7 | 46,07 |
| 39 | 72.50 | 37,9 | 47,29 | 43,4 | 48,87 | 40,2 | 47,97 | 44,3 | 49,02 | 46,2 | 49,75 | 42,1 | 48,49 | 37,1 | 47,12 | 40,8 | 49,36 | 38,7 | 47,48 |
| 40 | 75.00 | 41,7 | 48,73 | 50,5 | 50,30 | 45,5 | 49,41 | 50,0 | 50,48 | 54,3 | 51,25 | 48,6 | 49,97 | 39,8 | 48,55 | 47,1 | 50,76 | 42,9 | 48,90 |
| 41 | 77.50 | 47,0 | 50,18 | 56,0 | 51,72 | 50,8 | 50,84 | 55,7 | 51,95 | 61,8 | 52,76 | 55,1 | 51,44 | 44,7 | 49,98 | 50,8 | 52,15 | 47,3 | 50,31 |
| 42 | 80.00 | 53,4 | 51,63 | 60,9 | 53,14 | 56,6 | 52,27 | 61,0 | 53,41 | 65,9 | 54,27 | 60,1 | 52,92 | 51,9 | 51,41 | 56,5 | 53,55 | 53,8 | 51,73 |
| 43 | 82.50 | 59,5 | 53,08 | 67,2 | 54,57 | 62,8 | 53,71 | 64,0 | 54,88 | 73,4 | 55,77 | 66,3 | 54,39 | 58,3 | 52,84 | 61,3 | 54,94 | 59,6 | 53,14 |
| 44 | 85.00 | 65,2 | 54,53 | 69,4 | 55,99 | 67,0 | 55,14 | 69,7 | 56,34 | 76,9 | 57,28 | 69,6 | 55,87 | 66,3 | 54,27 | 62,3 | 56,34 | 64,6 | 54,56 |
| 45 | 87.50 | 71,3 | 55,97 | 76,5 | 57,42 | 73,5 | 56,58 | 75,4 | 57,81 | 82,7 | 58,78 | 75,3 | 57,34 | 72,7 | 55,70 | 70,7 | 57,73 | 71,9 | 55,97 |
| 46 | 90.00 | 75,3 | 57,42 | 80,6 | 58,84 | 77,6 | 58,01 | 82,9 | 59,27 | 86,1 | 60,29 | 80,0 | 58,82 | 75,4 | 57,13 | 75,4 | 59,12 | 75,4 | 57,39 |
| 47 | 92.50 | 80,4 | 58,87 | 86,1 | 60,27 | 82,8 | 59,45 | 87,3 | 60,74 | 91,9 | 61,80 | 86,8 | 60,29 | 78,4 | 58,55 | 80,6 | 60,52 | 79,3 | 58,80 |
| 48 | 95.00 | 85,0 | 60,32 | 90,7 | 61,69 | 87,4 | 60,88 | 94,3 | 62,20 | 95,4 | 63,30 | 90,8 | 61,77 | 83,0 | 59,98 | 86,4 | 61,91 | 84,4 | 60,21 |
| 49 | 97.50 | 92,3 | 61,76 | 96,2 | 63,11 | 94,0 | 62,32 |  |  | 97,7 | 64,81 | 95,8 | 63,24 | 90,5 | 61,41 | 94,8 | 63,31 | 92,3 | 61,63 |
| 50 | 100.00 | 100,0 | 63,21 | 100,0 | 64,54 | 100,0 | 63,75 | 100,0 | 63,67 | 100,0 | 66,32 | 100,0 | 64,72 | 100,0 | 62,84 | 100,0 |  | 100,0 | 63,04 |

Note: Calculation of scores was restricted to complete cases. RS = raw score; TRS = transformed raw score (range 0-100); PR = percentile; TS = T-score (M = 50, SD = 10). *These reference values should be selected when children **do not** receive medication/treatment and the respective scale is **not** applicable.

204

**Table 32  DISABKIDS smiley module (proxy-report) – DSM-P**

| DSM-P SMILEY'S SCORE PROXY-REPORT | | Total sample 4-7 (n = 362) | | Females 4-7 (n = 179) | | Males 4-7 (n = 183) | |
|---|---|---|---|---|---|---|---|
| RS | TRS | PR | TS | PR | TS | PR | TS |
| 6 | 0.00 | - | - | - | - | - | - |
| 7 | 4.17 | - | - | - | - | - | - |
| 8 | 8.33 | - | - | - | - | - | - |
| 9 | 12.50 | - | - | - | - | - | - |
| 10 | 16.67 | - | - | - | - | - | - |
| 11 | 20.83 | - | - | - | - | - | - |
| 12 | 25.00 | - | - | - | - | - | - |
| 13 | 29.17 | .3 | 17,93 | .6 | 19,00 | .5 | 19,91 |
| 14 | 33.33 | .6 | 21,14 | 1.7 | 22,39 | 1.1 | 26,02 |
| 15 | 37.50 | 1.4 | 24,35 | 1.7 | 22,39 | 1.1 | 26,02 |
| 16 | 41.67 | 1.7 | 27,56 | 4.5 | 29,18 | 1.6 | 29,07 |
| 17 | 45.83 | 7.2 | 30,76 | 6.1 | 32,57 | 9.8 | 32,13 |
| 18 | 50.00 | 9.7 | 33,97 | 10.1 | 35,96 | 13.1 | 35,18 |
| 19 | 54.17 | 13.5 | 37,18 | 13.4 | 39,35 | 16.9 | 38,23 |
| 20 | 58.33 | 18.5 | 40,39 | 25.7 | 42,74 | 23.5 | 41,29 |
| 21 | 62.50 | 26.8 | 43,60 | 41.3 | 46,13 | 27.9 | 44,34 |
| 22 | 66.67 | 40.1 | 46,81 | 57.5 | 49,53 | 38.8 | 47,40 |
| 23 | 70.83 | 55.8 | 50,02 | 68.2 | 52,92 | 54.1 | 50,45 |
| 24 | 75.00 | 68.5 | 53,23 | 79.9 | 56,31 | 68.9 | 53,50 |
| 25 | 79.17 | 80.1 | 56,44 | 88.3 | 59,70 | 80.3 | 56,56 |
| 26 | 83.33 | 87.8 | 59,64 | 92.7 | 63,09 | 87.4 | 59,61 |
| 27 | 87.50 | 93.6 | 62,85 | 95.5 | 66,48 | 94.5 | 62,67 |
| 28 | 91.67 | 96.4 | 66,06 | 98.9 | 69,88 | 97.3 | 65,72 |
| 29 | 95.83 | 98.6 | 69,27 | 100.0 | 73,27 | 98.4 | 68,78 |
| 30 | 100.00 | 100.0 | 72,48 | - | - | 100.0 | 71,83 |

Note: Calculation of scores was restricted to complete cases. RS = raw score; TRS = transformed raw score (range 0-100); PR = percentile; TS = T-score (M = 50, SD = 10).

**Table 33  DISABKIDS condition specific module asthma, sub-scales "impact" and "worry" (proxy-report) – DCSM-AsM-P**

### DCSM-AsM-P IMPACT PROXY-REPORT

| RS | TRS | Total sample 8-12 (n = 206) PR | TS | Total sample 13-16 (n = 104) PR | TS | Total sample Overall (n = 310) PR | TS |
|----|-------|------|-------|------|-------|------|-------|
| 6  | 0.00   | .5    | 19,06 | -    | -     | .3    | 20,18 |
| 7  | 4.17   | .5    | 19,06 | -    | -     | .3    | 20,18 |
| 8  | 8.33   | .5    | 19,06 | 1.0  | 25,20 | .6    | 24,07 |
| 9  | 12.50  | 2.4   | 19,06 | 1.9  | 27,27 | 1.0   | 26,02 |
| 10 | 16.67  | 3.4   | 26,81 | 3.8  | 29,34 | 2.9   | 27,97 |
| 11 | 20.83  | 3.4   | 28,75 | 5.8  | 31,40 | 4.2   | 29,92 |
| 12 | 25.00  | 6.3   | 30,69 | 6.7  | 33,47 | 4.5   | 31,86 |
| 13 | 29.17  | 8.7   | 32,62 | 10.6 | 35,53 | 7.7   | 33,81 |
| 14 | 33.33  | 11.7  | 34,56 | 15.4 | 37,60 | 11.0  | 35,76 |
| 15 | 37.50  | 15.0  | 36,49 | 16.3 | 39,67 | 13.2  | 37,71 |
| 16 | 41.67  | 20.4  | 38,43 | 20.2 | 41,73 | 16.8  | 39,66 |
| 17 | 45.83  | 26.2  | 40,37 | 25.0 | 43,80 | 21.9  | 41,60 |
| 18 | 50.00  | 32.5  | 42,31 | 37.5 | 45,87 | 30.0  | 43,55 |
| 19 | 54.17  | 36.9  | 44,24 | 47.1 | 47,93 | 37.4  | 45,50 |
| 20 | 58.33  | 44.7  | 46,18 | 55.8 | 50,00 | 43.2  | 47,45 |
| 21 | 62.50  | 51.9  | 48,12 | 62.5 | 52,07 | 50.6  | 49,40 |
| 22 | 66.67  | 57.3  | 50,06 | 68.3 | 54,13 | 57.4  | 51,34 |
| 23 | 70.83  | 65.0  | 51,99 | 74.0 | 56,20 | 62.9  | 53,29 |
| 24 | 75.00  | 70.4  | 53,93 | 79.8 | 58,27 | 70.0  | 55,24 |
| 25 | 79.17  | 77.2  | 55,87 | 86.5 | 60,33 | 75.8  | 57,19 |
| 26 | 83.33  | 83.5  | 57,81 | 92.3 | 62,40 | 82.3  | 59,14 |
| 27 | 87.50  | 89.8  | 59,74 | 96.2 | 64,47 | 87.7  | 61,09 |
| 28 | 91.67  | 94.2  | 61,68 | 96.2 | 64,47 | 91.9  | 63,03 |
| 29 | 95.83  |       | 63,62 | 97.1 | 68,60 | 95.2  | 64,98 |
| 30 | 100.00 | 100.0 | 65,56 | 100.0| 70,66 | 100.0 | 66,93 |

### DCSM-AsM-P WORRY PROXY-REPORT

| RS | TRS | Total sample 8-12 (n = 214) PR | TS | Total sample 13-16 (n = 108) PR | TS | Total sample Overall (n = 322) PR | TS |
|----|--------|------|-------|------|-------|------|-------|
| 5  | 0.00   | -    | -     | .9   | 8,60  | .3   | 6,41  |
| 6  | 5.00   | -    | -     | .9   | 8,60  | .3   | 6,41  |
| 7  | 10.00  | -    | -     | .9   | 8,60  | .3   | 6,41  |
| 8  | 15.00  | 1.4  | 13,15 | .9   | 8,60  | 1.2  | 14,43 |
| 9  | 20.00  | 1.9  | 15,86 | .9   | 8,60  | 1.6  | 17,11 |
| 10 | 25.00  | 2.3  | 18,58 | .9   | 8,60  | 1.9  | 19,78 |
| 11 | 30.00  | 2.8  | 21,29 | 1.9  | 24,37 | 2.5  | 22,46 |
| 12 | 35.00  | 3.3  | 24,00 | 2.8  | 27,00 | 3.1  | 25,13 |
| 13 | 40.00  | 3.7  | 26,72 | 4.6  | 29,63 | 4.0  | 27,80 |
| 14 | 45.00  | 3.7  | 26,72 | 6.5  | 32,26 | 4.7  | 30,48 |
| 15 | 50.00  | 5.6  | 32,14 | 10.2 | 34,88 | 7.1  | 33,15 |
| 16 | 55.00  | 9.8  | 34,86 | 14.8 | 37,51 | 11.5 | 35,83 |
| 17 | 60.00  | 12.1 | 37,57 | 18.5 | 40,14 | 14.3 | 38,50 |
| 18 | 65.00  | 17.3 | 40,29 | 22.2 | 42,77 | 18.9 | 41,17 |
| 19 | 70.00  | 24.8 | 43,00 | 32.4 | 45,40 | 27.3 | 43,85 |
| 20 | 75.00  | 33.6 | 45,71 | 42.6 | 48,03 | 36.6 | 46,52 |
| 21 | 80.00  | 39.7 | 48,43 | 50.0 | 50,66 | 43.2 | 49,19 |
| 22 | 85.00  | 49.1 | 51,14 | 58.3 | 53,29 | 52.2 | 51,87 |
| 23 | 90.00  | 58.9 | 53,86 | 70.4 | 55,91 | 62.7 | 54,54 |
| 24 | 95.00  | 72.0 | 56,57 | 84.3 | 58,54 | 76.1 | 57,22 |
| 25 | 100.00 | 100.0| 59,28 | 100.0| 61,17 | 100.0| 59,89 |

Note: Calculation of scores was restricted to complete cases. RS = raw score; TRS = transformed raw score (range 0-100); PR = percentile; TS = T-score (M = 50, SD = 10).

**Table 34  DISABKIDS condition specific module arthritis, sub-scales "impact" and "understanding" (proxy-report) – DCSM-ArM-P**

**DCSM-ArM-P IMPACT PROXY-REPORT**

| RS | TRS | Total sample 8-12 (n=62) | | Total sample 13-16 (n=58) | | Total sample Overall (n=120) | |
|---|---|---|---|---|---|---|---|
| | | PR | TS | PR | TS | PR | TS |
| 9 | 0.00 | - | - | - | - | - | - |
| 10 | 2.78 | - | - | - | - | - | - |
| 11 | 5.56 | - | - | - | - | - | - |
| 12 | 8.33 | - | - | - | - | - | - |
| 13 | 11.11 | - | - | - | - | - | - |
| 14 | 13.89 | 1.6 | 26,21 | 1.7 | 27,71 | 1.7 | 27,06 |
| 15 | 16.67 | 1.6 | 26,21 | 3.4 | 29,13 | 2.5 | 28,42 |
| 16 | 19.44 | 1.6 | 26,21 | 3.4 | 29,13 | 2.5 | 28,42 |
| 17 | 22.22 | 1.6 | 26,21 | 5.2 | 31,95 | 3.3 | 31,15 |
| 18 | 25.00 | 3.2 | 31,54 | 6.9 | 33,36 | 5.0 | 32,51 |
| 19 | 27.78 | 6.5 | 32,87 | 10.3 | 34,78 | 8.3 | 33,87 |
| 20 | 30.56 | 8.1 | 35,54 | 12.1 | 36,19 | 9.2 | 35,23 |
| 21 | 33.33 | 9.7 | 36,87 | 15.5 | 37,60 | 11.7 | 36,59 |
| 22 | 36.11 | 16.1 | 38,20 | 17.2 | 39,01 | 13.3 | 37,95 |
| 23 | 38.89 | 21.0 | 39,53 | 19.0 | 40,43 | 17.5 | 39,31 |
| 24 | 41.67 | 24.2 | 40,87 | 24.1 | 41,84 | 22.5 | 40,67 |
| 25 | 44.44 | 25.8 | 42,20 | 25.9 | 43,25 | 25.0 | 42,04 |
| 26 | 47.22 | 25.8 | 42,20 | 27.6 | 44,67 | 26.7 | 43,40 |
| 27 | 50.00 | 25.8 | 42,20 | 32.8 | 46,08 | 29.2 | 44,76 |
| 28 | 52.78 | 27.4 | 44,86 | 37.9 | 47,49 | 32.5 | 46,12 |
| 29 | 55.56 | 33.9 | 46,20 | 44.8 | 48,90 | 39.2 | 47,48 |
| 30 | 58.33 | 41.9 | 47,53 | 53.4 | 50,32 | 47.5 | 48,84 |
| 31 | 61.11 | 46.8 | 48,86 | 60.3 | 51,73 | 53.3 | 50,20 |
| 32 | 63.89 | 54.8 | 50,19 | 65.5 | 53,14 | 60.0 | 51,57 |
| 33 | 66.67 | 62.9 | 51,53 | 67.2 | 54,55 | 65.0 | 52,93 |
| 34 | 69.44 | 64.5 | 52,86 | 74.1 | 55,97 | 69.2 | 54,29 |
| 35 | 72.22 | 69.4 | 54,19 | 81.0 | 57,38 | 75.0 | 55,65 |
| 36 | 75.00 | 74.2 | 55,52 | 82.8 | 58,79 | 78.3 | 57,01 |
| 37 | 77.78 | 79.0 | 56,86 | 82.8 | 58,79 | 80.8 | 58,37 |
| 38 | 80.56 | 80.6 | 58,19 | 89.7 | 61,62 | 85.0 | 59,73 |
| 39 | 83.33 | 80.6 | 58,19 | 93.1 | 63,03 | 86.7 | 61,09 |
| 40 | 86.11 | 80.6 | 58,19 | 94.8 | 64,44 | 87.5 | 62,46 |
| 41 | 88.89 | 85.5 | 62,19 | 94.8 | 64,44 | 90.0 | 63,82 |
| 42 | 91.67 | 91.9 | 63,52 | 98.3 | 67,27 | 95.0 | 65,18 |
| 43 | 94.44 | 91.9 | 63,52 | 98.3 | 67,27 | 95.0 | 65,18 |
| 44 | 97.22 | 95.2 | 66,18 | 98.3 | 67,27 | 96.7 | 67,90 |
| 45 | 100.00 | 100.0 | 67,52 | 100.0 | 71,51 | 100.0 | 69,26 |

**DCSM-ArM-P UNDERSTANDING PROXY-REPORT**

| RS | TRS | Total sample 8-12 (n=67) | | Total sample 13-16 (n=59) | | Total sample Overall (n=126) | |
|---|---|---|---|---|---|---|---|
| | | PR | TS | PR | TS | PR | TS |
| 3 | 0.00 | - | - | 1.7 | 28,62 | 3.2 | 26,77 |
| 4 | 8.33 | 4.5 | 24,88 | 5.1 | 31,69 | 4.8 | 29,92 |
| 5 | 16.67 | 7.5 | 31,38 | 8.5 | 34,76 | 7.9 | 33,07 |
| 6 | 25.00 | 9.0 | 34,63 | 22.0 | 37,83 | 15.1 | 36,22 |
| 7 | 33.33 | 17.9 | 37,88 | 23.7 | 40,90 | 20.6 | 39,37 |
| 8 | 41.67 | 19.4 | 41,13 | 33.9 | 43,97 | 26.2 | 42,52 |
| 9 | 50.00 | 31.3 | 44,37 | 39.0 | 47,04 | 34.9 | 45,67 |
| 10 | 58.33 | 38.8 | 47,62 | 54.2 | 50,10 | 46.0 | 48,82 |
| 11 | 66.67 | 52.2 | 50,87 | 67.8 | 53,17 | 59.5 | 51,98 |
| 12 | 75.00 | 67.2 | 54,12 | 74.6 | 56,24 | 70.6 | 55,13 |
| 13 | 83.33 | 86.6 | 57,37 | 81.4 | 59,31 | 84.1 | 58,28 |
| 14 | 91.67 | 88.1 | 60,62 | 91.5 | 62,38 | 89.7 | 61,43 |
| 15 | 100.00 | 100.0 | 63,87 | 100.0 | 65,45 | 100.0 | 64,58 |

Note: Calculation of scores was restricted to complete cases. RS = raw score; TRS = transformed raw score (range 0-100); PR = percentile; TS = T-score (M = 50, SD = 10).

# Table 35 DISABKIDS condition specific module dermatitis, sub-scales "impact" and "stigma" (proxy-report) – DCSM-ADM-P

**DCSM-ADM-P IMPACT PROXY-REPORT**

| RS | TRS | Total sample 8-12 (n = 8) PR | TS | Total sample 13-16 (n = 24) PR | TS | Total sample Overall (n = 32) PR | TS |
|---|---|---|---|---|---|---|---|
| 8 | 0.00 | - | - | - | - | - | - |
| 9 | 3.13 | - | - | - | - | - | - |
| 10 | 6.25 | - | - | - | - | - | - |
| 11 | 9.38 | - | - | 4.2 | 32,93 | 3.1 | 33,74 |
| 12 | 12.5 | - | - | 4.2 | 32,93 | 3.1 | 33,74 |
| 13 | 15.63 | - | - | 8.3 | 36,57 | 6.3 | 36,81 |
| 14 | 18.75 | - | - | 12.5 | 38,39 | 9.4 | 38,34 |
| 15 | 21.88 | - | - | 12.5 | 38,39 | 9.4 | 38,34 |
| 16 | 25.00 | - | - | 20.8 | 42,03 | 15.6 | 41,41 |
| 17 | 28.13 | 25.0 | 40,03 | 25.0 | 43,85 | 25.0 | 42,95 |
| 18 | 31.25 | 25.0 | 40,03 | 37.5 | 45,68 | 34.4 | 44,48 |
| 19 | 34.38 | 37.5 | 42,45 | 54.2 | 47,50 | 50.0 | 46,02 |
| 20 | 37.50 | 37.5 | 42,45 | 66.7 | 49,32 | 59.4 | 47,55 |
| 21 | 40.63 | 50.0 | 44,86 | 75.0 | 51,14 | 68.8 | 49,09 |
| 22 | 43.75 | 50.0 | 44,86 | 75.0 | 51,14 | 68.8 | 49,09 |
| 23 | 46.88 | 50.0 | 44,86 | 75.0 | 51,14 | 68.8 | 49,09 |
| 24 | 50.00 | 62.5 | 48,49 | 75.0 | 51,14 | 71.9 | 53,69 |
| 25 | 53.13 | 62.5 | 48,49 | 79.2 | 58,42 | 75.0 | 55,23 |
| 26 | 56.25 | 62.5 | 48,49 | 83.3 | 60,24 | 78.1 | 56,76 |
| 27 | 59.38 | 62.5 | 48,49 | 91.7 | 62,06 | 84.4 | 58,30 |
| 28 | 62.5 | 62.5 | 48,49 | 91.7 | 62,06 | 84.4 | 58,30 |
| 29 | 65.63 | 62.5 | 48,49 | 91.7 | 62,06 | 84.4 | 58,30 |
| 30 | 68.75 | 62.5 | 48,49 | 91.7 | 62,06 | 84.4 | 58,30 |
| 31 | 71.88 | 62.5 | 48,49 | 91.7 | 62,06 | 84.4 | 58,30 |
| 32 | 75.00 | 75.0 | 58,16 | 95.8 | 71,17 | 90.6 | 65,97 |
| 33 | 78.13 | 75.0 | 58,16 | 100.0 | 72,99 | 93.8 | 67,51 |
| 34 | 81.25 | 87.5 | 60,57 | 100.0 | 72,99 | 96.9 | 69,04 |
| 35 | 84.38 | 87.5 | 60,57 | 100.0 | 72,99 | 96.9 | 69,04 |
| 36 | 87.50 | 87.5 | 60,57 | 100.0 | 72,99 | 96.9 | 69,04 |
| 37 | 90.63 | 87.5 | 60,57 | 100.0 | 72,99 | 96.9 | 69,04 |
| 38 | 93.75 | 100.0 | 65,41 | 100.0 | 72,99 | 100.0 | 75,18 |
| 39 | 96.88 | 100.0 | 65,41 | 100.0 | 72,99 | 100.0 | 75,18 |
| 40 | 100.00 | 100.0 | 65,41 | 100.0 | 72,99 | 100.0 | 75,18 |

**DCSM-ADM-P STIGMA PROXY-REPORT**

| RS | TRS | Total sample 8-12 (n = 6) PR | TS | Total sample 13-16 (n = 22) PR | TS | Total sample Overall (n = 28) PR | TS |
|---|---|---|---|---|---|---|---|
| 4 | 0.00 | - | - | 4.5 | 30,40 | 3.6 | 29,36 |
| 5 | 6.25 | - | - | 4.5 | 30,40 | 3.6 | 29,36 |
| 6 | 12.50 | - | - | 9.1 | 35,76 | 7.1 | 34,45 |
| 7 | 18.75 | - | - | 18.2 | 38,44 | 14.3 | 37,00 |
| 8 | 25.00 | - | - | 18.2 | 38,44 | 14.3 | 37,00 |
| 9 | 31.25 | - | - | 27.3 | 43,79 | 21.4 | 42,09 |
| 10 | 37.50 | - | - | 40.9 | 46,47 | 32.1 | 44,64 |
| 11 | 43.75 | 16.7 | 38,45 | 50.0 | 49,15 | 42.9 | 47,18 |
| 12 | 50.00 | 33.3 | 41,34 | 77.3 | 51,83 | 67.9 | 49,73 |
| 13 | 56.25 | 33.3 | 41,34 | 77.3 | 51,83 | 67.9 | 49,73 |
| 14 | 62.50 | 50.0 | 47,11 | 77.3 | 51,83 | 71.4 | 54,82 |
| 15 | 68.75 | 66.7 | 50,00 | 81.8 | 59,86 | 78.6 | 57,36 |
| 16 | 75.00 | 66.7 | 50,00 | 95.5 | 62,54 | 89.3 | 59,91 |
| 17 | 81.25 | 66.7 | 50,00 | 95.5 | 62,54 | 89.3 | 59,91 |
| 18 | 87.50 | 83.3 | 58,66 | 95.5 | 62,54 | 92.9 | 65,00 |
| 19 | 93.75 | 83.3 | 58,66 | 95.5 | 62,54 | 92.9 | 65,00 |
| 20 | 100.00 | 100.0 | 64,43 | 100.0 | 73,25 | 100.0 | 70,09 |

Note: Calculation of scores was restricted to complete cases. RS = raw score; TRS = transformed raw score (range 0-100); PR = percentile; TS = T-score (M = 50, SD = 10).

**Table 36  DISABKIDS condition specific module diabetes, sub-scales "impact" and "treatment" (proxy-report) – DCSM-DM-P**

| DCSM-DM-P IMPACT PROXY-REPORT | | Total sample 8-12 (n = 92) | | Total sample 13-16 (n = 87) | | Total sample Overall (n = 179) | |
|---|---|---|---|---|---|---|---|
| RS | TRS | PR | TS | PR | TS | PR | TS |
| 6 | 0.00 | - | - | - | - | - | - |
| 7 | 4.17 | - | - | - | - | - | - |
| 8 | 8.33 | 1.1 | 22,98 | - | - | .6 | 22,76 |
| 9 | 12.50 | 2.2 | 25,29 | - | - | 1.1 | 25,07 |
| 10 | 16.67 | 3.3 | 27,60 | - | - | 1.7 | 27,37 |
| 11 | 20.83 | 4.3 | 29,91 | 2.3 | 29,55 | 3.4 | 29,68 |
| 12 | 25.00 | 6.5 | 32,22 | 5.7 | 31,84 | 6.1 | 31,99 |
| 13 | 29.17 | 9.8 | 34,53 | 8.0 | 34,14 | 8.9 | 34,30 |
| 14 | 33.33 | 9.8 | 39,15 | 9.2 | 36,43 | 9.5 | 36,61 |
| 15 | 37.50 | 12.0 | 41,46 | 18.4 | 38,73 | 15.1 | 38,92 |
| 16 | 41.67 | 19.6 | 43,77 | 24.1 | 41,03 | 21.8 | 41,23 |
| 17 | 45.83 | 23.9 | 46,08 | 27.6 | 43,32 | 25.7 | 43,54 |
| 18 | 50.00 | 33.7 | 48,39 | 40.2 | 45,62 | 36.9 | 45,85 |
| 19 | 54.17 | 48.9 | 50,70 | 47.1 | 47,92 | 48.0 | 48,16 |
| 20 | 58.33 | 60.9 | 53,01 | 51.7 | 50,21 | 56.4 | 50,46 |
| 21 | 62.50 | 70.7 | 55,32 | 64.4 | 52,51 | 67.6 | 52,77 |
| 22 | 66.67 | 80.4 | 57,63 | 69.0 | 54,80 | 74.9 | 55,08 |
| 23 | 70.83 | 83.7 | 59,94 | 79.3 | 57,10 | 81.6 | 57,39 |
| 24 | 75.00 | 85.9 | 62,25 | 86.2 | 59,40 | 86.0 | 59,70 |
| 25 | 79.17 | 89.1 | 64,56 | 92.0 | 61,69 | 90.5 | 62,01 |
| 26 | 83.33 | 93.5 | 66,87 | 93.1 | 63,99 | 93.3 | 64,32 |
| 27 | 87.50 | 94.6 | 69,18 | 94.3 | 66,28 | 94.4 | 66,63 |
| 28 | 91.67 | 97.8 | 71,49 | 97.7 | 68,58 | 97.8 | 68,94 |
| 29 | 95.83 | 98.9 | 73,80 | 98.9 | 70,88 | 98.9 | 71,25 |
| 30 | 100.00 | 100.0 | 22,98 | 100.0 | 73,17 | 100.0 | 73,55 |

| DCSM-DM-P TREATMENT PROXY-REPORT | | Total sample 8-12 (n = 94) | | Total sample 13-16 (n = 86) | | Total sample Overall (n = 180) | |
|---|---|---|---|---|---|---|---|
| RS | TRS | PR | TS | PR | TS | PR | TS |
| 4 | 0.00 | 2.1 | 23,66 | 1.2 | 27,00 | 1.2 | 25,32 |
| 5 | 6.25 | 3.2 | 26,67 | 3.5 | 29,73 | 3.5 | 28,20 |
| 6 | 12.50 | 4.3 | 29,68 | 7.0 | 32,47 | 7.0 | 31,07 |
| 7 | 18.75 | 6.4 | 32,68 | 12.8 | 35,20 | 12.8 | 33,94 |
| 8 | 25.00 | 10.6 | 35,69 | 17.4 | 37,93 | 17.4 | 36,81 |
| 9 | 31.25 | 16.0 | 38,70 | 18.6 | 40,66 | 18.6 | 39,68 |
| 10 | 37.50 | 23.4 | 41,71 | 26.7 | 43,39 | 26.7 | 42,55 |
| 11 | 43.75 | 29.8 | 44,72 | 41.9 | 46,12 | 41.9 | 45,42 |
| 12 | 50.00 | 42.6 | 47,73 | 47.7 | 48,86 | 47.7 | 48,29 |
| 13 | 56.25 | 57.4 | 50,74 | 57.0 | 51,59 | 57.0 | 51,16 |
| 14 | 62.50 | 72.3 | 53,74 | 69.8 | 54,32 | 69.8 | 54,04 |
| 15 | 68.75 | 80.9 | 56,75 | 81.4 | 57,05 | 81.4 | 56,91 |
| 16 | 75.00 | 88.3 | 59,76 | 87.2 | 59,78 | 87.2 | 59,78 |
| 17 | 81.25 | 92.6 | 62,77 | 93.0 | 62,52 | 93.0 | 62,65 |
| 18 | 87.50 | 96.8 | 65,78 | 95.3 | 65,25 | 95.3 | 65,52 |
| 19 | 93.75 | 97.9 | 68,79 | 97.7 | 67,98 | 97.7 | 68,39 |
| 20 | 100.00 | 100.0 | 71,80 | 100.0 | 70,71 | 100.0 | 71,26 |

*Note: Calculation of scores was restricted to complete cases. RS = raw score; TRS = transformed raw score (range 0-100); PR = percentile; TS = T-score (M = 50, SD = 10).*

## Table 37 DISABKIDS condition specific module cerebral palsy, sub-scales "impact" and "communication" (proxy-report) – DCSM-CPM-P

### DCSM-CPM-P IMPACT PROXY-REPORT

| RS | TRS | Total sample 8-12 (n = 34) PR | TS | Total sample 13-16 (n = 30) PR | TS | Total sample Overall (n = 64) PR | PR |
|---|---|---|---|---|---|---|---|
| 10 | 0.00 | - | - | - | - | - | - |
| 11 | 2.50 | - | - | - | - | - | - |
| 12 | 5.00 | - | - | - | - | - | - |
| 13 | 7.50 | - | - | - | - | - | - |
| 14 | 10.00 | - | - | - | - | - | - |
| 15 | 12.50 | - | - | - | - | - | - |
| 16 | 15.00 | 2.9 | 24,96 | - | - | 1.6 | 21,82 |
| 17 | 17.50 | 2.9 | 24,96 | - | - | 1.6 | 21,82 |
| 18 | 20.00 | 2.9 | 24,96 | - | - | 1.6 | 21,82 |
| 19 | 22.50 | 2.9 | 24,96 | - | - | 1.6 | 21,82 |
| 20 | 25.00 | 2.9 | 24,96 | 3.3 | 27,84 | 3.1 | 27,84 |
| 21 | 27.50 | 2.9 | 24,96 | 3.3 | 27,84 | 3.1 | 27,84 |
| 22 | 30.00 | 2.9 | 24,96 | 3.3 | 27,84 | 3.1 | 27,84 |
| 23 | 32.50 | 5.9 | 34,36 | 3.3 | 27,84 | 4.7 | 32,35 |
| 24 | 35.00 | 11.8 | 35,70 | 3.3 | 27,84 | 7.8 | 33,85 |
| 25 | 37.50 | 11.8 | 35,70 | 6.7 | 35,36 | 9.4 | 35,36 |
| 26 | 40.00 | 11.8 | 35,70 | 10.0 | 36,86 | 10.9 | 36,86 |
| 27 | 42.50 | 14.7 | 39,73 | 10.0 | 36,86 | 12.5 | 38,37 |
| 28 | 45.00 | 17.6 | 41,07 | 10.0 | 36,86 | 14.1 | 39,87 |
| 29 | 47.50 | 17.6 | 41,07 | 13.3 | 41,37 | 15.6 | 41,37 |
| 30 | 50.00 | 29.4 | 43,76 | 23.3 | 42,88 | 26.6 | 42,88 |
| 31 | 52.50 | 32.4 | 45,10 | 26.7 | 44,38 | 29.7 | 44,38 |
| 32 | 55.00 | 41.2 | 46,45 | 36.7 | 45,89 | 39.1 | 45,89 |
| 33 | 57.50 | 47.1 | 47,79 | 40.0 | 47,39 | 43.8 | 47,39 |
| 34 | 60.00 | 50.0 | 49,13 | 53.3 | 48,90 | 51.6 | 48,90 |
| 35 | 62.50 | 52.9 | 50,47 | 53.3 | 48,90 | 53.1 | 50,40 |
| 36 | 65.00 | 55.9 | 51,82 | 53.3 | 48,90 | 54.7 | 51,90 |
| 37 | 67.50 | 64.7 | 53,16 | 56.7 | 53,41 | 60.9 | 53,41 |
| 38 | 70.00 | 67.6 | 54,50 | 66.7 | 54,91 | 67.2 | 54,91 |
| 39 | 72.50 | 73.5 | 55,85 | 76.7 | 56,42 | 75.0 | 56,42 |
| 40 | 75.00 | 82.4 | 57,19 | 80.0 | 57,92 | 81.3 | 57,92 |
| 41 | 77.50 | 82.4 | 57,19 | 86.7 | 59,42 | 84.4 | 59,42 |
| 42 | 80.00 | 88.2 | 59,87 | 96.7 | 60,93 | 92.2 | 60,93 |
| 43 | 82.50 | 91.2 | 61,22 | 100.0 | 62,43 | 95.3 | 62,43 |
| 44 | 85.00 | 94.1 | 62,56 | 100.0 | 62,43 | 96.9 | 63,94 |
| 45 | 87.50 | 94.1 | 62,56 | 100.0 | 62,43 | 96.9 | 63,94 |
| 46 | 90.00 | 94.1 | 62,56 | 100.0 | 62,43 | 96.9 | 63,94 |
| 47 | 92.50 | 94.1 | 62,56 | 100.0 | 62,43 | 96.9 | 63,94 |
| 48 | 95.00 | 94.1 | 62,56 | 100.0 | 62,43 | 96.9 | 63,94 |
| 49 | 97.50 | 94.1 | 62,56 | 100.0 | 62,43 | 96.9 | 63,94 |
| 50 | 100.00 | 100.0 | 70,62 | 100.0 | 62,43 | 100.0 | 72,96 |

### DCSM-CPM-P COMMUNICATION PROXY-REPORT

| RS | TRS | Total sample 8-12 (n = 36) PR | TS | Total sample 13-16 (n = 31) PR | TS | Total sample Overall (n = 67) PR | PR |
|---|---|---|---|---|---|---|---|
| 2 | 0.00 | 2.8 | 23,10 | - | - | 1.5 | 22,02 |
| 3 | 12.50 | 5.6 | 27,45 | 3.2 | 25,76 | 4.5 | 26,53 |
| 4 | 25.00 | 8.3 | 31,79 | 9.7 | 30,40 | 9.0 | 31,03 |
| 5 | 37.50 | 13.9 | 36,13 | 12.9 | 35,04 | 13.4 | 35,54 |
| 6 | 50.00 | 27.8 | 40,47 | 25.8 | 39,68 | 26.9 | 40,05 |
| 7 | 62.50 | 30.6 | 44,81 | 29.0 | 44,31 | 29.9 | 44,55 |
| 8 | 75.00 | 36.1 | 49,16 | 38.7 | 48,95 | 37.3 | 49,06 |
| 9 | 87.50 | 55.6 | 53,50 | 58.1 | 53,59 | 56.7 | 53,56 |
| 10 | 100.00 | 100.0 | 57,84 | 100.0 | 58,23 | 100.0 | 58,07 |

Note: Calculation of scores was restricted to complete cases. RS = raw score; TRS = transformed raw score (range 0-100); PR = percentile; TS = T-score (M = 50, SD = 10).

**Table 38** DISABKIDS condition specific module cystic fibrosis, sub-scales "impact" and "treatment" (proxy-report) – DCSM-CFM-P

| DCSM-CFM-P IMPACT PROXY-REPORT | | Total sample 8-12 (n = 13) | | Total sample 13-16 (n = 8) | | Total sample Overall (n = 21) | |
|---|---|---|---|---|---|---|---|
| RS | TRS | PR | TS | PR | TS | PR | TS |
| 4 | 0.00 | - | - | - | - | - | - |
| 5 | 6.25 | - | - | - | - | - | - |
| 6 | 12.50 | - | - | - | - | - | - |
| 7 | 18.75 | - | - | - | - | - | - |
| 8 | 25.00 | - | - | - | - | - | - |
| 9 | 31.25 | - | - | - | - | - | - |
| 10 | 37.50 | 15.4 | 35,65 | - | - | 9.5 | 34,32 |
| 11 | 43.75 | 23.1 | 39,04 | 12.5 | 36,63 | 19.0 | 37,94 |
| 12 | 50.00 | 30.8 | 42,43 | 37.5 | 40,45 | 33.3 | 41,55 |
| 13 | 56.25 | 38.5 | 45,83 | 37.5 | 40,45 | 38.1 | 45,17 |
| 14 | 62.50 | 53.8 | 49,22 | 50.0 | 48,09 | 52.4 | 48,79 |
| 15 | 68.75 | 69.2 | 52,61 | 50.0 | 48,09 | 61.9 | 52,41 |
| 16 | 75.00 | 69.2 | 52,61 | 75.0 | 55,73 | 71.4 | 56,03 |
| 17 | 81.25 | 76.9 | 59,39 | 87.5 | 59,55 | 81.0 | 59,65 |
| 18 | 87.50 | 100.0 | 62,78 | 100.0 | 63,37 | 100.0 | 63,27 |
| 19 | 93.75 | 100.0 | 62,78 | 100.0 | 63,37 | 100.0 | 63,27 |
| 20 | 100.00 | 100.0 | 62,78 | 100.0 | 63,37 | 100.0 | 63,27 |

| DCSM-CFM-P TREATMENT PROXY-REPORT | | Total sample 8-12 (n = 12) | | Total sample 13-16 (n = 9) | | Total sample Overall (n = 21) | |
|---|---|---|---|---|---|---|---|
| RS | TRS | PR | TS | PR | TS | PR | TS |
| 6 | 0.00 | - | - | - | - | - | - |
| 7 | 4.17 | - | - | - | - | - | - |
| 8 | 8.33 | 8.3 | 34,61 | 11.1 | 30,25 | 4.8 | 31,43 |
| 9 | 12.50 | 16.7 | 36,49 | 11.1 | 30,25 | 9.5 | 33,51 |
| 10 | 16.67 | 16.7 | 36,49 | 11.1 | 30,25 | 14.3 | 35,58 |
| 11 | 20.83 | 25.0 | 40,26 | 11.1 | 30,25 | 14.3 | 35,58 |
| 12 | 25.00 | 25.0 | 40,26 | 11.1 | 30,25 | 19.0 | 39,73 |
| 13 | 29.17 | 41.7 | 44,03 | 22.2 | 41,64 | 23.8 | 41,80 |
| 14 | 33.33 | 41.7 | 44,03 | 22.2 | 41,64 | 33.3 | 43,88 |
| 15 | 37.50 | 41.7 | 44,03 | 33.3 | 46,20 | 38.1 | 45,95 |
| 16 | 41.67 | 41.7 | 44,03 | 55.6 | 48,48 | 47.6 | 48,02 |
| 17 | 45.83 | 41.7 | 44,03 | 55.6 | 48,48 | 47.6 | 48,02 |
| 18 | 50.00 | 50.0 | 51,57 | 55.6 | 48,48 | 52.4 | 52,17 |
| 19 | 54.17 | 66.7 | 53,46 | 55.6 | 48,48 | 61.9 | 54,25 |
| 20 | 58.33 | 75.0 | 55,34 | 88.9 | 57,60 | 81.0 | 56,32 |
| 21 | 62.50 | 75.0 | 55,34 | 88.9 | 57,60 | 81.0 | 56,32 |
| 22 | 66.67 | 75.0 | 55,34 | 100.0 | 62,16 | 85.7 | 60,47 |
| 23 | 70.83 | 91.7 | 60,99 | 100.0 | 62,16 | 95.2 | 62,54 |
| 24 | 75.00 | 100.0 | 64,76 | 100.0 | 62,16 | 100.0 | 66,69 |
| 25 | 79.17 | 100.0 | 64,76 | 100.0 | 62,16 | 100.0 | 66,69 |
| 26 | 83.33 | 100.0 | 64,76 | 100.0 | 62,16 | 100.0 | 66,69 |
| 27 | 87.50 | 100.0 | 64,76 | 100.0 | 62,16 | 100.0 | 66,69 |
| 28 | 91.67 | 100.0 | 64,76 | 100.0 | 62,16 | 100.0 | 66,69 |
| 29 | 95.83 | 100.0 | 64,76 | 100.0 | 62,16 | 100.0 | 66,69 |
| 30 | 100.00 | 100.0 | 64,76 | 100.0 | 62,16 | 100.0 | 66,69 |

*Note: Calculation of scores was restricted to complete cases. RS = raw score; TRS = transformed raw score (range 0-100); PR = percentile; TS = T-score (M = 50, SD = 10).*

**Table 39  DISABKIDS condition specific module epilepsy, sub-scales "impact" and "social" (proxy-report) – DCSM-EM-P**

### DCSM-EM-P IMPACT PROXY-REPORT

| RS | TRS | Total sample 8-12 (n = 54) | | Total sample 13-16 (n = 53) | | Total sample Overall (n = 107) | |
|---|---|---|---|---|---|---|---|
| | | PR | TS | PR | TS | PR | TS |
| 5 | 0.00 | 1.9 | 22,84 | 1.9 | 24,87 | 1.9 | 23,88 |
| 6 | 5.00 | 3.7 | 24,74 | 1.9 | 24,87 | 2.8 | 25,78 |
| 7 | 10.00 | 3.7 | 24,74 | 3.8 | 28,70 | 3.7 | 27,69 |
| 8 | 15.00 | 3.7 | 24,74 | 5.7 | 30,61 | 4.7 | 29,59 |
| 9 | 20.00 | 5.6 | 30,45 | 7.5 | 32,53 | 6.5 | 31,50 |
| 10 | 25.00 | 5.6 | 30,45 | 13.2 | 34,44 | 9.3 | 33,40 |
| 11 | 30.00 | 5.6 | 36,16 | 15.1 | 36,35 | 10.3 | 35,31 |
| 12 | 35.00 | 7.4 | 36,16 | 15.1 | 36,35 | 11.2 | 37,21 |
| 13 | 40.00 | 16.7 | 38,06 | 17.0 | 40,18 | 16.8 | 39,12 |
| 14 | 45.00 | 24.1 | 39,96 | 20.8 | 42,09 | 22.4 | 41,03 |
| 15 | 50.00 | 25.9 | 41,86 | 26.4 | 44,01 | 26.2 | 42,93 |
| 16 | 55.00 | 27.8 | 43,77 | 32.1 | 45,92 | 29.9 | 44,84 |
| 17 | 60.00 | 31.5 | 45,67 | 45.3 | 47,83 | 38.3 | 46,74 |
| 18 | 65.00 | 37.0 | 47,57 | 49.1 | 49,75 | 43.0 | 48,65 |
| 19 | 70.00 | 46.3 | 49,47 | 52.8 | 51,66 | 49.5 | 50,55 |
| 20 | 75.00 | 53.7 | 51,37 | 56.6 | 53,57 | 55.1 | 52,46 |
| 21 | 80.00 | 63.0 | 53,28 | 75.5 | 55,49 | 69.2 | 54,36 |
| 22 | 85.00 | 66.7 | 55,18 | 77.4 | 57,40 | 72.0 | 56,27 |
| 23 | 90.00 | 70.4 | 57,08 | 83.0 | 59,32 | 76.6 | 58,17 |
| 24 | 95.00 | 72.2 | 58,98 | 86.8 | 61,23 | 79.4 | 60,08 |
| 25 | 100.00 | 100.0 | 60,88 | 100.0 | 63,14 | 100.0 | 61,98 |

### DCSM-EM-P SOCIAL PROXY-REPORT

| RS | TRS | Total sample 8-12 (n = 51) | | Total sample 13-16 (n = 51) | | Total sample Overall (n = 102) | |
|---|---|---|---|---|---|---|---|
| | | PR | TS | PR | TS | PR | TS |
| 5 | 0.00 | – | – | 2.0 | 23,15 | 1.0 | 19,95 |
| 6 | 5.00 | – | – | 3.9 | 25,11 | 2.0 | 22,07 |
| 7 | 10.00 | – | – | 3.9 | 25,11 | 2.0 | 22,07 |
| 8 | 15.00 | – | – | 3.9 | 25,11 | 2.0 | 22,07 |
| 9 | 20.00 | – | – | 3.9 | 25,11 | 2.0 | 22,07 |
| 10 | 25.00 | – | – | 5.9 | 31,00 | 2.9 | 28,43 |
| 11 | 30.00 | 2.0 | 27,53 | 7.8 | 32,96 | 4.9 | 30,55 |
| 12 | 35.00 | 3.9 | 29,86 | 9.8 | 34,92 | 6.9 | 32,67 |
| 13 | 40.00 | 9.8 | 32,19 | 11.8 | 36,88 | 10.8 | 34,80 |
| 14 | 45.00 | 9.8 | 32,19 | 17.6 | 38,84 | 13.7 | 36,92 |
| 15 | 50.00 | 15.7 | 36,85 | 19.6 | 40,81 | 17.6 | 39,04 |
| 16 | 55.00 | 21.6 | 39,18 | 21.6 | 42,77 | 21.6 | 41,16 |
| 17 | 60.00 | 25.5 | 41,51 | 33.3 | 44,73 | 29.4 | 43,28 |
| 18 | 65.00 | 29.4 | 43,83 | 39.2 | 46,69 | 34.3 | 45,40 |
| 19 | 70.00 | 37.3 | 46,16 | 43.1 | 48,65 | 40.2 | 47,52 |
| 20 | 75.00 | 45.1 | 48,49 | 51.0 | 50,62 | 48.0 | 49,65 |
| 21 | 80.00 | 49.0 | 50,82 | 52.9 | 52,58 | 51.0 | 51,77 |
| 22 | 85.00 | 54.9 | 53,15 | 62.7 | 54,54 | 58.8 | 53,89 |
| 23 | 90.00 | 62.7 | 55,48 | 66.7 | 56,50 | 64.7 | 56,01 |
| 24 | 95.00 | 68.6 | 57,81 | 74.5 | 58,46 | 71.6 | 58,13 |
| 25 | 100.00 | 100.0 | 60,14 | 100.0 | 60,43 | 100.0 | 60,25 |

Note: Calculation of scores was restricted to complete cases. RS = raw score; TRS = transformed raw score (range 0-100); PR = percentile; TS = T-score (M = 50, SD = 10).